Ensuring a Sustainable Future

ENSURING A SUSTAINABLE FUTURE

Making Progress on Environment and Equity

Edited by Jody Heymann

   and

Magda Barrera

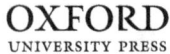

OXFORD
UNIVERSITY PRESS

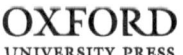

OXFORD
UNIVERSITY PRESS

Oxford University Press is a department of the University of Oxford.
It furthers the University's objective of excellence in research, scholarship,
and education by publishing worldwide.

Oxford   New York
Auckland   Cape Town   Dar es Salaam   Hong Kong   Karachi
Kuala Lumpur   Madrid   Melbourne   Mexico City   Nairobi
New Delhi   Shanghai   Taipei   Toronto

With offices in
Argentina   Austria   Brazil   Chile   Czech Republic   France   Greece
Guatemala   Hungary   Italy   Japan   Poland   Portugal   Singapore
South Korea   Switzerland   Thailand   Turkey   Ukraine   Vietnam

Oxford is a registered trademark of Oxford University Press in
the UK and certain other countries.

Published in the United States of America by
Oxford University Press
198 Madison Avenue, New York, NY 10016

© Oxford University Press 2014

Library of Congress Cataloging-in-Publication Data
Ensuring a sustainable future (2014)
Ensuring a sustainable future : making progress on environment and equity / edited by
Jody Heymann and Magda Barrera.
    p. ; cm.
Includes bibliographical references.
ISBN 978-0-19-997470-2 (alk. paper)
I. Heymann, Jody, 1959-   II. Barrera, Magda.   III. Title.
[DNLM: 1. Environmental Health.   2. Conservation of Natural Resources.
3. Health Policy.   4. Socioeconomic Factors. WA 30.5]
RA427.8
362.1—dc23
2013023768

9 8 7 6 5 4 3 2 1
Printed in the United States of America
on acid-free paper

To everyone who takes the time in their daily actions and in their work to support the health of the environment we all share

CONTENTS

Acknowledgments   ix

About the Editors   xi

About the Authors   xiii

Introduction: The Environment and the Economy: Finding Equitable and Effective Solutions   xix
Magda Barrera and Jody Heymann

SECTION ONE: Moving Forward on the Environment and the Economy: Creating Jobs, Building Healthy Communities

1. The Essential Connection: Environmental Sustainability, Community Stability, and Equitable Development in Struggling Cities in High-Income Countries   3
   Ted Howard

2. Community Action in Informal Settlements: Strategies for Improved Environmental Health and Equity in Low- and Middle-Income Countries   26
   David Satterthwaite

3. Achieving Environmental Equity: Race, Place, and the Movement to Build Healthy Communities in the United States   48
   Angela Glover Blackwell

4. Building Income and Social Equity through Urban Sustainability: Lessons from Vancouver's Downtown Eastside   69
   Mitra Thompson

5. New Skills for the Green Economy: Two Training Programs for Job Seekers in the United States   92
   Cosmin Paduraru and Kara Quennell

6. Green Social Entrepreneurship as a Poverty-Reduction Strategy: TIDE India's Use of Technological Innovation for Healthier and More Sustainable Communities   112
   Shannon Lockhart

**SECTION TWO: Addressing Specific Environmental Challenges
in an Economically Sustainable Way**

7. Moving Toward Sustainable Urban Transport: How Can We Integrate
   Environmental, Health, and Equity Objectives Globally?   *135*
   David Banister and James Woodcock

8. The New Challenges of Rapid Urban Growth: Imperatives and Strategies
   for Transport in India   *167*
   Madhav Badami

9. Healthy and Sustainable Agriculture: Working with Farmers to
   Transform Food Production in Latin America   *189*
   Donald Cole, Gordon Prain, and Willy Pradel

10. Access to Healthy Foods in Urban Settings: A Comprehensive
    Strategy for Low-Income Communities in Montreal   *221*
    Lise Bertrand

11. Water for Development: Investing in Health and Economic
    Well-Being Globally   *246*
    William Cosgrove and Håkan Tropp

12. The Potential of Clean Energy for Equity in Remote
    Communities in the North   *275*
    Tim Weis

13. Remote Indigenous Populations and Climate Change: Reducing
    the Impacts on Health and Well-Being   *299*
    James Ford and Peter Adams

Index   *321*

ACKNOWLEDGMENTS

Our work on *Ensuring a Sustainable Future* resulted from a major 5-year initiative, Moving from Research to Effective Action, which conducted evidence-based research on policies addressing health and socioeconomic inequalities around the world. We are deeply appreciative of the generous support of Allan Northcott, David Elton, and Ralph Strother at the Max Bell Foundation, which made this initiative possible. We are also deeply indebted to Heather Munroe-Blum, Anthony Masi, Rose Goldstein, Arnold Steinberg, Rich Levin, and Chris Manfredi at McGill University for their support for a program devoted to the intersection of research and action, which was crucial in enabling us to make it a reality.

We were extremely fortunate to be able to count on the contributions of a wonderful team when developing this book. Jennifer Proudfoot and Brittany Lambert's outstanding outreach skills proved an invaluable contribution to the project, as they searched for and brought together leading experts and practitioners to provide contributions on environmental equity. During the initial steps of the research, David Baumann, Leo Perez, and Chris Connolly along with 10 Institute Policy Fellows conducted a comprehensive search for innovative programs addressing environment and equity, and examined hundreds of potential case studies. Tinka Markham Piper's stellar management of the Policy Fellowship program was instrumental in facilitating the work of the Policy Fellows and allowing us to acquire knowledge on how to implement effective change. In-depth background research is a necessity for any research initiative of this size. This project would not have been the same without the meticulous research conducted by Denise Maines and Institute for Health and Social Policy interns Hope Bigda-Peyton and Annette Slonim.

There are many decisions we each make every day in how we live our lives that affect the environment and equity. Most of us do some things—recycling when it's readily available, reducing energy use if it means turning down the heat—and not others. We could all do far more both as individuals and as societies. This book is dedicated to the ability of each of us, in the daily steps we take as well as in our work, to support the health of the environment we all share.

ABOUT THE EDITORS

Jody Heymann is Dean and Distinguished Professor of Epidemiology at the UCLA Fielding School of Public Health. Heymann was the Founding Director of the Institute for Health and Social Policy at McGill University and the Project on Global Working Families at Harvard University. She is a fellow of the Canadian Academy of Health Sciences and held a Canada Research Chair in Global Health and Social Policy. Heymann has authored and edited 15 books, including *Children's Chances* (Harvard University Press, 2013), *Profit at the Bottom of the Ladder* (Harvard Business Press, 2009), *Raising the Global Floor* (Stanford University Press, 2009), and *Forgotten Families* (Oxford University Press, 2006).

Heymann established and leads the WORLD Policy Analysis Centre, the first global initiative to examine public policy in all 193 UN nations. This initiative provides an in-depth look at how social and environmental policies affect the ability of individuals, families and communities to meet their health, human development, and financial needs across the political, economic, and social spectrum worldwide. Deeply committed to translating research into policies and programs that will improve individual and population health, Heymann has worked with leaders in North American, European, African, and Latin American governments as well as a wide range of intergovernmental organizations, including the World Health Organization, the International Labor Organization, UNICEF, and UNESCO. Central to her efforts are bridging the gap between research and policy makers, and Heymann's research has been presented to heads of state and senior policy makers around the world. She has worked closely on the development of legislation with the US Congress as well as with UN agencies on the implications of her team's results for global policy.

Magda Barrera received her BA in Economics from Williams College and her MA from Carleton University's Norman Paterson School of International Affairs. For the past 6 years she has been working at McGill University's Institute for Health and Social Policy conducting research and writing on how to effectively improve social conditions in an economically sustainable manner. She has co-led a fellowship program designed to examine policies and programs around the world on topics such as urban sustainability and environmental equity.

ABOUT THE AUTHORS

Peter Adams is a policy analyst for Acclimatise, a climate risk management consultancy. Previously, Adams was a member of McGill University's Climate Change Adaptation Research Group, where he studied impacts of climate change in Arctic Canada and Greenland. As part of this, Adams conducted an intensive field research mission in Nunavut, Canada, working with local institutions to understand climate change impacts and adaptation strategies in vulnerable northern communities. He has worked with the US Peace Corps in China, as a teacher in Tibet, and as a researcher studying climate change and water policy in India and Bangladesh. Adams obtained a Masters in Geography from McGill University.

Madhav Badami has a joint faculty appointment in the School of Urban Planning and the School of Environment at McGill University. After having studied mechanical engineering at the Indian Institute of Technology, Madras, he spent 9 years in diesel engine development in the Indian truck and bus industry. He obtained a PhD in environmental policy and planning at the University of British Columbia. He has led extensive research into urban transportation in fast-growing cities in India and urban transport policy. His teaching and research interests are in the areas of environmental policy and planning; urban infrastructure and services; urban transport; alternative transport fuels; and environment and development.

David Banister is Professor of Transport Studies at Oxford University and Director of the Transport Studies Unit. Until 2006, he was Professor of Transport Planning at University College London. He has also been a Research Fellow at the Warren Centre in the University of Sydney (2001–2002) on the Sustainable Transport for a Sustainable City project, was Visiting VSB Professor at the Tinbergen Institute in Amsterdam (1994–1997), and Visiting Professor at the University of Bodenkultur in Vienna in 2007. He is currently the first holder of the Benelux BIVET-GIBET Transport Chair (2012–2013). He has published 23 books, either as author or editor, and some 200 papers in refereed scientific journals. He is editor of two major international journals, *Transport Reviews* and *Built Environment* (jointly), and he is on the editorial board of seven other journals.

Lise Bertrand is Chef d'équipe développement social at the Direction de santé publique, Agence de la santé et des services sociaux de Montréal, and a Researcher at the Centre Léa Roback. Bertrand completed a master's degree in Public Health at the University of California at Berkeley. Her current role involves partnering with government and community groups to advocate for policies and programs that enhance health, improve nutrition, and address social inequalities at the regional level. Bertrand currently oversees 16 initiatives that involve partnerships with citizens as well as community groups, decision makers, and borough administrators to improve food access, healthy eating, and sustainable food systems. She conducts research on disparities in access to food in Montreal, and on food consumption monitoring.

Angela Glover Blackwell is the Founder and Chief Executive Officer of PolicyLink, a leading voice in the movement to use public policy to improve access and opportunity for all low-income people and communities of color, particularly in the areas of health, housing, transportation, education, and infrastructure. Glover Blackwell is the coauthor of the recently published *Uncommon Common Ground: Race and America's Future* (W.W. Norton & Co., 2010) and contributed to *Ending Poverty in America: How to Restore the American Dream* (The New Press, 2007) and *The Covenant with Black America* (Third World Press, 2006). She earned a law degree from the University of California at Berkeley. Glover Blackwell is a former senior vice president at the Rockefeller Foundation. She served as cochair of the task force on poverty for the Center for American Progress.

Donald Cole is the Interim Head, Global Health Division at the Dalla Lana School of Public Health and Interim Director of a new Institute for Global Health Equity and Innovation at the University of Toronto. Cole practiced primary care, public health, occupational health, and environmental health in a variety of settings in Canada and low- and middle-income countries. He developed a long-standing relationship with the International Potato Center around agriculture and health research for development, with a particular focus on pesticides, urban agriculture, and nutrition. As a tenured Associate Professor, he currently teaches, mentors, does research, and contributes research evidence in Canada and internationally. As cochair of the Capacity Development Program Area of the Canadian Coalition for Global Health Research (CCGHR), he has a particular interest in evaluation of health research capacity strengthening.

William Cosgrove is President of Ecoconsult Inc. and is currently Senior Adviser for the fourth edition of the UN World Water Development Report and the World Water Scenarios Project of the UN World Water Assessment Program. Cosgrove received his M. Eng. Sanitary Engineering and an Honorary Doctorate of Science from McGill University. From 2005 to 2008 he was

President of the Bureau d'audiences publiques sur l'environnement in Québec. Cosgrove is a former vice president of the World Bank, past-president of the World Water Council, and served as chairman of the International Steering Committee of the Dialogue on Water and Climate.

James Ford is an assistant professor in geography at McGill University. He works with indigenous communities on climate change vulnerability assessment and adaptation planning, and he received a Young Innovator Award from the Canadian government for his innovative community-based research. Ford was a contributing author to the IPCC fourth assessment report and is currently co-leading the Indigenous Health Adaptation to Climate Change project, a 5-year initiative examining the vulnerability of remote indigenous health systems in the Arctic, Peru, and Uganda to climate change. Ford's research team is also developing novel approaches to track climate change adaptation at global and regional levels, and exploring ways to effectively communicate research to stakeholders and the public at large.

Ted Howard is the founder and Executive Director of The Democracy Collaborative at the University of Maryland. In July 2010, Howard was appointed as the Steven Minter Senior Fellow for Social Justice at The Cleveland Foundation. In this position, he has been responsible for developing a comprehensive job creation and wealth building strategy that has resulted in the Evergreen Cooperative Initiative, based in part on the Mondragon Cooperatives in the Basque Region of Spain. From 1998 to 2007, Howard served as Chairman of the Board of Search for Common Ground, the world's largest conflict resolution nongovernmental organization. He is chairman of the board of ocean advocacy group Blue Frontier. For the past three decades, Howard has worked in the not-for-profit sector, including agencies of the UN system and The Hunger Project, where he was Global Communications Director and Chief Operating Office.

Shannon Lockhart is a medical student studying at the University of British Columbia. She interned with the William J. Clinton Foundation working to facilitate the social initiatives of college students and has currently focused her research on the effects of incorporating physical exercise into medical education curricula. Shannon Lockhart was a policy fellow at the Institute for Health and Social Policy and conducted a case study on TIDE India (Technology Informatics Design Endeavor), an organization that promotes the use of technological innovation for sustainable development.

Cosmin Paduraru is currently finishing his PhD in artificial intelligence at McGill University, focusing on automated decision making in complex environments. He completed his MSc in computer science at the University of Alberta. His primary focus continues to be on applying his analytical skills to health, equity, and environmental sustainability. Paduraru was a Policy

Fellow at the Institute for Health and Social Policy and conducted a case study on Casa Verde Builders in Austin, a green job training program targeting disadvantaged youth.

Willy Pradel is a researcher at the International Potato Center, working on agricultural and health-related projects with a focus on rural nutrition in Andean countries as well as evaluating the risks of pesticide use in Latin America and Africa. Pradel holds a M.Sc. in Agricultural Development Economics. Pradel has experience in environmental valuation techniques of potato diversity in Andean countries, and he is responsible for the design, capacity building, and analysis of results related to monitoring and evaluation methodologies using participatory evaluation approaches and standard and innovative quantitative methods.

Gordon Prain is a Senior Scientist in Social and Health Sciences at the International Potato Center, and the Global Coordinator for Urban Harvest-Consultative Group on International Agricultural Research. He is one of the editors of African Urban Harvest: Agriculture in the Cities of Cameroon, Kenya, and Uganda.

Kara Quennell is currently completing her M.A. in Medical Anthropology at the University of Toronto. Quennell was a Policy Fellow at the McGill Institute for Health and Social Policy, conducting a case study on a green jobs training program in the South Bronx. Her research continues to address the relationships between social, economic, and health-related inequalities. Her current projects focus on chronic disease and racialized conceptions of care in Canada.

David Satterthwaite is a Senior Fellow at the International Institute for Environment and Development, Visiting Professor at University College London (the Development Planning Unit), and Honorary Professor, University of Hull. He currently serves as the Editor of the international journal *Environment and Urbanization*. He has worked with numerous organizations in informal settlements around the world, leading research into urban challenges in cities in low- and middle-income countries. Satterthwaite holds a PhD from the London School of Economics and is the author of numerous publications, including *Squatter Citizen* (with Jorge E. Hardoy) and *The Earthscan Reader on Sustainable Cities*. He has contributed to the IPCC's Third and Fourth Assessments and is the lead author for the chapter on Adapting Cities in the IPCC's Fifth Assessment.

Mitra Thompson is currently based in Ottawa and is an analyst at one of Canada's leading public opinion and market research organizations. She obtained an MA in Political Science from McGill University. She was a Policy

Fellow at the McGill Institute for Health and Social Policy and conducted research on United We Can in Vancouver, an organization fostering job creation through recycling in one of Canada's poorest neighborhoods.

Håkan Tropp works in developing the water governance concept and its practical application in a development context. He spearheaded and leads the Water Governance Facility (WGF), a demand-driven program that assists governments in water governance reform and its implementation. WGF is an initiative by the United Nations Development Program (UNDP) and implemented by the Stockholm International Water Institute (SIWI). Tropp previously worked with Agenda 21 at the United Nations Department for Economic and Social Affairs and as a Water Specialist at the UNDP. He is a founding member of the Water Integrity Network and was its first Chair (2006–2010). Tropp received degrees in political science and political economy from Lund University, and he holds a PhD from the Department of Water and Environmental Studies, Linköping University.

Tim Weis is a professional engineer and the director of renewable energy and efficiency policy at the Pembina Institute in Canada. Weis specializes in clean energy policy design, research, and strategic decision making. He has assisted more than 20 communities at various stages of development of renewable energy projects and has written extensively on sustainable energy technical and policy issues at national, provincial, and municipal levels, as well as opportunities specific to off-grid communities. Weis holds a PhD from the Université du Québec à Rimouski in environmental sciences, with a focus on wind energy development in remote communities.

James Woodcock is a public health researcher at the Centre for Diet and Activity Research (CEDAR), University of Cambridge. Woodcock's research focuses on how to improve health and well-being during the transition to a low-carbon transport system. He has led the development of macro-simulation health exposure and impact models for physical activity and road traffic injuries. His health impact modelling of transport has led to highly cited publications in the *Lancet* and presentations to international audiences of policy makers. Current research includes working with London policy makers to model the health impacts of the London hire bikes and other active travel initiatives, and a UK research council (ESRC) funded project "Changing Commutes" in which he is using agent-based modeling to investigate how a transition to mass cycle commuting in English cities could be achieved.

Introduction: The Environment and the Economy: Finding Equitable and Effective Solutions

MAGDA BARRERA AND JODY HEYMANN

SEEKING SOLUTIONS TO ENVIRONMENTAL EQUITY

When we started to work on this book, we had a central question: could we find feasible solutions to the critical challenge of addressing environmental sustainability and the economy while increasing equity? To answer this question, we approached a wide range of experts to ask them for examples of innovative and proven strategies and initiatives. The people we approached had diverse backgrounds: they came from and had worked in regions around the world; they had experience working with community organizations, governments, international organizations, and the private sector; and they had expertise in a wide range of areas related to environmental equity, including water, climate change, transportation, energy, and housing.

In addition to asking experts in the field for their contributions, we conducted case studies on a number of initiatives that addressed environmental challenges while disproportionately benefiting poor and marginalized populations. Case studies were selected according to three criteria: they had to have environmental benefits; they needed to promote greater equity; and they had to be economically feasible. Over 150 innovative programs were reviewed. Ten were selected for in-depth field studies. Three of the resulting case studies are presented in this volume.

The contributors address the environment, economy, and equity in both marginalized parts of high-income countries and in low-income countries. While we believe environmental equity challenges must be addressed in countries at every level of income, the debate on environmental challenges has often been pushed by high-income countries while failing to adequately address their own shortcomings in environmental conditions for low-income communities.

ENVIRONMENT AND (IN)EQUITY: BURDEN DISPROPORTIONATELY FELT BY THE POOR

While all of humanity would suffer from the deterioration of conditions in the natural and built environments, poor and marginalized adults and children around the world already bear the brunt of these effects, absent solutions. From extreme weather events to pollution, from limited transportation options to the inadequate availability of healthy food, poor populations are disadvantaged by the environments in which they live and work. This is the case at the macro level, in terms of inequities between rich and poor countries, as well as the micro level, between the rich and the poor within countries.

The accelerating pace of urbanization is playing a key role in the pressure on natural resources and growing energy demand. Studies of the impact of urbanization found that at the current pace, natural resources and ecosystems could be severely damaged by 2030.[1] Rapid rates of urbanization, while increasing pressure on the natural environment and its resources, can also create challenges within the built environment. When large numbers of people move to cities within a relatively short period of time, it fuels the development of informal settlements and slums. The fastest rates of urbanization are currently taking place in cities in Asia and Africa. The number of people living in slums in low- and middle-income countries has risen from 657 million in 1990 to 767 million in 2000 and 828 million in 2010,[2] with recent estimates suggesting that over 30 percent of the world's urban population currently live in slums.[3]

It is almost exclusively the poor who live in the worst environmental conditions prevalent in informal settlements, settling in marginal areas that are prone to flooding or landslides or are closest to industrial areas.[4] In addition, informal settlements tend to have high levels of pollution, poor access to water and sanitation facilities, and poor-quality housing conditions. As a result, residents of informal settlements tend to experience stark inequalities in health outcomes compared to city and national averages. A study by the African Population and Health Research Centre found that child health outcomes in Nairobi's informal settlements were far worse than outcomes for the remainder of Kenya's urban and rural populations. Infant mortality rates in informal settlements averaged 91 per 1,000, compared to 76 in rural areas, and 39 in Nairobi overall.[5] Recognizing the magnitude of the problem of poor living conditions in informal settlements, Target 7 of the Millennium Development Goals included: "By 2020, to have achieved a significant improvement in the lives of at least 100 million slum dwellers." However, progress has been slow as informal settlements continue to grow.

Deep inequalities in neighborhood environmental conditions remain a concern for low-income urban residents outside informal settlements. The frequent proximity of poor residential areas to industry leads to exposure to harmful chemical and biological agents in addition to noise pollution. The Bhopal disaster resulted in 2,000 people dying and 20,000 being poisoned; the majority of exposed individuals were low income, with incomes close to the government-defined poverty level of US$12/month.[6] Poor-quality housing is a key challenge in middle- and low-income countries, with over 900 million people in cities in Africa, Asia, and Latin America and the Caribbean living in poor-quality structures, with inadequate provision of water and sanitation, and insecure tenure.[7] Lower income groups in high-income countries also experience inequalities in access to adequate housing. In 2009, 8.5 percent of householders in the United States earning below $25,000 in annual salary were living in inadequate housing, compared to 2.4 percent of higher income householders.

The distribution and availability of healthy foods, such as fresh fruit and vegetables, is a key element of a healthy living environment. Again, it is the poor who are living in the worst circumstances. Studies have shown that the availability of healthy foods is reduced in lower income neighborhoods.[8,9,10] The ability of lower income households to make healthy food choices is constrained by the lack of local supermarkets and limited public transportation to larger grocery stores. The smaller neighborhood stores that tend to be available are less likely to stock a good variety of healthy foods and also charge higher prices, further constraining options.[11] More than 23.5 million people in low-income communities in the United States have no supermarket or large grocery store within a mile of their homes.[12] In California, lower income communities have 20 percent fewer healthy food sources than higher income ones.[13]

Urbanization and changes in dietary habits have had an impact on environmental health well beyond cities. While developments in food production in the 20th century made it easier for farmers to increase yields, respond to urban food demands, and reap economic benefits, they often involve a greater use of pesticides and chemicals. While benefiting yields, these developments in agricultural production have had harmful impacts on the health of people working in the sector, as well as problematic environmental consequences for the natural resources used in agricultural production.[14,15,16,17] In low- and middle-income countries, agricultural workers are among the poorest members of the population and are the ones most affected by the harmful health effects of pesticides used in agricultural production.[18]

At the same time as urbanization is increasing pressures on natural resources, climate change is presenting new challenges in ensuring environmental sustainability. Average global temperature from 1850 to 2005 increased by about 0.76°C, with a further increase of 1.4°C to 5.8°C projected by 2100.[19] Climate change is projected to have severe environmental impacts, including sea level rise, variations in rainfall patterns, strain on water resources, desertification, and droughts. These will have negative consequences for a range of issues essential to human life such as water supply, food prices, and prevalence of infectious diseases. The average rate of sea level rise grew from 1.8 mm per year between 1961 and 2003 to 3.1 mm per year between 1993 and 2003. Sea level is predicted to rise between 180mm and 590mm over the course of the 21st century.[20] Sea level rise will have particularly severe impacts for the low-elevation coastal zone (coastal areas that are less than 10 m above sea level), which contains 10 percent of the world's population. Climate change is already having severe impacts on health. For example, the heat wave of summer 2003 in Europe led to more than 70,000 excess deaths.[21] A World Health Organization (WHO) assessment, examining a subset of the possible health impacts, concluded that global climate change that has occurred since the 1970s was already causing over 140,000 excess deaths annually by the year 2004.[22]

Climate change presents a particularly strong example of the unequal distribution of the burden of environmental harm. Though they have contributed much less to climate change than higher income countries, lower income countries will suffer the brunt of its consequences. Low- and middle-income countries, constituting 80 percent of the world's population, have contributed only 23 percent of cumulative global emissions since the mid-18th century.[23] Nevertheless, low-income countries are more affected by climate change due to a combination of factors, including geographic location and higher reliance on agriculture and natural resources. Within countries, the effects of climate change similarly disadvantage the poor, who bear the double burden of higher vulnerability to the negative impacts of climate change and fewer resources with which to adapt. As the Intergovernmental Panel on Climate Change's (IPCC) 4th assessment report summarizes: "Poor communities can be especially vulnerable, in particular those concentrated in high-risk areas. They tend to have more limited adaptive capacities, and are more dependent on climate-sensitive resources such as local water and food supplies."[24] Low-income populations are more likely to suffer from climate change–related risks such as increasing exposure to infectious diseases, exacerbated water and food insecurity, and natural disasters.

Extreme weather events have a greater impact on low-income households, which possess fewer assets that they can use to cope with natural disasters. Residents of informal settlements in low- and middle-income countries are particularly vulnerable to extreme weather events, since they live in hazardous areas with poor-quality housing with high levels of overcrowding and limited infrastructure. A study of flood-related mortality in Nepal, for instance, found that poor households had six times higher risk than their better-off neighbors.[25] But the heightened risk is not limited to poor families in low-income countries. During Hurricane Katrina in New Orleans, low-income residents were disproportionately affected. Residents who lacked cars and financial resources to evacuate were left behind, while many of the lowest income residents lived in the hardest hit low-lying neighborhoods.[26] Low-income households lack the resources to cope with the direct and indirect costs of illness and injuries as the result of extreme weather events, with often devastating economic consequences.[27]

Increasing demand for water resources combined with climate change means that water stress is likely to increase; in the absence of new measures, an estimated 3.9 billion people will be living under conditions of severe water stress by 2030.[28] During the last century, mean precipitation has tended to decrease in all the world's main arid and semiarid regions; these trends imply that water stress will become increasingly severe in the regions where it is already a limited resource.[29] Again, the poor suffer disproportionately. Within India's urban population, 81.5 percent of the poorest quartile did not have access to piped water at home in 2005–2006, compared to 38 percent for the urban population overall.[30] In urban areas in many low- and middle-income countries, the price of water in different areas within the same city can differ 4- to 10-fold; counterintuitively, it is generally the wealthier areas that pay the least.[31,32]

Air quality also manifests itself inequitably. Urban air pollution results in an estimated 800,000 additional deaths annually, with the burden taking place disproportionately in low- and middle-income countries.[33] Lower income populations are consistently exposed to higher levels of air pollution,[34,35,36,37] and studies have found disproportionately high rates of respiratory diseases in low-income and minority populations.[38,39,40,41,42] For example, a study of particulate air pollution across different districts in Hong Kong found that the lower the average monthly household income, the higher the ambient air pollution index levels. The same study found that people in lower income neighborhoods were up to five times as likely to be hospitalized for respiratory illnesses as people in higher income neighborhoods.[43] Low-income neighborhoods are more likely to experience high traffic density, and low-income communities tend to live closer to factories and industries producing high levels of pollutants.[44,45] Outdoor air pollution may disproportionately affect low-income workers. In a comparative study in Mexico City, exposure levels to air pollution were far higher among outdoor laborers: outdoor workers who were either vendors or taxi drivers had median occupational exposures to benzene, toluene, and other pollutants that were 1.5–2.5 times higher than indoor workers who were office workers.[46]

Energy poverty is directly linked to inequalities in air quality. The availability of energy is a key element of quality of life in modern times. When modern energy sources are not available, households are forced to use other alternatives—an estimated 1.4 billion people around the world continue to depend on solid fuels, including biomass fuels and coal, for their energy needs. Eighty-five percent of these people live in rural areas.[47] Solid fuels are used by low-income households that cannot afford cleaner sources such as natural gas or electricity.[48] Reliance on solid fuels for energy needs has serious health implications. Indoor air pollution is linked to respiratory problems, including pneumonia, chronic obstructive lung disease, and asthma, and is also associated with elevated risk of low birth weight, cancer, and cardiovascular failure.[49] According to WHO estimates, indoor air pollution from cooking with solid fuels is responsible for 1.5 million deaths every year.[50] Indoor air pollution from solid fuel use causes about 21 percent of lower respiratory infection deaths worldwide, 35 percent of chronic obstructive pulmonary deaths, and about 3 percent of lung cancer deaths. Of these deaths, an estimated 64 percent occur in low-income countries, especially in South-East Asia and Africa.[51] The use of solid fuels also has detrimental environmental impacts, with an estimated 2 million tons of biomass consumed every day.[52]

Road traffic is a major contributor to air pollution. Additionally, motor vehicles create physical risks, especially in cities with poorly designed road systems, insufficient enforcement of road safety rules, and overcrowded and unsafe public transportation. Road traffic is a major cause of injuries and fatalities worldwide—the World Health Organization estimated that 1.2 million people were killed and 50 million people injured by road traffic crashes in just 1 year.[53] The poor in low-income, middle-income, and high-income countries alike are disproportionately affected by road traffic injuries and fatalities since they are more likely to walk or use nonmotorized transport, and less able to cope with the associated expenses and income losses.[54] In the United Kingdom, fatal injury rates for child pedestrians from the lowest socioeconomic group are 21 times higher than those for the top socioeconomic group, while child cyclists from the lowest socioeconomic group have fatal injury rates almost 28 times higher.[55] Low-income populations in low- and middle-income countries are particularly disadvantaged, since choices of transport mode are linked to socioeconomic status and vulnerable road users (pedestrians, cyclists, and those using motorized two- or three-wheel vehicles) experience higher injury and fatality rates.[56] Research from Bangalore, India, found that mortality from road traffic injuries was 13.1 and 48.1 per 100,000 in lower income urban and rural socioeconomic groups, compared to 7.8 and 26.1 for more affluent groups.[57]

Lack of equitable access to transportation helps perpetuate poverty. The United Kingdom's Social Exclusion Unit found that two out of five job seekers stated that lack of transport constituted a barrier to getting a job, while the two most common problems experienced by young job seekers were "lack of personal transport" and "no job nearby."[58] In the United Kingdom, the Sustainable Development Commission found that public spending on transport is strongly biased toward higher income groups, since a greater proportion of public spending on transport goes to road and rail travel rather than to bus services, which are the most often utilized transportation means in poorer households.[59]

BARRIERS TO ACTION: ARE THE ECONOMY AND THE ENVIRONMENT COMPLEMENTARY?

It is clear that, for the sake of a healthy, equitable, and sustainable future, action must be taken to address environmental challenges. However, a long-standing barrier to action on environmental issues has been concern over potential negative economic consequences. The perceived existence of a tradeoff between environmental protection and economic growth has been the subject of much discussion.[60,61,62,63] Economic growth has historically both required and led to greater use of energy and natural resources, with a resulting increase in carbon emissions. As stated by the United Nations Development Program in its 2011 Human Development report, "recent progress in the [Human Development Index] has come at the cost of global warming," with carbon dioxide emissions per capita growing faster in countries advancing faster in the HDI.[64] As incomes rose in many middle-income countries, energy use, natural resource demands, and carbon footprints increased. Yet the link is not inevitable. Transportation is crucial for economic development; it can but does not have to be one of the main contributors to air pollution. Rising incomes have also led to improvements in environmental issues such as inadequate water supply, sanitation, and solid waste management.[65,66]

While there are few who would currently argue that environmental improvements can never occur without financial loss, concerns about potential negative economic consequences continue to be an obstacle to progress on environmental issues. In political decision making, frequently environmental sustainability is perceived as desirable, but growth limiting and therefore postponed. In discussions on climate change, concerns over economic growth are a frequently cited obstacle, with emerging economies arguing that setting targets for emissions reductions will constrain their economic development.[67] Lower income countries have long expressed the view that their primary concern must be economic growth and development, with environmental protection a secondary concern to be addressed at a later stage.[68] In the words of a United Nations Environment Program officer, "Environment is still perceived by some countries as a luxury. Policymakers in developing countries want more employment, higher income. They tend to say: 'Don't come talk to us now. Developed countries have already gone through this process. When we reach a similar stage, we will look at the environment.' "[69]

The 2008 economic crisis increased concerns over the negative impacts of environmental concerns in emerging economies and higher income countries alike. This led to changes in policy priorities, with environmental issues taking a backseat to economic fears. For instance, before 2008, China's new environmental agenda had led to the closing of factories with heavy pollution problems; once the recession began in 2008, there were reports that these environmental regulations were much less strictly enforced due to concerns over job losses in a slowing economy.[70] Parallel concerns are raised in high-income countries. In Canada in 2009, opposition by environmental groups to proposed new energy projects was dubbed by the Minister of Natural Resources as "undermin[ing] Canada's national economic interest."[71] At a European Union summit in 2008, Eastern European countries and Italy expressed concerns about the affordability of a climate change plan agreed upon in 2007 that targeted 20 percent reductions from 1990 levels by the year 2020.[72] In the United States, both proponents and opponents of climate-change legislation agreed that the odds of passing new legislation were significantly diminished by the 2008 economic crisis. In the words of Senator James Inhofe, an opponent of climate-change action, "Financial realities will make it much more difficult for the new administration or Congress to put forth a very aggressive, economy-wide climate bill."[73]

Yet, contrary to rhetoric that pits economic growth against environmental protection, substantial evidence underscores the economic threats posed by environmental degradation. Environmental degradation has been estimated to cost between 4 and 8 percent of gross domestic product (GDP) in many low- and middle-income countries through the loss of economically productive natural resources in addition to the health costs of lack of safe water and sanitation and air pollution.[74] Natural resources are a major source of livelihood for large portions of the population around the world, with an estimated 40 percent of the economically active population undertaking resource-dependent economic activities such as agriculture, fishing, and forestry. If unaddressed, environmental trends will undermine progress in reducing poverty.[75,76] In sub-Saharan Africa, over US$28 billion, or 5 percent of GDP, are lost each year to the consequences of poor water and sanitation; this amounts to more than the total aid flows and debt relief the region receives.[77] Natural disasters, on the rise as a result of climate change, resulted in an estimated US$366.1 billion in economic damages in 2011 alone, as well as 30,773 deaths and 244.7 million affected worldwide.[78]

LEARNING FROM EFFECTIVE EXAMPLES

Having asked our contributors for solutions to environmental sustainability and equity challenges, they came back to us with examples of how one could achieve three interrelated objectives: (1) how to improve the environment while improving equity; (2) how to improve the environment while improving conditions for the poor; and (3) how to improve the environment while creating jobs.

The chapters in this volume help to answer the key question of how we can solve environmental and equity challenges simultaneously in the face of economic constraints. The first section presents examples of how to address these overarching challenges across environmental areas. The first three chapters examine the role of community ownership of initiatives, particularly important in communities that in addition to economic marginalization and environmental erosion have had little say in their own futures. Ted Howard presents an innovative plan for asset building in marginalized urban neighborhoods through the creation of green enterprises that are owned by their employees. Angela Glover Blackwell examines initiatives that address the interconnections between environmental, social, and economic inequalities in vulnerable communities by giving these communities a voice in generating solutions in high-income countries. David Satterthwaite raises the importance of involving the urban poor in planning for the improvement of informal settlements in low- and middle-income countries.

The next three chapters focus on how to address environment and equity challenges while setting in place income-generating opportunities. Mitra Thompson focuses on the impact of a recycling initiative that creates jobs for members of a highly marginalized population, substance users in British Columbia. Cosmin paduraru and Kara Quennell address strategies to promote training and participation in green jobs as a poverty reduction strategy in high unemployment communities in New York and Texas. Shannon Lockhart examines how green entrepreneurship can provide income-generating opportunities to poor rural communities in India.

The next section of the book focuses on specific areas that experience environmental, economic, and equity obstacles, and presents promising strategies for addressing them. David Banister and James Woodcock offer approaches for moving toward more sustainable transportation for health and equity on a global scale. Madhav Badami addresses policies for sustainable transportation in the specific case of India, a rapidly growing economy. Donald Cole, Gordon Prain, and Willy Pradel focus on how to achieve environmentally and economically sustainable farming techniques in the Andean region. Lise Bertrand examines how the municipal government has partnered with communities to promote increased access to healthy foods for low-income populations in high-income countries. Bill Cosgrove and Hakan Tropp examine how government and IGOs can partner in cost-effective water interventions. Tim Weis presents policy options for achieving more equitable energy access for remote communities in Canada. James Ford looks at the increasing challenges presented by climate change, and how its impacts on the health and well-being of indigenous communities can be reduced.

Ensuring a Sustainable Future is neither a map of all solutions nor a consensus statement. The contributors came to the table with diverse perspectives, each informed by his or her experiences and backgrounds. Like all books, by necessity, this volume presents a limited number of examples. What contributors to this volume have achieved, both individually and collectively, is to present answers to two critical questions: Does action on environmental issues have to put economic development at risk? Is it inevitable that environmental problems disproportionately affect the poor? The solutions proposed by contributors to this volume answer these questions with a clear no. Their chapters show that it is feasible to solve this puzzle and that there is a pressing need for greater engagement in moving toward a sustainable future.

NOTES

1. R. McDonald, "The Implications of Current and Future Urbanization for Global Protected Areas and Biodiversity Conservation," *Biological Conservation* 141 (2008): 1695–703.
2. *Millenium Development Goals Report 2010,* United Nations, accessed June 20, 2011, http://www.un.org/millenniumgoals/pdf/MDG%20Report%202010%20 En%20r15%20-low%20res%2020100615%20-.pdf
3. U. N. Habitat, *Cities and Climate Change: Global Report on Human Settlements 2011,* (London, England: Earthscan, 2011).
4. T. Campbell and A. Campbell, "Emerging Disease Burdens and the Poor in Cities of the Developing World," *Journal of Urban Health* 84, sup. 1 (2007): i54–i164.
5. African Population and Health Research Centre, *Population and Health Dynamics in Nairobi's Informal Settlements: Report of the Nairobi Cross-Sectional slums Survey 2000* (Nairobi, Kenya: APHRC, 2002).
6. V. R. Dhara and R. Dhara, "The Union Carbide Disaster in Bhopal: A Review of Health Effects". *Archives of Environmental and Occupational Health* 57, no. 5 (2002): 391–404.
7. U. N. Habitat, *The Challenge of Slums: Global Report on Human Settlements 2003,* (London, England: Earthscan, 2003).
8. K. Morland, "Disparities in the Availability of Fruits and Vegetables Between Racially Segregated Urban Neighbourhoods," *Public Health Nutrition* 10, no. 12 (2007): 1481–9.
9. A. Shaffer, *The Persistence of L.A.'s Grocery Gap: The Need for a New Food Policy and Approach to Market Development* (Los Angeles, CA: Center for Food and Justice, Urban and Environmental Policy Institute, Occidental College, 2002).
10. K. Morland et al., "Neighborhood Characteristics Associated with the Location of Food Stores and Food Service Places," *American Journal of Preventive Medicine* 22, no. 1 (2002): 23–9.
11. R. Flournoy and S. Treuhaft, *Healthy Foods, Healthy Communities: Improving Access and Opportunities through Food Retailing,* Policy Link, accessed June 20, 2011, http://www.policylink.org/atf/cf/%7B97C6D565-BB43-406D-A6D5-ECA3BBF35AF0%7D/HEALTHYFOOD.pdf
12. USDA Economic Research Service, *Access to Affordable and Nutritious Food: Measuring and Understanding Food Deserts and Their Consequences. Report to Congress.* (Washington, DC: US Department of Agriculture, 2009).
13. California Center for Public Health Advocacy, PolicyLink, and the UCLA Center for Health Policy Research, *Designed for Disease: The Link Between Local Food*

Environments and Obesity and Diabetes (Oakland, CA: PolicyLink, 2008), accessed June 20, 2011, http://www.policylink.org/documents/DesignedforDisease.pdf

14. P. L. Pingali and P. A. Roger, *Impact of Pesticides on Farmers' Health and the Rice Environment* (Dordrecht, The Netherlands: Kluwer, 1995).

15. J. Pretty et al., "An Assessment of the Total External Costs of UK Agriculture," *Agricultural Systems* 65, no. 2 (2000): 113–36.

16. E. M. Tegtmeier and M. D. Duffy, "External Costs of Agricultural Production in the US," *International Journal of Agriculture and Sustainability* 2 (2004): 1–20.

17. N. Uphoff, *Agroecological Innovations* (London, England: Earthscan, 2002).

18. *Agricultural Waged Workers*, FAO and ILO Working Together, accessed October 21, 2012, http://www.fao-ilo.org/more/fao-ilo-ruralworkers/en/.

19. *Climate Change Fact Sheet*, Convention on Biological Diversity, accessed July 11, 2012, http://www.cbd.int/iyb/doc/prints/factsheets/iyb-cbd-factsheet-cc-en. pdf

20. *Climate Change 2007: Synthesis Report. An Assessment of the Intergovernmental Panel on Climate Change*, IGPCC, accessed July 11, 2012, http://www.ipcc.ch/pdf/ assessment-report/ar4/syr/ar4_syr.pdf

21. *Climate Change and Health: Fact sheet No. 266*, World Health Organization, accessed June 20, 2012, http://www.who.int/mediacentre/factsheets/fs266/en/

22. World Health Organization, *Global Health Risks: Mortality and Burden of Disease Attributable to Selected Major Risks* (Geneva, Switzerland: World Health Organization, 2009).

23. M. R. Raupach et al., "Global and Regional Drivers of Accelerating CO2 Emissions," *Proceedings of the National Academy of Sciences USA* 104, no. 24 (2007): 10288–93.

24. *Climate Change 2007: Synthesis Report...*

25. E. K. Pradhan et al., "Risk of Flood-Related Mortality in Nepal," *Disasters* 31, no. 1, (2007): 57–70.

26. U. N. Habitat, *The State of the World's Cities 2006/2007*, (London, England: Earthscan, 2007).

27. R. A. Gosselin et al., "Injuries: The Neglected Burden in Developing Countries," *Bulletin of the World Health Organization* 87 (2009): 246.

28. *Managing Water for All: An OECD Perspective on Pricing and Financing, Key Messages for Policy Makers*, Organisation for Economic Co-Operation and Development, accessed August 11, 2012, http://www.oecd.org/env/42350563. pdf

29. D. Satterthwaite et al., "Adapting to Climate Change in Urban Areas: The Possibilities and Constraints in Low- and Middle-Income Nations (Human Settlements Discussion Paper Series IIED, London: 2007).

30. S. Agarwal, "The State of Urban Health in India; Comparing the Poorest Quartile to the Rest of the Urban Population in Selected States and Cities," *Environment and Urbanization* 23 (2011): 13.

31. U. N. Habitat, *The Challenge of Slums...*

32. J. Thompson et al., "Waiting at the Tap: Changes in Urban Water Use in East Africa over Three Decades. *Environment and Urbanization* 12, no. 2 (2000): 37–52.

33. A. J. Cohen, "The Global Burden of Disease Due to Outdoor Air Pollution," *Journal of Toxicology and Environmental Health, Part A* 68 (2005): 1301–7.

34. M. S. O'Neill, P. L. Kinney, and A. J. Cohen, "Environmental Equity in Air Quality Management: Local and International Implications for Human Health

and Climate Change," *Journal of Toxicology and Environmental Health, Part A* 71 (2008): 570–7.

35. P. L. Kinney and M. S. O'Neill, "Environmental Equity," in *WHO Air Quality Guidelines for Particulate Matter, Ozone, Nitrogen Dioxide and Sulfur Dioxide: Global Update 2005,* accessed May 6, 2013, http://www.euro.who.int/__data/assets/pdf_file/0005/78638/E90038.pdf

36. M. M. Finkelstein et al., "Relation between Income, Air Pollution and Mortality: A Cohort Study," *Canadian Medical Association Journal* 169 (2003): 397–402.

37. R. S. Green et al., "Proximity of California Public Schools to Busy Roads," *Environmental Health Perspectives* 112 (2004): 61–6.

38. F. P. Perera et al., "The Challenge of Preventing Environmentally Related Disease in Young Children: Community-Based Research in New York City," *Environmental Health Perspectives* volume 110, no. 2 (2002): 197–204.

39. O'Neill et al., "Environmental Equity in Air Quality. . ."

40. Kinney and O'Neill, "Environmental Equity."

41. Finkelstein et al., "Relation Between Income, Air Pollution. . ."

42. Green et al., "Proximity of California Public Schools. . ."

43. R. E. Stern, "Hong Kong Haze: Air Pollution as a Social Class Issue," *Asian Survey* 43, no. 5 (2003); 780–800.

44. D. Houston et al., "Structural Disparities of Urban Traffic in Southern California: Implications for Vehicle-related Air Pollution Exposure in Minority and High-Poverty Neighborhoods," *Journal of Urban Affairs* 26, no. 5 (2004): 565–92.

45. G. McGranahan, L. Leitmann, and C. Surjadi, *Understanding Environmental Problems in Disadvantaged Neighborhoods: Broad Spectrum Surveys, Participatory Appraisal and Contingent Valuation* (working paper no. 16, UNDP/UNCHS, World Bank, Washington, DC, 1997).

46. H. Tovalin-Ahumada and L. Whitehead, "Personal Exposures to Volatile Organic Compounds among Outdoor and Indoor Workers in Two Mexican Cities," *Science of the Total Environment* 376, no. 1–3 (2007): 60–71.

47. *Energy Poverty: How to Make Modern Energy Access Universal?* (special excerpt, The World Energy Outlook 2010 for the U. N. General Assembly on Millenium Development Goals, International Energy Agency, Geneva, Switzerland, 2010).

48. A. Sverdlik, "Ill-Health and Poverty: A Literature Review on Health in Informal Settlements," *Environment and Urbanization,* 23 (2011): 123.

49. Ibid.

50. *Fuel for Life: Household Energy and Health,* World Health Organization, accessed May 11, 2012, http://www.who.int/indoorair/publications/fuelforlife.pdf.

51. World Health Organization, *Global Health Risks: Mortality and Burden of Disease Attributable to Selected Major Risks* (Geneva, Switzerland: WHO, 2009).

52. *Fuel for Life. . .*

53. M. Peden et al., *World Report on Road Traffic Injury Prevention* (Geneva, Switzerland: World Health Organization, 2004).

54. *Global Status Report on Road Safety: Time for Action,* World Health Organization, accessed May 6, 2013, http://www.un.org/ar/roadsafety/pdf/roadsafetyreport.pdf

55. P. Edwards et al. "Deaths from Injury in Children and Employment Status in Family: Analysis of Trends in Class Specifi c Death Rates," *British Medical Journal,* doi:10.1136/bmj.38875.757488.4F.

56. *Global Status Report on Road Safety. . .*

57. A. Aeron-Thomas et al., *The Involvement and Impact of Road Crashes on the Poor: Bangladesh and India Case Studies,* accessed May 11, 2012, http://www.dfid.gov.uk/r4d/pdf/outputs/R7780.pdf

58. *Making the Connections: Final Report on Transport and Social Exclusion,* Social Exclusion Unit,, accessed May 10, 2013. http://assets.dft.gov.uk/statistics/series/accessibility/making-the-connections.pdf

59. *Fairness in a Car Dependent Society,* Sustainable Development Commission, London, accessed October 20, 2012, http://www.sd-commission.org.uk/data/files/publications/fairness_car_dependant.pdf.

60. E. Neumayer, "Is Economic Growth the Environment's Best Friend?" *Journal of Environmental Law and Policy* 2/98 (1998) 161–76.

61. W. Beckerman, *Economic Development and the Environment—Conflict or Complementarity?* (working paper no. 961, World Bank, Washington, DC, 1992).

62. G. Grossman and A. B. Krueger, "Economic Growth and the Environment," *The Quarterly Journal of Economics* 110 (1995): 353–77.

63. F. A. G. Den Butter and H. Verbruggen, "Measuring the Trade-Off Between Economic Growth and a Clean Environment," *Environmental and Resource Economics* 4 (1994): 187–208.

64. U. N. Development Programme, *Human Development Report 2011: Sustainability and Equity: A Better Future For All* (UNDP: New York, 2011).

65. Commission of the European Communities, "Protecting the Environment and Economic Growth: Trade-Off or Growth-Enhancing Structural Adjustment," chap. 6 in *The EU Economy 2004 Review,* accessed May 6, 2013, http://ec.europa.eu/economy_finance/publications/publication451_en.pdf

66. U. N. Development Programme, *Human Development Report 2011...*

67. B. C. Parks and R. J. Timmons, "Inequality and the Global Climate Regime: Breaking the North-South Impasse," *Cambridge Review of International Affairs* 21, no. 4 (2008): 621–628.

68. J. M. Broder, "Climate Talks in Durban Yield Limited Agreement," *The New York Times,* December 11, 2011, accessed http://www.nytimes.com/2011/12/12/science/earth/countries-at-un-conference-agree-to-draft-new-emissions-treaty.html?_r=1

69. Director, Economics and Trade Branch, Division of Technology, Industry and Economics, UNEP, quoted in *Challenges in Decision-Making: From Barriers to Synergies,* The Health and Environment Linkages Initiative (HELI), accessed November 21, 2012, http://www.who.int/heli/decisions/barriers/en/index.html

70. A. Eunjung Cha A, "As Global Recession Threatens, China Pulls Back on Environmental Efforts," *Washington Post Foreign Service,* November 19, 2008, accessed http://www.washingtonpost.com/wp-dyn/content/article/2008/11/18/AR2008111803625.html

71. "An Open Letter from the Honourable Joe Oliver, Minister of Natural Resources, on Canada's Commitment to Diversify Our Energy Markets and the Need to Further Streamline the Regulatory Process in Order to Advance Canada's National Economic Interest, January 9, 2009, accessed October 15, 2012, http://www.joeoliver.ca/news/an-open-letter-from-the-honourable-joe-oliver-minister-of-natural-resources-on-canada%E2%80%99s-commitment-to-diversify-our-energy-markets-and-the-need-to-further-streamline-the-regulatory-process/

72. S. Castle, "European Nations Seek to Revise Agreement on Emissions Cuts," *The New York Times,* October 16, 2008, accessed http://www.nytimes.com/2008/10/17/world/europe/17union.html?_r=0.

73. M. Kriz, "Financial Crisis Dims Chances for U.S. Climate Legislation," *Yale Environment 360,* October 6, 2008, accessed http://e360.yale.edu/feature/financial_crisis_dims_chances_for_us_climate_legislation/2070/

74. *Environment Matters,* World Bank, accessed August 8, 2012, http://www-wds.worldbank.org/external/default/WDSContentServer/WDSP/IB/2006/11/16/000310607_20061116144825/Rendered/PDF/380060Environment0matters0EM0601PUBLIC1.pdf

75. E. B. Barbier. "Poverty, Development, and Environment," *Environment and Development Economics* 15, special issue 6 (2010): 635–60.

76. U. N. Development Programme, *Human Development Report 2011...*

77. UN Development Programme. *Human Development Report 2006. Beyond Scarcity: Power, poverty and the global water crisis.* (UNDP: New York, 2006).

78. D. Guha-Sapir et al., *Annual Disaster Statistical Review 2011: The Numbers and Trends* (Brussels, Belgium: CRED, 2012).

Moving Forward on the Environment and the Economy: Creating Jobs, Building Healthy Communities

CHAPTER 1

The Essential Connection

Environmental Sustainability, Community Stability, and Equitable Development in Struggling Cities in High-Income Countries

TED HOWARD

Barry Commoner, one of the founders of the global environmental movement, described the first law of ecology as "Everything is connected to everything else."[1] Likewise, this chapter will draw a close and compelling linkage between environmental sustainability, community stabilization, and equitable development. That is to say, the environment, place, and equity are intimately and inextricably interconnected. Given these linkages, building healthy communities must necessarily include both addressing environmental problems and building wealth and assets. Other chapters will examine in detail how environmental problems disproportionately impact the poor, leading to inequalities in health and quality of life as well as development opportunities. This chapter examines the central role of community initiatives in furthering equitable economic growth and thereby promoting greater environmental sustainability. The chapter first explores the largely untapped potential of anchor institutions in fostering locally rooted economic growth. It then considers the potential of combining the growing green economy with community wealth-building strategies, to pursue the notion that healthy, sustainable communities need to include both economic growth and environmental quality.

A community that is not economically sustainable cannot be ecologically sustainable. But a community that is at the mercy of the investment decisions made by distant corporations concerned with their bottom line—not the fate of the community in which their business is located—can neither be certain of its economic future nor self-confident enough to undertake an aggressive sustainability initiative at the local level. Tremendous economic instability is faced by American cities whose economic futures are dependent on decisions made by mobile investors of capital and by market forces beyond their control.

As a result, we have "throw-away cities" with crumbling infrastructure, the flight of jobs and productive capital, and people left behind, trapped in intergenerational poverty. These communities that are left behind experience the consequences of rising inequalities, including worse health outcomes, inferior education, and a lack of job opportunities.

Arresting these trends will require major efforts to, first, improve the quality of life in cities and end the gaping social disparities between suburbs and cities; second, reduce gaping social disparities *within* cities (a major cause of "urban decline" of the past half century); and third, stabilize the economic underpinnings of cities—that is, the job base. The best laid sustainability plans cannot work when jobs and people continue to flee our cities.

American poverty remains disproportionately concentrated in urban areas, a core cause of sprawl and its related ecologically harmful consequences. Dealing with that problem necessitates a serious strategy to provide stable, living wage employment in every community and every neighborhood in the country.

Enhancing community stability requires bolstering the economic core of our cities by:

- promoting and nurturing community-rooted enterprises that can create and sustain long-term employment;
- leveraging local institutional purchasing to support community-rooted enterprises;
- financing larger scale public investments in the new urban infrastructure to support a low-carbon economy;
- using national policy to build up domestic capacity in key green industries; and
- allocating public capital and investment to cities threatened by private disinvestment.

Implementing a broad strategy that integrates these various elements would permit a dramatic break with the past practice of allowing cities to wither and decay as market forces dictate. It would allow us to stop throwing away our cities.

A central part of a community-stabilizing strategy must be using existing and new streams of public investment to build up stable, community-based enterprise. Whenever possible, the billions of dollars now being invested in green jobs, for instance, should be targeted toward community-stabilizing organizations rather than becoming just another profit opportunity for large corporations. Even in economically struggling cities, existing anchor institutions such as hospitals and educational facilities can be leveraged to generate support for community-based enterprise. An important example is taking place in Cleveland, Ohio, where a network of worker-owned businesses—the Evergreen Cooperatives—has been launched in low-income, inner-city neighborhoods. The cooperatives will initially provide services to anchor institutions, particularly local hospitals and universities. Rather than allowing vast streams of money to leak out of the community or be captured by distant companies, existing local spending can be used to support place-based enterprise. Cleveland is but one example. There are many others.

As John Fullerton, a former managing director of the investment firm J.P. Morgan and founder of the Capital Institute has written:

> The conceivers of the Evergreen Cooperatives see the challenge of economic development and sustainable prosperity…through the lens that renowned urban activist and unconventional economist Jane Jacobs articulated so well, identifying cities rather than nations as the core organizing instruments of economies, and drawing parallels between healthy, place-based economies and healthy ecosystems. Central to Jacob's framing is the resilient demand creation of local anchor institutions—the hospitals, universities, and government agencies that all have a strategic long-term interest in the health of their local communities. The properly harnessed energy of these anchor institutions is a vital source of resiliency in place-based economies. And resilient place-based economies provide the strong foundation that is the necessary pre-condition for successfully engaging in the competitive global economy.[2]

POVERTY, WEALTH INEQUALITY, AND THE DECLINE OF AMERICA'S CITIES

In September 2011, the US Census Bureau released new statistics about poverty in the United States. According to the Bureau's analysis, fully 25 percent of very young children in America are now living in poverty. Furthermore, the Bureau announced that 46.2 million Americans lived in poverty in 2010—the most since the agency began tracking poverty levels in the 1950s.[3]

US Supreme Court Justice Louis Brandeis famously said: "We can have democracy in this country, or we can have great wealth concentrated in the hands of a few, but we can't have both."[4] Accompanying the growth in poverty has been the escalating concentration of wealth in American society:

- The top 5 percent of Americans own 70 percent of all financial wealth.
- The top 1 percent of Americans now claim more income per year than the bottom 100 million Americans taken together.

- Over the last three decades, the top 1 percent of the country has received 36 percent of all the gains in household income.
- The average family of color owns less than 10 cents for every dollar held by a white family.
- Two of five American children are raised in asset-poor households, including one of every two Latino children and one of every two African American children.[5]

One does not need to be an organizer with Occupy Wall Street to be astonished by this fact: just 400 individuals in the United States own more wealth than the bottom 150 million Americans.[6] My colleague, political economist Gar Alperovitz, characterizes this concentration of wealth as "medieval"—which he means not rhetorically, but in actual fact in terms of wealth-holding patterns between our time and that of Medieval Europe. As Timothy Noah observed in his essay "The Great Divergence," "Economically speaking, the richest nation on earth is starting to resemble a banana republic."[7]

Nor have the past several decades been good ones for many American cities, particularly our older industrial—or "weak market"—cities. Many communities have experienced extraordinary distress. The foreclosure crisis of recent years is but the most recent disaster to hit these urban areas. Since the 1970s, many of America's cities have seen declining populations (from 2000 to 2010, for example, Detroit lost 25 percent of its population and Cleveland 17 percent), the flight of capital and millions of jobs, stressed city services, and endemic poverty.[8]

According to the US Census Bureau, even before the Great Recession hit, in 2007 Detroit had a poverty rate of 33.8 percent, Cleveland 29.5 percent, and Buffalo 28.7 percent. The level of pain in our smaller cities is even greater: in 2007, Bloomington, Indiana, led the list with a poverty rate of 41.6 percent.[9]

The growing distress and destabilization of many of our cities has been fueled in great measure by the loss of much of the country's manufacturing strength. Between 1980 and 2009, the United States lost 7.1 million manufacturing jobs, 38 percent of the total manufacturing base. More than 61 percent of these lost jobs were in 114 industrial metropolitan areas—urban centers that strongly specialized in manufacturing through the 1970s.[10]

As capital becomes increasingly mobile, these jobs have been relocated to other regions or countries with the lowest wages. The result: a destabilized economic base in American communities as jobs are displaced, the local tax base erodes, and falling revenues result in cuts in needed neighborhood social services. Existing infrastructure is allowed to crumble as cities are depopulated, in effect throwing away billions of dollars of our existing urban infrastructure. Concurrently, Sun Belt cities like Phoenix and Houston experience dramatic expansion as billions of dollars are invested in new construction at great environmental cost.

COMMUNITY WEALTH BUILDING: A NEW PARADIGM OF
SUSTAINABLE AND EQUITABLE ECONOMIC DEVELOPMENT

In the face of these destabilizing trends, how might we begin to address the "essential connection" among environmental sustainability, community stability, and equitable development? Some of the most exciting and dynamic experimentation is occurring across the United States at the community level, as cities and residents beset by pain and decades of failed promises and disinvestment are charting dynamic new approaches to rebuilding their communities.

Although largely unnoticed by the media, over the past few decades there has been a steady buildup of new forms of community-supportive economic enterprises. These ideas, now being implemented in communities across the country, are beginning to define the underlying structural building blocks of a democratic political-economic system—a new "model"—that is different in fundamental ways from both traditional capitalism and socialism.

Increasingly, this approach is known as *community wealth building*. It is a form of development that puts wealth in the hands of locally rooted forms of business enterprise (with ownership vested in community stakeholders), not simply investor-driven corporations. These anchored businesses (both for-profit and nonprofit) in turn reinvest in their local neighborhoods, building wealth in asset-poor communities. As such, they contribute to local economic stability and stop the leakage of dollars from communities, which in turn reinforces environmental sustainability and equitable development.

Community wealth-building strategies spread the benefits of business ownership widely, thus improving the ability of communities and their residents to own assets, anchor jobs, expand public services, and ensure local economic stability. The field is comprised of a broad array of locally anchored economic institutions that have the potential to be powerful agents to build both individual and commonly held assets. Their activities range along a continuum from efforts focused solely on building modest levels of assets for low-income individuals to establishing urban land trusts, community-benefiting businesses, municipal enterprises, nonprofit financial institutions, cooperatives, social enterprises, and employee-owned companies. Also included in the mix is a range of new asset-development policy proposals that are winning support in city and state governments.

Forty years ago, there were fewer than 200 employee-owned companies in the United States. The community development finance industry did not yet exist. Likewise, few community development corporations (CDCs) and no significant community land trusts existed. State public pension funds did not employ economically targeted investments.

Today, the National Center for Employee Ownership reports that 13.7 million Americans work at roughly 11,400 businesses where they own all or part of the company through employee stock option plans, with an ownership stake of $922.5 billion as of the end of 2006. There are now over 4,600 CDCs nationwide that develop on average 86,000 units of affordable housing and 8.75 million square feet of commercial real estate a year. Between 1998 and 2005, CDC business development efforts helped create an estimated 527,000 jobs.

Community development financial institutions (CDFIs) manage assets of over $25 billion. In 2006 these groups financed affordable housing for 69,000 housing units and helped create or maintain 35,000 jobs. More than half of all states now allocate a portion of their pension funds to economically targeted investments, which now total $10 billion. Additionally, older forms of community ownership continue to thrive—everything from the 2,000-plus publicly owned utility companies spanning the nation to a cooperative movement in which 130 million Americans participate, which has $3 trillion in assets, generates $650 billion in annual revenue, and employs over 850,000.[11,12,13,14,15,16]

What these institutional forms of community wealth building offer is a perspective that assists communities to build upon their own assets. They make asset accumulation and community/shared ownership central to local economic development. In so doing, community wealth building provides a new direction to begin to heal the economic opportunity divide between haves and have-nots at its source: providing low- and moderate-income communities the tools necessary to build their own wealth.

National policy can promote the community wealth-building paradigm by developing an integrated strategy and set of activities and processes that foster economic regeneration through:

- advancing shared-ownership mechanisms (including employee ownership, cooperatives community development corporations and financial institutions, community land trusts, and social enterprise) to create local economic stability;
- linking land use planning and stewardship to transportation access, energy use, affordable housing, and local job creation and economic development;
- increasing economic multipliers to spur locally oriented economic growth;
- leveraging anchor institutions (such as place-bound large nonprofit universities and hospitals) to focus their procurement, investment, and other economic activities toward local ends; and
- expanding investment opportunities and asset creation for low- and moderate-income Americans.

While a strategy to scale up community wealth-building strategies and mechanisms will face many challenges, a pair of unusual openings exist that, if seized upon, can greatly strengthen the effort. In particular, momentum and scale can be achieved by (1) aligning wealth building efforts with the growing movement among place-based anchor institutions to participate in community building and economic development, and (2) capitalizing on the growing interest in building a green economy and green jobs.

ANCHOR INSTITUTIONS AS COMMUNITY-STABILIZING ENTITIES

Anchor institutions are place-based enterprises, firmly rooted in their locales. In addition to universities and hospitals (often referred to as "eds and meds"), anchors may include cultural institutions (such as museums), health care facilities (such as nursing and retirement homes), community foundations, faith-based institutions, public utilities, and municipal governments. Typically, anchors tend to be nonprofit corporations. Because they are rooted in place (unlike for-profit corporations that may relocate for a variety of reasons, such as lower labor costs, pursuing subsidies, avoiding environmental regulations, and so on), anchors have, at least in principle, an economic self-interest in helping ensure that the communities in which they are based are safe, vibrant, healthy, and stable.

A key strategic issue is how to leverage the vast resources that flow through these institutions to build community wealth by such means as targeted local purchasing, hiring, real estate development, and investment. Importantly, both within the higher education and health care sectors, institutions are increasingly committed to defined and measurable environmental goals—such as shrinking their carbon footprints—which help reinforce a focus on localizing their procurement, investment, and other business practices.

Stable, community-anchoring jobs cannot be relocated and moved to different localities (or even different countries). The most obvious examples of such stable jobs are those provided by colleges and universities, hospitals, and government operations.

Cities with a large proportion of jobs in these community-anchored sectors will be more stable over time and thus be much more capable of achieving carbon emissions reduction targets. A study of 62 cities over two decades (1980 to 1999) that were home to state capitals and/or state flagship universities and had moderate population levels (25,000 to 250,000) bears out this point about the stabilizing effect of community-based institutions. Of these 62 cities, nearly two-thirds enjoyed stable populations or moderate growth, while another 21 percent had population growth of greater than 20 percent—a marked contrast with the population decline faced by many US cities during this period.[17]

City governments are also obviously anchors. It is no accident that Austin, Texas—often called the greenest city in America—is itself both a state capital and host to a major state university, both of which anchor and stabilize the local economy in a manner not currently possible in many cities. The city's low crime rate and high quality of life (Austin regularly is near the top of "best city to live in" rankings) also means green issues have a higher saliency to local residents than cities facing more significant public safety and economic problems. Critically, policy makers in Austin do not have to spend much time worrying about whether the economic basis of the city will disappear. Most other localities in the United States are not so fortunate.

Over the past decade a great deal of momentum has been built around engaging anchor institutions in local community and economic development. It is now widely recognized that place-based anchors are important economic engines in many cities and regions, including their role as significant employers. For example, a 1999 Brookings Institution report found that in the 20 largest US cities, universities and hospitals accounted for 35 percent of the workforce employed by the top 10 private employers.[18]

Nationwide, universities employ over 2 million full-time workers and another million part-time workers. In 2006 alone, the nation's colleges and universities purchased over $373 billion in goods and services—or more than 2 percent of the nation's gross domestic product—and their endowment investments exceeded $411 billion before the stock market bubble and, even post bubble remain well above $300 billion. Hospitals have an even greater economic impact; for example, their annual purchasing now exceeds $750 billion and the total number of hospital employees in 2009 exceeded 5.4 million. Despite the prominence of for-profit hospitals, roughly 86 percent of hospital beds are either in nonprofit (70 percent) or publicly owned hospitals (16 percent).[19]

The potential for anchor institutions to leverage this purchasing power in order to generate local jobs is substantial. The University of Pennsylvania example is illustrative: in fiscal year 2008 alone, Penn purchased approximately $89.6 million (approximately 11 percent of its total purchase order spending) from West Philadelphia suppliers; when Penn began its effort in 1986, its local spending was only $1.3 million. Determining economic impact is an inexact science, but given that Penn has shifted more than $85 million of its spending to West Philadelphia, a very conservative estimate would suggest that minimally Penn's effort has generated 160 additional local jobs and $5 million more in local wages than if old spending patterns had stayed in place.[20]

Another innovative example of an anchor institution using its economic power to directly benefit the community recently occurred in northeast Ohio.

In 2005, University Hospitals announced a path-breaking, 5-year strategic growth plan called *Vision 2010*. The most visible feature of Vision 2010 was new construction of five major facilities, as well as outpatient health centers and expansion of a number of other facilities. The total cost of the plan was $1.2 billion, of which about $750 million was in construction.

In implementing Vision 2010, University Hospitals made a decision to intentionally target and leverage its expenditures to directly benefit the residents of Cleveland and the overall economy of northeast Ohio. For example, Vision 2010 included diversity goals (minority and female business targets were set and monitored), procurement of products and services offered by local companies, hiring of local residents, and other targeted initiatives. These goals were linked both to the construction phase and the ongoing operation of the new facilities once opened.

Specific Vision 2010 expenditure targets included the following:

- Five percent of contractors working on Vision 2010 projects were to be female-owned businesses.
- Fifteen percent of contractors were to be minority-owned businesses.
- Twenty percent of all workers on Vision 2010–related projects were to be residents of the City of Cleveland.
- Eighty percent of businesses that received contracts were to be locally based companies.

Over the 5-year course of the initiative, UH exceeded all of these targets except for the residency goal (e.g., more than 100 minority- and female-owned businesses were engaged through UH's efforts; more than 90 percent of all businesses that participated in Vision 2010 were locally based, far exceeding the target). To realize its objectives, UH instituted internal administrative changes to its traditional business practices to give preference to local residents and vendors, and to ensure that its "spend" would be leveraged to produce a multiplier effect in the region.

The Vision 2010 goal of using regionally based companies encouraged nonlocal companies to open offices and to employ northeast Ohio residents. For example, a non-Ohio company could meet the regionalism goal by opening a Cleveland office and employing Cleveland residents. This portion of Vision 2010 sought to introduce new, hospital-related businesses to the region.

To encourage wealth building among traditionally disadvantaged residents of the region, Vision 2010 also included diversity goals for minority and female business participation in contracts.

Finally, in order to maintain diversity standards following the completion of Vision 2010, UH contributed funds to training programs that targeted diversity job creation for years after the completion of Vision 2010.

Because the model explicitly sought to multiply the effect of the Vision 2010 expenditures through localizing procurement to improve the economy in northeast Ohio, its impact is anticipated to be long term. It is noteworthy that the hospital system has voluntarily decided to follow on the success of Vision 2010 by reorienting its entire supply chain (beyond construction projects), with local targets now set for all purchases over $20,000. Given that

University Hospitals' annual spending is in excess of $800 million, this should produce considerable local economic value and job creation in a region that has been hard hit by loss of manufacturing jobs, population decrease, and the foreclosure crisis.

As an example of how an anchor institution can focus its business practices to produce lasting economic benefit for local communities, Vision 2010 represents an important model for hospitals and other types of anchor institutions across the country.[21,22]

Another concerted effort to leverage anchor institution purchasing could have an even greater impact in northeast Ohio. For example, a study of northeast Ohio food spending (which totaled roughly $15 billion) found that a shift of 25 percent of food production to local production in a 16-county Northeast Ohio region "could create 27,664 new jobs, providing work for about one in eight unemployed residents. It could increase annual regional output by $4.2 billion and expand state and local tax collections by $126 million." In northeast Ohio, institutional buyers such as schools, universities, hospitals, and nursing homes combined make more than 9 percent of total food purchases. In other words, even if supermarket and restaurant buyers in Northeast Ohio failed to shift *any* of their purchasing, a shift of 25 percent of anchor institution food purchases alone would create over 2,500 new jobs, increase regional output by nearly $400 million, and expand state and local tax collections by nearly $12 million. Additionally, anchor institutions, because of their scale and visibility, often prod others into action. Indeed, the northeast Ohio study authors cited precisely this demonstration effect in describing the "25 percent shift" goal of their study: "Locally, institutions such as Oberlin College, which now purchases 30–40 percent of its food locally, have demonstrated that a shift of this magnitude is possible."[23]

Despite increased efforts in recent years, anchor institutions remain a largely untapped resource for local job creation and equitable economic development. Properly focused and leveraged, anchor institution procurement, investment, and hiring can generate a significant and beneficial local economic impact, far exceeding what is currently achieved. What is required is a much deeper level of institutional engagement in which anchors commit themselves to consciously apply their place-based economic power, in combination with their human and intellectual resources, to better the long-term welfare of the places in which they reside, including for low-income residents of urban areas.

FROM GREEN JOBS TO GREEN OWNERSHIP

The growth of the green economy presents another potential source of urban renewal. Over the past several years, the vision of a new and transformative green American economy—one capable of employing millions of workers in renewable energy, green construction, clean transportation, recycling, reuse, waste management, land use, and more—has exploded across the nation. Unions, business groups, and activists are all strong advocates of public investment in this green new world.

The green economy is growing in the United States despite a lack of consistent policy focus and investment. A 2009 study by the Pew Charitable Trust attributes more than 770,000 jobs generated by nearly 70,000 businesses to this sector. A study written 3 years earlier for the US Conference of Mayors arrived at a similar estimate and projects that, by 2038, an estimated 4.2 million jobs can be created, representing 10 percent of new job growth. Although green jobs represent only half of 1 percent of all jobs today, their growth outpaces overall job growth; according to Pew, between 1998 and 2007, green jobs grew at an annual rate of 9.1 percent versus overall growth of 3.7 percent.[24,25,26]

To date, green jobs have been seen primarily as a new employment strategy and workforce development opportunity. The jobs that are envisioned are little different in quality from the economy's traditional employment opportunities: some of the new jobs will be high wage, but most will not; some will be unionized, but most will not; virtually all of the companies in the green sector will either be privately held or owned by outside investors. While many billions of dollars in public monies will be devoted to building the green economy and its jobs, little discussion has been held about whom, in the end, will be the beneficiaries of the vast wealth that will be created through this investment. The hope has been for jobs, pure and simple.

Given the central role that taxpayer-financed public investment will play in building the green economy, should we not—as a matter of public policy— attempt whenever possible to ensure that these investments are targeted in such a way as to create wealth and financial security for America's workers, and economic stability for the communities in which green businesses are located?

The emerging green economy is an opportunity not only to create a significant number—perhaps millions—of new, green jobs. It also represents an historic moment to organize those jobs so that they significantly broaden ownership over wealth and capital. In short: *green jobs you can own.*

By building on numerous practical precedents and expanding our vision beyond green jobs to green ownership, we can offer America's workers living wage (or better) employment and the chance to build their wealth and assets through an equity stake in the businesses in which they work. Joining the vision of the green economy with practical and well-established mechanisms and strategies of community wealth building and broadly shared ownership can also result in new community-stabilizing strategies—innovations that can begin to turn back the tide of disinvestment that has overwhelmed our urban areas in recent decades.

Without such a strategy, the advent of the green economy may result in business as usual: that is, the use of public funds to subsidize large corporations that invest in green industries and technology. That may help reduce the nation's reliance on fossil fuels, but the promise of a more equitable and community-stabilizing green economy will have been squandered.

There are a growing number of examples of real-life green jobs and ownership strategies now spreading across the United States, and, indeed, in other countries as well. Encouragingly, they include electric cooperatives that invest in renewables, municipal utilities that support solar ownership, employee-owned businesses that engage in green manufacturing, worker co-ops that install solar panels and grow fresh produce in urban settings, social enterprises that dominate the recycling industry in their communities, and nonprofit developers that are taking the lead on greening affordable housing.

Many of these efforts are in an early stage of development, and only a few have moved to a significant scale or are in the manufacturing sector, where jobs are typically higher paid and there are true career paths. Nonetheless, building forward on the basis of current experience, there is now a real opportunity to create significant momentum around a genuinely new model of large-scale worker and community-benefiting green enterprises that are broadly owned and locally rooted.

There is a real and historic opening at this time to expand economic opportunity and reduce wealth and income disparities, while advancing environmental sustainability. Among these opportunities are the following:

- *Community ownership of wind production.* In Denmark today, roughly 5 percent of the population (which would be the equivalent of 15 million people in the United States) owns a stake in a windmill guild or cooperative. This ownership pattern requires a "feed-in tariff" system that provides guaranteed prices for renewable energy. Such a policy regime can be duplicated in the United States. Indeed, in 2009, Gainesville, Florida, and the state of Vermont both passed laws establishing feed-in-tariff policies.[27]
- *Public and co-op power company procurement of renewable energy.* Today, more than a quarter of all US electricity is distributed via cooperative or public power companies. These entities can use their market power to promote sustainability, with the profits generated supporting their members. In Austin, Texas, for instance, Austin Energy has shifted 12 percent of its energy purchasing to renewables. In other cases, co-ops and municipal energy companies have become direct renewable energy producers.[28]
- *Employee ownership in solar energy and recycling.* Solar energy is a growing field in which community-oriented forms of business have excelled. For instance, Boulder-based Namasté Solar is a 100 percent, employee-owned company that has gained an estimated 20 percent share of the Colorado solar installation market. Recycling also has strong employee-owned examples. Employee-owned Recology, based in San

Francisco, is a recycling industry leader that serves more than 50 communities in California.[29]

- *Leveraging existing employee-owned company assets.* Employee stock ownership plan (ESOP) companies today employ 13.7 million Americans or roughly 9 percent of the total labor force. They represent a much higher concentration of workers engaged in manufacturing. These businesses have over $900 billion in assets which can be reinvested in growing "green" sectors of the economy, capturing the economic benefits for their employee owners. For example, in Sharon Heights, Ohio, the EBO Group whose work once focused almost entirely on providing drive systems for the coal industry, now does nearly half of its business in the clean transportation, solar, recycling, and medical equipment sectors.[30]
- *Developing cooperative networks.* Network building is a proven strategy for supporting community enterprise. In the San Francisco Bay area, Women's Action for Gains in Economic Security (WAGES) has developed a network of five worker co-ops that provide housecleaning services that avoid petrochemical cleaning agents, while providing living wages and ownership dividends to their immigrant women owners.[31]

THE EVERGREEN COOPERATIVES OF CLEVELAND, OHIO

One of the most innovative examples of the "essential connection"—the nexus of environmental sustainability, community stabilization, and equitable development—that leverages community wealth-building strategies involving anchor institutions and green ownership is the Evergreen Cooperative business network in Cleveland, Ohio.[32,33,34] This network of green worker cooperative businesses aims to generate wealth for its workers while promoting area-wide sustainability goals. Each of the Evergreen cooperatives is closely linked to the procurement needs of the city's major educational and health sector institutions.

Already, the "Cleveland model"—as many have come to label the initiative—has spread beyond Cleveland, with efforts now gathering early momentum in places as diverse as Amarillo, Texas; Atlanta, Georgia; Milwaukee, Wisconsin; Pittsburgh, Pennsylvania; Richmond, California; Springfield, Massachusetts; and Washington, DC.

The Evergreen Cooperative Initiative is centered in Cleveland's University Circle area, home to many of the city's wealthiest and most important anchor institutions that are a legacy of the city's industrial past and former manufacturing strength. These include, for example, the Cleveland Clinic, Case Western Reserve University, the University Hospitals, the Veterans Administration Medical Center, and numerous cultural organizations. Together, they employ more than 50,000 people and represent one of the leading economic engines of northeast Ohio.

Yet the neighborhoods (Glenville, Hough, Fairfax, Buckeye/Shaker, Little Italy, and the eastern portion of East Cleveland) surrounding these multi-billion-dollar institutions are among the most disadvantaged in the city. Annual median household income is below $18,500 and fully 40 percent of the population lives below the poverty line. There is a paucity of retail and service outlets in the neighborhoods, as well as many other amenities. Unemployment is high, educational attainment is low, housing is distressed, and relatively few job opportunities exist within the neighborhoods. Individual families are in general asset poor, as are the neighborhoods as a whole.

In 2005, the Cleveland Foundation catalyzed a partnership of Cleveland's major anchors, community-based organizations, and other civic leaders to form the Greater University Circle Initiative. Over time, the Initiative has become a comprehensive community-building and development strategy designed to transform Greater University Circle by breaking down barriers between institutions and neighborhoods. The goal of this anchor-based effort is to stabilize and revitalize the neighborhoods of Greater University Circle and similar areas of Cleveland.

The Initiative works on a number of fronts: new transportation projects and transit-oriented commercial development are being implemented; an employer-assisted housing program open to all employees of area nonprofits is encouraging people to move back into the city's neighborhoods; an education transformation plan has been developed in partnership with the city government; and community engagement and outreach efforts are promoting resident involvement. The most recent strategic development has been the launch in 2007 of an economic inclusion program known as the Evergreen Cooperative Initiative.

The Initiative's audacious goal is to spur an economic breakthrough in Cleveland by creating living wage jobs and asset building opportunities in six low-income neighborhoods with 43,000 residents. Rather than a trickle-down strategy, Evergreen focuses on economic inclusion and building a local economy from the ground up; rather than offering public subsidy to induce corporations to bring what are often low-wage jobs into the city, the Evergreen strategy is catalyzing new businesses that are owned by their employees; rather than concentrate on workforce training for employment opportunities that are largely unavailable to low-skill and low-income workers, the Evergreen Initiative first creates the jobs, and then recruits and trains local residents to take them.

While drawing on precedents and experience gained in cities around the country, it represents a powerful mechanism to bring together anchor institution economic power to create widely shared and owned assets and capital in low-income neighborhoods. It creates green jobs that not only pay a decent wage and benefits but also, unlike most green job efforts, build assets and wealth for employees through ownership mechanisms.

Although still in its early stages of implementation, the Evergreen Cooperative Initiative is already drawing substantial support, including multi-million-dollar financial investments from the federal government (particularly the US Department of Housing and Urban Development) and from major institutional actors in Cleveland.

The strategic pillars on which the Initiative is built are as follows: (1) leveraging a portion of the multi-billion-dollar annual business expenditures of anchor institutions into the surrounding neighborhoods; (2) establishing a robust network of Evergreen Cooperative enterprises based on community wealth building and ownership models designed to service these institutional needs; (3) building on the growing momentum to create environmentally sustainable energy and green collar jobs (and, concurrently, support area anchor institutions in achieving their own environmental goals to shrink their carbon footprints); (4) linking the entire effort to expanding sectors of the economy (e.g., health and sustainable energy) that are recipients of large-scale public investment; and (5) developing the financing and management capacities that can take this effort to scale (that is, to move beyond a few boutique projects or models to have significant municipal impact).

To date, Evergreen has created approximately 75 jobs for low-income residents of Cleveland. The near-term goal (over the next 5 to 10 years) is to catalyze the creation of up to 10 new for-profit, worker-owned cooperatives that can provide family-supporting, living wage jobs for 1,000 workers. The ultimate goal is to stabilize and revitalize Greater University Circle's neighborhoods.

The first two businesses—the Evergreen Cooperative Laundry (ECL) and Ohio Cooperative Solar (OCS)—launched in October 2009:

- ECL is the greenest commercial-scale health care bed linen laundry in Ohio. When working at full capacity, it will clean 10 to 12 million pounds of health care linen a year, and it will employ 50 residents of GUC neighborhoods. The laundry is the greenest in northeast Ohio; it is based in a LEED Gold building, requires less than one-quarter of the amount of water used by competitors to clean each pound of bed linen, and produces considerable carbon emission savings through reduced energy consumption.
- Ohio Cooperative Solar is a community-based clean energy and weatherization company that will ultimately employ as many as 50 residents. In addition to home weatherization, OCS installs, owns, and maintains large-scale solar generators (panels) on the roofs of the city's biggest nonprofit health and education buildings. The institutions, in turn, purchase the generated electricity from OCS over a 15-year period. Within 3 years, OCS likely will have more than doubled the total installed solar in the entire state of Ohio.

A third business, Green City Growers, was launched in 2012. Green City Growers is a year-round, large-scale, food production hydroponic greenhouse.

The greenhouse is sited on 10 acres in the heart of Cleveland, with 3.25 acres under glass (making it the largest food production facility in a core urban area in America, and one of the largest "local food" initiatives in the country). GCG will produce approximately 3 million heads of lettuce per year, along with several hundred thousand pounds of basil and other herbs. GCG will employ approximately 45 people. Construction on the greenhouse began in September 2011, and the first leafy greens were harvested in early 2013. Importantly, virtually every head of lettuce consumed in northeast Ohio is trucked from California and Arizona. By growing its product locally, Green City Growers will save more than 2,000 miles of transportation—and the resulting carbon emissions—on each head of lettuce it sells.

Beyond these three specific businesses, the Evergreen Cooperative Corporation acts as a research-and-development vehicle for new business creation tied to specific needs of area anchor institutions. Through this process, a pipeline of next generation businesses is being developed.

An anchor institution strategy like the one in Cleveland can be a powerful job creation engine, not simply by localizing production but also by forging a local business development strategy that effectively meets many of the anchor institutions' own needs, which the existing market may not be equipped to handle. Or, put more succinctly, anchor institutions have the potential to not only support local job creation but also to shape local markets.

BASIC PRINCIPLES FOR A NEW DIRECTION

The community wealth-building approach to community and economic development is based on a set of design criteria that emphasize the following principles:[35]

1. Anchor local ownership by:

- identifying and leveraging existing community assets; and
- focusing on building local equity and ownership.

The concept of anchoring local ownership is simple: community ownership of business pays big dividends by anchoring jobs and building business assets locally. For instance, as of the end of 2006, the average ownership stake for an employee at a company with an ESOP was over $67,000—more than the average worker's 401(k) holdings.[36] Local ownership also helps "anchor" businesses in communities—an important feature in these days of globalization, when nonanchored companies can and do often change location, leaving considerable economic dislocation in their wake.

2. Increase local economic multipliers to spur locally oriented economic growth by:

- concentrating on increasing the local circulation of goods and services;
- working with existing anchor institutions (universities, hospitals, churches, museums, public utilities) to support community economic development strategy;
- leveraging funding from local foundations, anchor institutions, and existing city and chamber of commerce business development programs to support wealth building;
- complementing systematic local-preference procurement policies at major institutions (such as hospitals, universities, local government, utilities, and major corporations); and
- building "buy local" campaigns directed at households and small businesses.

A number of studies have demonstrated that local firms, when they sell a product in their local market, tend to spend a larger proportion of their income on local wages and procurement, while chain stores are more likely to divert revenues abroad and import from abroad. For instance, a 2007 study of San Francisco found that every $1 million spent at local bookstores created $321,000 in additional economic activity in the area, including $119,000 in wages paid to local employees, while the same $1 million spent at chain bookstores generated only $188,000 in local economic activity, including $71,000 in local wages. The study further found that if residents shifted 10 percent of their spending from chains to local businesses, this would generate $192 million in additional economic activity in San Francisco and almost 1,300 new jobs.[37]

3. Build local community economic development capacity by:

- helping retiring owners sell their businesses to their workers through promoting greater use of ESOPs;
- working across sectoral lines to build comprehensive strategies that can unite different community groups to support common community wealth-building goals (and build community awareness of the need for a comprehensive wealth-building approach);
- expanding community development corporation (CDC) capacity to generate income through property management and business ownership
- developing nonprofit trusts that own land to ensure permanent low- and moderate-income housing, stabilize neighborhoods, and avoid gentrification; and
- attacking efforts that strip assets away from communities or otherwise have wealth-reducing effects (e.g., predatory lending).

Building a support system for CDCs and related community groups is one important step. The 15-year, $1 billion effort by LISC, Enterprise, and Living Cities between 1991 and 2005 helped leverage a total of over $14 billion in community investment. However, outreach capacity for community development organizations is equally important, as has been made painfully obvious by the wave of foreclosures, many of which might have been prevented had community groups been able to reach those in need in time. Outreach is needed in other areas as well, such as employee ownership. A 2008 article in the *Milwaukee Business Times* points out that "As the baby boom generation ages over the next 20 years, the owners of most of Wisconsin's 150,000 businesses will retire or will start seriously planning for retirement. More than 75 percent of American middle-market business owners," the article adds, "anticipate selling within a few years."[38] Nationally, economist Robert Avery wrote in a 2006 paper that "The majority of boomer wealth is held in 12 million privately owned businesses, of which more than 70 percent are expected to change hands in the next 10–15 years." Avery further estimated that the wealth transfer over the next 20 years would total $4.8 trillion.[39] As John Logue, the founder of the Ohio Employee Ownership Center, has noted, "The failure to plan for business succession is the number one cause of preventable job loss in this country."[40,41] For the majority of family businesses that lack an obvious successor, an ESOP or a worker cooperative can be a valuable, tax-advantaged way to exit, but it will only happen if business owners are aware of the availability of this alternative.

4. Expand investment opportunities for Americans of modest means by:

- augmenting funding for individual development accounts (IDAs) and other related mechanisms that help low- and moderate-income individuals save and acquire wealth;
- developing investment opportunities for low-income people by promoting shared-equity housing and affordable equity shares in community-owned enterprises; and
- working across the asset-development continuum to devise mechanisms that integrate individual or family asset accumulation with community wealth-building strategies.

Coupled with the place-based strategies identified earlier, successful community wealth building also requires direct efforts to boost the savings and wealth-building abilities of individuals. The range of available strategies is broad. For instance, worker co-ops are rarely considered as a wealth-building strategy. However, the 1,500 worker-owners at Cooperative Home Care Associates in the Bronx, in addition to earning higher wages and enjoying better working conditions, have accumulated ownership stakes in the company that are collectively now worth more than $400,000, as well as having 401(k) holdings that collectively exceed $2.5 million. Venture investments are certainly a wealth-building strategy, but not usually for employees. However, SJF Ventures, a community development venture firm, promotes employee ownership in the companies in which it invests. When SJF Ventures exited from one firm in its portfolio, the firm employees earned between $700 and $5,500.[42,43]

Cleveland's Evergreen Initiative provides worker-owners with the opportunity to build equity in their firms by allocating dividends into each employee's patronage account. In addition, Evergreen is now developing a set of individual asset accumulation products (such as matched savings and employer-assisted housing programs) that will be made available to workers within the cooperatives. In San Diego, the Market Creek Plaza commercial development project has offered local residents an ownership stake in the project through an innovative community-development initial public offering (CD-IPO). Today, more than 400 residents of nearby low- and moderate-income neighborhoods own 20 percent of the development. The goal is to transfer complete ownership to local residents and the community over the next decade or so.[44]

CONCLUSION

In order for us to create a sustainable, green economy, it has to be an integral part of what we do every day. It has to be what we do as a community...being green is not just about producing green products. It's about how we run our economy.

Mayor Frank Jackson, Cleveland, Ohio, August 2009[45]

Reinforcing goals of environmental sustainability, community stability, and equitable development will require that the central cities and older suburbs of metropolitan areas across the United States are well anchored economically by a stable job base.

A second part of the strategy must involve targeting new public investment in infrastructure to cities and older suburbs. Public flows of investment in green jobs, health care, education, and general government represent an enormous opportunity to expand community stability and nurture community-based ownership (or "green community wealth building.") Looking at ways to capitalize upon existing and forthcoming public investments so as to maximize their community-stabilizing and wealth-building potential is the logical place to start.

By reinforcing the essential connection between sustainability, community, and equity, we can begin to create a more sustainable environmental and economic path—one that not only meets national energy efficiency, renewable energy production, and carbon emissions reduction objectives, but that also promotes long-sought goals of equality, justice, and a more equitable distribution of income, ownership, and wealth.

These considerations point to the need to develop comprehensive strategies aimed at stabilizing jobs and capital in America's urban areas. The primary strategies for achieving this end include:

- developing place-based forms of green community wealth building that are inherently rooted in the community;
- tapping into resource flows generated by public spending as well as quasi-public institutions (anchor institutions such as hospitals and universities) to nurture and support place-based ownership; and
- larger order green development policies that place top priority on preserving communities and their productive capacities.

Such a strategy presents a particular opportunity in urban areas to create lasting forms of community-based ownership that assure that jobs have staying power, that communities capture the full benefits of the new economic activity, and that environmental sustainability is at the heart of each city's economic development vision.

ACKNOWLEDGMENTS

This chapter draws in part on research reports previously published by The Democracy Collaborative, including "Climate Change, Community Stabilization and the Next 150 Million Americans" (Thad Williamson, Steve Dubb, and Gar Alperovitz), "Building a Green Economy for All" (Deborah Warren and Steve Dubb), and "Rebuilding America's Communities" (Gar Alperovitz, Steve Dubb, and Ted Howard.) All are available as pdf downloads at http://www.Community-Wealth.org.

NOTES

1. B. Commoner, *The Closing Circle: Nature, Man and Technology* (New York: Alfred Knopf, 1971).
2. *Evergreen Cooperatives Field Study, No. 2*, Capital Institute, accessed April 26, 2013, http://www.capitalinstitute.org/sites/capitalinstitute.org/files/docs/FS2-Evergreen%20full%20article.pdf
3. "One in Four Young U.S. Children Living in Poverty, Study Finds" *HuffingtonPost*, September 23, 2011. Accessed May 23, 2013, http://www.huffingtonpost.com/2011/09/22/children-in-poverty-us_n_976868.html
4. T. Noah, "The Great Divergence," *Slate*, September 3, 2010. Accessed May 23, 2013, http://www.slate.com/articles/news_and_politics/the_great_divergence/features/2010/the_united_states_of_inequality/introducing_the_great_divergence.html

5. G. Alperovitz, *America Beyond Capitalism: Reclaiming Our Wealth, Our Liberty, and Our Democracy* (New York: Democracy Collaborative Press, 2011)

6. "Michael Moore Says 400 Americans Have More Wealth Than Half of All Americans Combined," *Politifact*, March 5, 2011. Accessed May 23, 2013, http://www.politifact.com/wisconsin/statements/2011/mar/10/michael-moore/michael-moore-says-400-americans-have-more-wealth-/

7. T. Noah, "The Great Divergence," *Slate*, September 3, 2010. Accessed May 23, 2013, http://www.slate.com/articles/news_and_politics/the_great_divergence/features/2010/the_united_states_of_inequality/introducing_the_great_divergence.html

8. P. Mackun and S. Wilson, *U.S. Census Bureau, Population Distribution and Change: 2000–2010.* (Washington, DC: Office of the Census, 2011).

9. G. Alperovitz, S. Dubb, and T. Howard, *Rebuilding America's Communities: A Comprehensive Community Wealth Building Federal Policy Proposal.* (The Democracy Collaborative at the University of Maryland, 2010). Accessed May 23, 2013, http://www.community-wealth.org/_pdfs/news/recent-articles/04-10/report-alperovitz-et-al.pdf

10. A. Friedhoff, H. Wial, and H. Wolman, *The Consequences of Metropolitan Manufacturing Decline: Testing Conventional Wisdom* (Washington, DC: Brookings Institution, 2010).

11. National Center for Employee Ownership, *A Statistical Profile of Employee Ownership* (Oakland, CA: NCEO), last modified February 2009, http://www.nceo.org/library/eo_stat.html, accessed July 9, 2009.

12. S. Deller, A. Hoyt, B. Hueth, and R. Sundaram-Stukel, *Research on the Economic Impact of Cooperatives* (Madison, WI: University of Wisconsin Center for Cooperatives, 2009), 11.

13. The Democracy Collaborative, *Building Wealth: The New Asset-Based Approach to Solving Social and Economic Problems* (Washington, DC: The Aspen Institute, 2005), 97–103.

14. Social Investment Forum, *2007 Report on Socially Responsible Investing Trends in the United States: Executive Summary* (Washington, DC: Social Investment Forum, 2007), iv.

15. CDFI Data Project, *Community Development Financial Institutions: Providing Capital, Building Communities, Creating Impact, FY 2006 Data*, 6th Ed. (Philadelphia, PA: Opportunity Finance Network, 2008), 2.

16. National Congress for Community Economic Development, *Reaching New Heights: Trends and Achievements of Community-Based Development Organizations. 5th National Community Development Census* (Washington, DC: NCCED, 2006), 4–15.

17. T. Williamson, D. Imbroscio, and G. Alperovitz, *Making a Place for Community: Local Democracy in a Global Era* (New York: Routledge, 2002), 17–19.

18. I. Harkavy and H. Zuckerman, *Eds and Meds: Cities' Hidden Assets* (Washington, DC: Brookings Institution, 1999), 1.

19. S. Dubb and T. Howard, *Leveraging Anchor Institutions for Local Job Creation and Wealth Building* (Berkeley, CA: Institute for Research on Labor and Employment, University of California, 2012).

20. I. Harkavy et al., "Anchor Institutions as Partners in Building Successful Communities and Local Economies." Chap 8 in *Retooling HUD for a Catalytic Federal Government: A Report to Secretary Shaun Donovan* (Philadelphia, PA: Penn Institute for Urban Research, University of Pennsylvania, 2009).

21. S. Standley (Chief Administrative Officer, University Hospitals), interview February 27, 2012.
22. F. Serang, J. P. Thompson and T. Howard, *The Anchor Mission: Leveraging the Power of Anchor Institutions to Build Community Wealth*, College Park, MD: The Democracy Collaborative at the University of Maryland, February 2, 2013.
23. B. Masi et al., *The 25% Shift: The Benefits of Food Localization for Northeast Ohio & How to Realize Them* (Cleveland, OH and Silver Spring, MD: Cleveland Foundation, ParkWorks, Kent State University Cleveland Urban Design Collaborative, Neighborhood Progress Inc., and Cleveland-Cuyahoga County Food Policy Coalition, 2010).
24. Pew Charitable Trust, *The CleanEnergy Economy: Repowering Jobs, Businesses and Investments Across America*. (Philadelphia, PA: Pew, 2009), accessed Sept. 12, 2009, http://www.pewcenteronthestates.org/uploadedFiles/Clean_Economy_Report_Web.pdf
25. Global Insight, *Green Jobs in U.S. Metro Areas* (Lexington, MA: Global Insight, 2008).
26. R. Pollin, J. Wicks-Lim, and H. Garrett-Peltier, *Green Prosperity: How Clean-Energy Policies Can Fight Poverty and Raise Living Standards in the United States* (Amherst, MA: PERI, 2009).
27. D. Warren and S. Dubb, *Growing a Green Economy for All: From Green Jobs to Green Ownership* (The Democracy Collaborative at the University of Maryland, July 2010). Accessed May 23, 2013, http://evergreencooperatives.com/wp-content/uploads/2011/12/Evergreen-2.042-GrowingGreenEconomy.pdf
28. Ibid.
29. Ibid.
30. Ibid.
31. Ibid.
32. Capital Institute, *Evergreen Cooperatives Field Study, No. 2*, E. Want and N. A. Filion, The Cleveland Evergreen Cooperatives: Building Community Wealth through Worker-Owned Businesses, Institute for Sustainable Communities, 2011.
33. S. Arterian Chang, "Best Job in the Neighborhood—and They Own It." *Yes!* Fall 2011.
34. T. Howard, L. Kuri, and I. Pierce Lee. *A Sense of Place: Place-Based Grantmaking in Practice. Neighborhood Funders Group Special Report.* (Cleveland, OH: The Evergreen Cooperative Initiative of Cleveland, Ohio, 2010).
35. Alperovitz, Dubb, and Howard, *Rebuilding America's Communities...*
36. National Center for Employee Ownership, *A Statistical Profile...*
37. Civic Economics, *The San Francisco Retail Diversity Study*, report prepared for the San Francisco Locally Owned Merchants Alliance (Chicago, IL and Austin, TX: Civic Economics, 2007).
38. Metis Associates, *The Cities Program; Follow-the-Money Report, Living Cities: The National Community Development Initiative–Analyzing How Funds Are Used for Real Estate Investment and Production* (New York, NY: Metis Associates, 2006), 6.
39. Cited by: J. Leonetti, *Exiting Your Business, Protecting Your Wealth: A Strategic Guide for Owner's and Their Advisors* (Hoboken, NJ: John Wiley & Sons, 2008), 11, 38.
40. E. Decker, "What's Your Exit Strategy?" *Milwaukee Business-Times*, February 22, 2008. Accessed May 23, 2013, http://www.promcp.com/News/presssrel/SBT%202-22-08%20What%27s%20Your%20Exit%20Strategy.pdf

41. John Logue (Executive Director, Ohio Employee Ownership Center of Kent, OH), interview by Steve Dubb, May 2008, transcript, The Democracy Collaborative, College Park, MD.
42. S. Sutcliffe and A. C. Broughton, interventions, December 2, 2008, Annie E. Casey Foundation Conference on Expanding Asset Building Opportunities Through Shared Ownership: National Discussion.
43. H. McCulloch, *Building Assets While Building Communities: Expanding Savings & Investment Opportunities for Low-Income Bay Area Residents*, report for the Walter and Elise Haas Fund (San Francisco, CA: Asset Building Strategies, 2006).
44. Jacobs Center for Neighborhood Innovation, *Market Creek Plaza*, accessed April 11, 2010, http://www.marketcreekplaza.com
45. J. Funk, "Sustainability is the Future of Cleveland, Mayor Frank Jackson Says." *Cleveland Plain Dealer*, August 12, 2009.

CHAPTER 2

Community Action in Informal Settlements

Strategies for Improved Environmental Health

and Equity in Low- and Middle-Income Countries

DAVID SATTERTHWAITE

This chapter looks at the potential for community organizations in informal settlements to address environmental health and equity challenges, and to provide alternatives to aid projects that are developed without local ownership or participation. Whereas the next chapter focuses on marginalized neighborhoods in high-income settings, this chapter addresses the challenges facing some of the poorest communities in low- and middle-income countries. The chapter begins by considering several of the serious environmental health and equity challenges facing urban populations in low- and middle-income nations. This includes inequalities in health outcomes and in their determinants between nations and within nations and cities. It then reviews some of the strategies used by low-income groups and their organizations to address the environmental health challenges they face and considers where and how international funding can support this. The chapter draws from the experiences of organizations in informal settlements to examine the potential impact of community-led initiatives on environmental health inequalities. Finally, the chapter addresses the present emphasis on channeling development aid through national governments and international organizations, where the poor have limited voice and representation.

Discussions of environmental health issues in urban areas in low- and middle-income nations usually focus on the particular problems faced by those living in specific settlements, for instance, in the problems of overcrowding and inadequate provision for water and sanitation in tenements or cheap boarding houses or in informal or illegal settlements[1,2,3] (or what some authorities or researchers may term "slums"[4]). For most urban settings, this means ignoring higher income groups because they do not face these problems.

Looking at the most serious equity challenges means considering environmental health issues across the whole population. This means looking at the differentials within urban populations in regard to who enjoys good health outcomes or healthy living and working conditions and who does not. This focus on equity also means considering the differentials in income and the means to obtain healthy living and working conditions. This has importance because it highlights the scale of the environmental health disadvantage suffered by low-income groups. It also provides examples of where this disadvantage has been much reduced, that is, cities where low-income groups do not suffer profound environmental health disadvantages. In addition to income, differentials associated with other factors, including discrimination based on gender or race, influence health outcomes or health determinants.

Figure 2.1 lists many influences on health outcomes in urban settings. Differentials in health outcomes (for instance, premature death, including infant, child, and maternal mortality and illness or injury where data are available) provide the most direct measures of inequalities in health. Differentials can also be studied in environmental health determinants (including housing size and quality, safety of site, quality of provision for water, sanitation, solid waste collection, and drainage) and in the quality and accessibility of health care and other social services. Differentials can also be studied for many other factors listed in Figure 2.1.

Considering environmental health differentials means focusing on the differentials between defined population groups. These groups are often classified according to their wealth. For instance, it is common for surveys of households to include questions on their asset portfolios so health outcomes or health determinants can be compared between those with the largest and smallest asset portfolios.[5] Asset portfolios are considered a more accurate way of classifying households by their wealth than by households responding to questions on their income levels. Comparisons may also be made between population groups on the basis of geographic area—that is, comparing health outcomes or health determinants for those living in different provinces or different cities or different settlements within cities (for instance, comparing informal settlements with the rest of the city).

Differentials relating to what are termed "intermediary factors" in Figure 2.1 also have importance for understanding health outcomes. These include population groups' capacity to participate in and influence local government and service providers[6] and the strength and support of social networks; both may have significant influences on health outcomes and on living and working conditions and access to services. There are also the larger scale city or municipal-level

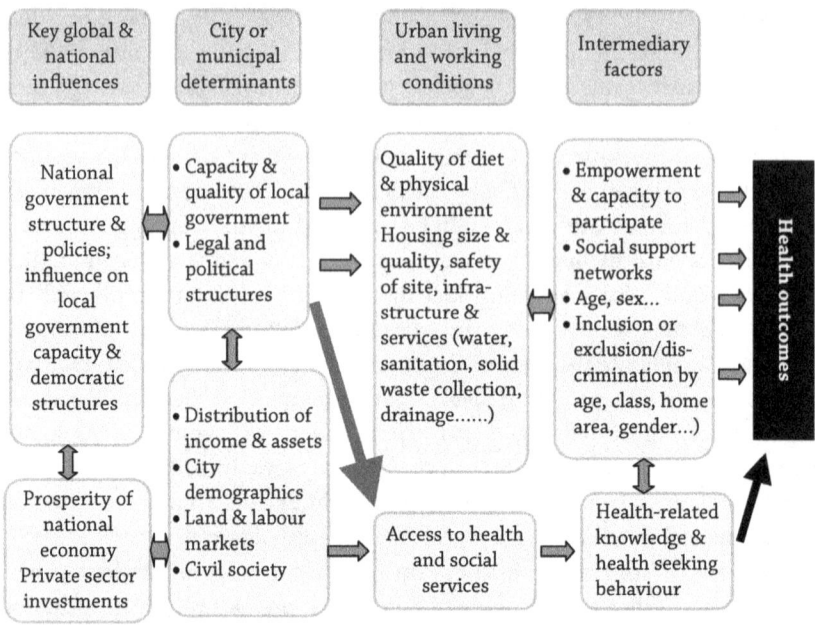

Key global & national influences	City or municipal determinants	Urban living and working conditions	Intermediary factors

National government structure & policies; influence on local government capacity & democratic structures

• Capacity & quality of local government
• Legal and political structures

Quality of diet & physical environment Housing size & quality, safety of site, infra-structure & services (water, sanitation, solid waste collection, drainage......)

• Empowerment & capacity to participate
• Social support networks
• Age, sex...
• Inclusion or exclusion/dis-crimination by age, class, home area, gender...)

• Distribution of income & assets
• City demographics
• Land & labour markets
• Civil society

Prosperity of national economy Private sector investments

Access to health and social services

Health-related knowledge & health seeking behaviour

Health outcomes

Figure 2.1:
The many influences on health outcomes in urban settings. (From D. Mitlin and D. Satterthwaite, *Urban Poverty in the Global South: Scale and Nature* [Abingdon, UK: Routledge, 2013]. It draws on figures in T. Kjellstrom and S. Mercado, "Towards Action on Social Determinants for Health Equity in Urban Settings," *Environment and Urbanization* 20, no. 2 [2008]: 551–574, and S. Cairncross, J. E. Hardoy, and D. Satterthwaite, "The Urban Context," in *The Poor Die Young: Housing and Health in Third World Cities*, J. E. Hardoy, S. Cairncross, and D. Satterthwaite, eds. [London: Earthscan Publications, 1990], 1–24.)

determinants. One of the most important determinants is the quality and capacity of local government, whether it can and does meet its responsibilities for all the infrastructure and services that fall under its jurisdiction, which in turn have strong influences on housing and living conditions and health care. Other important city determinants include land markets (and whether low-income groups can find or afford land for housing), labor markets (with its influence on income levels and income distribution), and the actions and capacities of civil society organizations. These determinants are influenced by national and international factors, including the prosperity of the national economy and the structure and policies of national government. In many nations, they are influenced by what aid agencies and development banks provide and prioritize (and, of course, by what they ignore).

INEQUALITIES IN ENVIRONMENTAL HEALTH BETWEEN COUNTRIES

There are many dramatic examples of inequalities in environmental health determinants within the 3.8 billion people that make up the global urban population—and in many of the health outcomes that are strongly influenced by environmental factors. A review of studies on provisions for water found that the prices paid per liter by urban populations in countries around the world varied by a factor of 500[7]—although, of course, this is based on the two most extreme cases found in the studies reviewed, the lowest price paid by households with a connection to a piped supply in Cairo, and the highest price paid for water from a tanker in a peripheral settlement in Luanda. Mortality rates for children under 5 years of age vary by a factor of 40 if we compare cities with the lowest rates with low-income settlements in particular cities with the highest rates.[8] There are dramatic differentials in housing size and quality between urban populations across the world, for instance, between households that have 1 square meter of indoor space per person (the pavement dwellers in Mumbai have even less than this) and high-income households that enjoy 100 or more square meters per person. There are also dramatic differentials in the quality of provision for sanitation around the world—whether measured by convenience (time taken to get access), accessibility (for those dependent on public toilets, hours open and level of safety using them, including use at night), cost, and risk levels for fecal contamination. There are also dramatic differentials within the global urban population in most of the health determinants listed in Figure 2.1.

INEQUALITIES IN ENVIRONMENTAL HEALTH WITHIN CITIES

Many dramatic examples of inequality in the determinants of environmental health or in health outcomes can be found within a city as well. Within many cities in low- and middle-income nations, studies of water use by different income groups or by populations in different districts show 4- to 10-fold differences in the price of water and it is usually the wealthier groups served by water piped to their homes that get the cheapest water.[9,10] A study in Nairobi showed that mortality rates for children 5 years and younger in the worst performing informal settlements were around 20 times those in wealthy areas.[11] It is likely that there are comparable differentials within many more cities, but neither national governments nor international funding agencies have prioritized documentation that gives detailed data on municipal-level inequalities, in large part because they have shown little interest in urban poverty. The dramatic differentials evident within the global urban population when it comes to the quality of provision for sanitation is also present within most urban centers in the Global South. A proportion of the population in urban centers in the Global South have high-quality provision within their homes, while other groups within the same cities have no provision within their homes and very inadequate public provision with many resorting to open defecation.[12,13] However, the scale and nature of the differentials in provision for sanitation are masked by the lack of detail in the statistics collected. For instance, in the

World Health Organization (WHO) global dataset used to monitor trends in sanitation, urban populations are classified by whether they have improved or unimproved sanitation, with improved sanitation, including toilets with flush or pour flush to sewers, a septic tank or a pit latrine, a ventilated improved pit latrine, a pit latrine with a slab, or a composting toilet.[14] What is needed is more disaggregation between these very different services. This same source chooses to classify all public toilets as unimproved. But here the differentials in any city with public toilets would range from those served by public toilets that are easily accessible with little or no queuing time, clean, cheap, open most or all the time, and safe for all family members to use at night to those that only have public toilets that are distant, dirty, and expensive, with long queues, restricted opening hours, and are unsafe to journey to at night.

Of course, the scale of these differentials depends on which groups are compared. For data from household surveys, the largest differentials are evident when there is the largest disaggregation, for instance, comparing the top 2 and the bottom 2 percent rather than the top and bottom quartile or quintile. For differentials based on geographic areas, the smaller the geographic areas, the larger the likely differentials. For instance, in Buenos Aires, an analysis of infant and child mortality rates in the early 1990s showed significant differentials between municipalities, but if this analysis could have been done with smaller geographic units (i.e., below municipality), the differentials would have been much higher.[15] However, for some of the key determinants of health, there may be no differentials in some cities; for instance, in almost all cities in high-income nations and some in middle-income nations, even low-income households have water of drinking quality piped into their homes 24 hours a day.

One important issue here is when and where environmental health inequalities have been reduced or removed for low-income groups. In high-income nations, all or very nearly all the urban population live in housing served by piped water, toilets, drains, and solid waste removal. They also have access to health care and emergency services (including ambulances and fire fighting services). Nearly all live in buildings that conform to health and safety regulations and are served by piped water, all-weather roads, electricity, and drains 24 hours a day. The urban centers they live in usually have elected governments, and there are channels for complaints if needed, for instance, local politicians or lawyers, ombudsmen, consumer groups, and watchdogs. While coverage for some services may be substandard and some groups ill served or excluded, the scale of the differentials in provision for many key health determinants and the proportion of the population affected has been reduced. This is also the case in some key health determinants in many cities in middle-income nations, for instance, in provision for piped water supplies into homes and sewer connections. This is not to diminish the importance of addressing health equity issues in high-income nations since there are still some dramatic differentials, for instance, in life expectancy at birth or in infant and child mortality rates.[16] While provision of basic services such as water and sanitation have for the most part been addressed, differentials in exposure to factors such as pollution, toxins, and violence remain and result in significant differences in health indicators across income levels. In the United States, the life expectancy for Asian females in an affluent county of the New York City metropolitan area is 91 years, while a Native American male in areas of South Dakota has a life expectancy of 58 years.[17] Even in the same city, differences can be striking: male life expectancy in the Glaswegian neighborhood of Calton is 54 years, whereas in Lenzie, 7 miles away, male life expectancy is 82 years.[18] While these inequalities are significant, they impact a smaller proportion of the population than health equity issues in low- and middle-income nations. For instance, the proportion of urban households that have to rely on public standpipes, wells, water vendors, or kiosks and that have no toilet in their home often represents 20–80 percent of the population in low- and middle-income nations but is extremely low in high-income nations. The deficiencies in provision for water and sanitation are generally highest in low-income nations. Figure 2.2 illustrates this by showing the range in the proportion of the urban population that has piped water on their premises. For the 173 nations for which data was available for 2010, 18 nations had less than a quarter of their urban population with water piped to their premises; most are in sub-Saharan Africa but they also include Bangladesh, Myanmar, Afghanistan, and Haiti. This figure probably understates the scale of the problem because data on water and sanitation were not available for some low-income nations that are likely to have very low levels of provision. Among the nations for which data are available, 35 had *decreases* in the proportion of their urban population with water piped to the premises between 1990 and 2010. Some nations had dramatic drops. Congo DR was reported to have 51 percent of its urban population with water piped to the premises in 1990 and 21 percent in 2010. Coverage of this for urban areas in the Sudan dropped from 76 to 47 percent in these two decades. Fourteen other nations had urban coverage dropping by more than 20 percentage points. There is also a large cluster of middle-income nations where 90 or more percent of the population have piped water to their premises. In regard to sanitation, in sub-Saharan Africa, most urban centres have no sewers at all, and for many of those that do, only a small percentage of the total population is served.[19,20]

Similarly, the proportion of urban dwellers living in buildings that do not meet building standards and where occupation of the land or its development is illegal is 20–70 percent in many cities in low- and middle-income nations and very low in high-income nations. In most high-income nations, almost every urban dweller has access to schools, health care, and emergency services (even if some groups may face poor quality or difficult access); in most low- and middle-income nations, many urban dwellers cannot access these services at all.

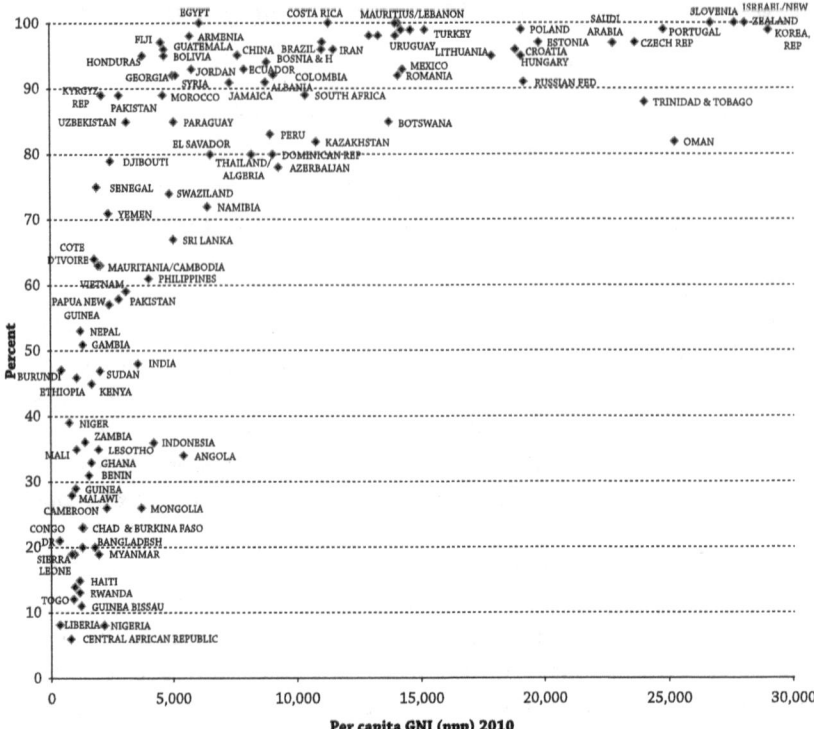

Figure 2.2:
The percent of nations' urban population with water piped to their premises in 2010. This figure does not include the many nations that have more than US$30,000 gross national income (GNI) per capita since all of them have 99 or 100 percent coverage. This graph shows the strong association between the proportion of the urban population with water piped to their premises and per capita GNI—but it also shows the large differences in this proportion between nations with similar per capita GNI. In 2010, for nations with per capita incomes below $2,000, it was still common for 60–85 percent of the urban population in low-income nations *not* to have water piped to their premises; this was also the case for some nations with above $2,000, including Nigeria, Indonesia, and Angola. Above a per capita income of $5,500, in almost all nations, 80–100 percent of the urban population had water piped to their premises. There is also a remarkable spread in the proportion of the urban population so served for nations with per capita incomes between $2,000 and $5,500, which suggests a significant role of political determinants. Note that having water piped to the premises does not mean that it is necessarily available or available regularly or of drinking quality. (From UNICEF and WHO, Progress on Drinking Water and Sanitation; 2012 Update, Joint Monitoring Programme for Water Supply and Sanitation [New York and Geneva: UNICEF and WHO, 2012].)

INEQUALITIES IN ECOLOGICAL IMPACTS

A focus on equity also means that wherever there are limits—for instance, limited resources—the issue of who has access to these resources and who does not becomes a key issue. So an interest in equity would include an interest in whether differentials were influenced by scarcities, for instance, differentials in access to fresh water supplies and productive land on which crops could be grown. There may be local ecological limits that need consideration. Wetlands provide an important component of flood risk reduction for many cities, and if these are being encroached by urban development, this can be putting the whole city at risk; however, it is usually informal settlements with a high concentration of low-income groups that face the largest risks.[21]

There are also global ecological limits to be considered, as in the limited capacity of planetary sinks to absorb or break down greenhouse gases. All human-induced greenhouse gas emissions can be traced back to individual or household consumption, and there are obvious equity issues in regard to whose consumption is contributing most to global warming. Global warming can be considered as the largest transfer of environmental health risks from rich groups (whose consumption patterns drive human-induced climate change) to poor groups (who contribute very little but who include the majority of those most at risk from climate change's impacts). Within the global urban population, there are dramatic differentials in individuals' greenhouse gas emissions resulting from consumption patterns. Although the exact scale is not yet known, there is likely to be a 1,000-fold difference between the wealthiest 2 percent and poorest 2 percent.[22] There are urban population groups that have such low incomes and low levels of consumption that they may contribute almost nothing to greenhouse gas emissions.[23] If their livelihoods are within the informal waste economy, the greenhouse gas emissions avoided as a result of their work (for instance, collecting and sorting waste so it can be reused or recycled) may be more than the greenhouse gas emissions caused by their consumption. There are also dramatic differentials evident within nations or within cities. This is especially so in prosperous cities in the global South, where the highest income groups may have consumption levels that imply greenhouse gas emissions per person comparable to the wealthiest in London or New York while a significant proportion of residents have very low emissions.

WHAT ASPECTS OF INEQUALITY NEED ATTENTION?

If we are interested in inequalities within cities (or within national urban populations), there are at least six categories that deserve attention:

- Inequalities in material conditions in homes, residential neighborhoods, and workplaces (including housing quality and size, quality of provision for water, sanitation, drainage, energy, roads and paths, solid waste collection, and air pollution). Climate change increases the importance of reducing differentials in risk and vulnerability to extreme weather.
- Inequalities in health outcomes (premature death for infants, children, mothers, youth; injury, illness, nutritional status)
- Inequalities in wealth (as incomes and assets provide the means to acquire better living conditions and health care)

- Inequalities in public entitlements and services (health care, emergency services, education, social wage, pension)
- Inequalities in voice, in social networks, and in social status (for instance, the inequalities faced by those unable to get onto the voter's register or to get access to government schools and health care services)
- Inequalities in the contribution of individuals or households to the depletion of scarce resources and ecological capital and to greenhouse gas emissions[24]

While there is considerable literature on each of the aforementioned factors, there is one aspect of inequality that rarely gets attention: the inequalities in influence over how aid is used. The needs of "the poor" are the basis for legitimizing the operations and funding of all official development assistance agencies and all charities that work in development. But what influence do "the poor" have on how this spending is allocated and to whom? Official development assistance from bilateral agencies is complicated by the fact that it comes from governments in one nation (that are accountable to that nation's voters) and is provided to governments in the recipient nations. The funding and how it is used is strongly influenced by the bilateral agency (and the government from which it gets funding and the citizens who make up the electorate in that country), but it is not influenced by or accountable to "the poor" in the recipient nation. The many measures by which governments reduced inequalities in health outcomes or health determinants in what are today high-income nations were influenced by (and often driven by) organizations in which low-income groups were active, including trade unions, social movements, and political parties. These measures were also accountable to voters. So there were important links between what was done and those with inadequate incomes who had votes and could mobilize to get more political influence. But the low-income groups living in very poor conditions in informal settlements in Mumbai or Dhaka or Dar es Salaam or Nairobi cannot mobilize to influence aid allocations made by national governments in high-income nations. The same is true for the multilateral aid agencies and development banks that are accountable to member governments. It is also true of international charities and who they are accountable to, although a few do have a strong engagement with urban poor organizations.

This lack of engagement by aid agencies, development banks, and international charities with urban poor groups can be seen in any analysis of the processes by which decisions are made about priorities in any aid agency or development bank, for instance, which countries and sectoral priorities are supported.[25,26] There is little or no scope for the poor to present their case for priorities. Indeed, the discussions and documents about priorities are usually in the language of the aid agency, not the languages spoken by the poor. The poor have at best very limited and usually no possibility of holding the aid agency to account for their decisions.

This lack of engagement with poor groups can also be seen in the flow of funding. Aid agencies and development banks do not actually address needs directly; they fund others to do so. Most funding goes to national government agencies, some to international nongovernmental organizations (NGOs), and a very small proportion to local NGOs. So an aid agency or development bank is only as effective as the intermediaries that it funds. Do these intermediary institutions provide scope for the poor to influence their decisions? Are they accountable to the poor? At least in regard to the urban poor, the answer is no. Aid agencies generally need to spend large sums of money quickly. They allocate large chunks of money to national governments or to other international development assistance agencies. Both multilateral banks and bilateral agencies are under pressure to keep down staff costs, and this helps explain the lack of staff on the ground with a capacity to engage with the poor. If the very large sums of funding made available each year for development are not influenced by or accountable to "the poor," it is difficult to see them becoming more effective in poverty reduction. Aid agencies may suggest that this accountability to the poor should be provided by recipient governments, but this is clearly not happening in many nations that get very substantial aid funding.

ADDRESSING ENVIRONMENTAL HEALTH INEQUITIES FROM THE BOTTOM UP

Over the last 20 years, there has been a growing number of representative organizations and federations or networks of the urban poor. These grassroot organizations are making significant headway in improving environmental health for those who are worst off. Some are organized around their livelihoods, for instance, as waste pickers and recyclers[27] or as self-employed (see, for instance, Self-Employed Women's Association, or SEWA,in India). Others are organized around their settlement, including slum and shack dweller federations or homeless people's federations. For example, there is now an international network of the slum/shack dwellers federations that support and learn from each other. These federations and the local NGOs that work closely with them have formed their own international umbrella organization, Slum/Shack Dwellers International (SDI). SDI also supports them in negotiating for external support by having a presence in global discussions of funding and the management of such funding. SDI was initially formed by six of the federations that had long been active in nations such as India,[28,29] Thailand,[30,31] and South Africa.[32,33] Table 2.1 gives details of the most established federations.

The foundation for all these federations are savings groups formed by slum or shack dwellers in which the savings group manager visits all savers and potential savers each day. Most savers and most savings managers are women. Despite the diversity in what the different national federations do (reflecting

Table 2.1. EXAMPLES OF THE SCALE OF THE SAVINGS AND WORK PROGRAMS OF SOME OF THE URBAN POOR FEDERATIONS THAT ARE MEMBERS OF SLUM/SHACK DWELLERS INTERNATIONAL (SDI)

	Date[a]	No. of Cities with a Process[b]	Active Savers[c]	Savings (US$)[d]	Houses Built	Tenure Secured (no. of families)
India	1986	57	130,000	1.2 million	6,000[e]	80,000
South Africa	1991	45	21,927	491,652	13,500	15,000
Namibia[f]	1992	84	19,168	1.69 million	2,272	4,554
Phillipines	1994	15	25,901	2.81 million	1,759	4,500
Zimbabwe[f]	1995	53	42,665	324,000	966	14,450
Nepal	1998	6	15,694	110,000	283	26,000
Sri Lanka	1998	24	52,735	5.03 million	63	93
Kenya	2000	11	61,000	1.13 million	120	25,000
Zambia	2002	28	45,000	131,000	95	95
Ghana[f]	2003	5	12,663	227,000	31	6,500
Uganda	2003	6	21,880	184,000	5	300
Malawi	2004	28	9,745	178,000	757	3,076
Brazil	2004	4	771	16,162	–	7,000
Tanzania	2004	6	5,878	105,000	10	500
Swaziland	2005	2	200	–	–	–
Bolivia[f]	2010	2	103	1,850	–	–
Sierra Leone	2008	2	1,492	9,788	–	–

a. The year in which significant savings scheme activity began; this may predate the year when the federation was established.

b. Within any city, there will be a number of settlements where grassroots activities are taking place to build collective capacity and catalyse grassroots-led development.

c. The second indicator of scale—the number of people who save regularly.

d. Local currency values converted to US$; includes daily savings and Urban Poor Fund savings.

e. A further 30,000 households in India have obtained new housing not constructed by the federations.

f. Updated in February 2011 for Bolivia, Ghana, Namibia, and Zimbabwe.
More details of the work of all these federations can be obtained from http://www.sdinet.org/

Source: D. Mitlin, *Urban Poor Funds; Development by the People for the People*, Poverty Reduction in Urban Areas Working Paper, London: IIED, 2008, updated with data from http://www.sdinet.org; this updated table was published in D. Mitlin, D. Satterthwaite, and S. Bartlett, *Capital, Capacities and Collaboration; the Multiple Roles of Community Savings in Addressing Urban Poverty*, IIED Working Paper (London: Human Settlements Group, IIED, 2011).

what is possible within their own particular national and local contexts), all the federations that are members of SDI use a common set of organizing methodologies and practices: support to community-based daily savings groups; active engagement in information gathering through settlement profiles, mapping, and enumerations; peer learning (between savings groups with a federation, between federations); seeking dialogue; and, where possible, partnership with government agencies. All the federations have projects and initiatives to support member savings groups in building homes (in cases where they can access land) or upgrading homes, or building or improving services such as community toilets. The federations also seek to engage with governments and where feasible international funding agencies. They are unusual in that they do not seek to influence government by protest but by offering partnerships with (usually local) government and using their own initiatives to show government their capacities.[34,35,36] For instance, many national federations have prepared city-wide surveys and careful enumerations/censuses and maps of informal settlements—the documentation needed for acting to improve conditions and install or improve infrastructure.[37,38,39,40,41,42,43,44,45,46]

Over the last two decades, more than 150,000 families within these federations have secured land tenure or negotiated land on which they have built good quality housing. Most federations have initiatives under way for upgrading or for developing new housing supported by local government, including in India, South Africa, Thailand, Namibia, Malawi, Kenya, the Philippines, and Zimbabwe.[47,48,49,50,51] In Thailand, savings groups formed by slum or shack dwellers have been supported by a national agency (the Community Organizations Development Institute, or CODI) in implementing a highly ambitious upgrading initiative centered on partnerships between community organizations and government. CODI channels government funds in the form of infrastructure subsidies and housing loans directly to community organizations formed by low-income inhabitants in informal settlements who plan and carry out improvements to their housing or develop new housing and work with local governments or utilities to provide or improve infrastructure and services. From 2003 to 2010, within the *Baan Mankong* (secure housing) program, CODI approved 745 projects in 1,319 communities covering 80,201 households,[52] and it plans a considerable expansion in the program within the next few years. Overall, CODI (and the organization out of which it developed, the Urban Community Development Office) has provided loans and grants to community organizations that reached 2.4 million households between 1992 and 2007, thereby promoting community-led urban development.[53,54]

Similarly, in India, the women's savings groups that make up *Mahila Milan* (the federation of women savings groups) have designed, built, and managed community toilets that serve hundreds of thousands of people in cities in India.[55,56] They first designed and built some community toilets to show government what they were capable of achieving. This then led to partnerships between government agencies and the federation to work on a much larger scale.[57] Today, hundreds of thousands of people in low-income urban areas in India have much better quality toilets and washing facilities because of government-community partnerships.[58,59] In Mumbai, *Mahila Milan* and the National Slum Dwellers Federation persuaded the police to work with them to set up police stations in dozens of informal settlements that are joint ventures between the police and community representatives.[60]

Grassroots organizations not only create healthier, more liveable spaces for the urban poor, but they can also make significant impact in terms of disaster risk reductions and disaster response. Box 2.1 gives one example from the growing number of partnerships between the Homeless People's Federation and municipal governments in the Philippines.[61]

Box 2.1: THE PARTNERSHIP BETWEEN COMMUNITY ORGANI-ZATIONS AND THE CITY GOVERNMENT OF ILOILO

In the city of Iloilo, established partnerships between local and national government, grassroots organizations, and the Homeless People's Federation of the Philippines were strengthened after the devastation caused by Typhoon Frank in 2008. The city government recognized that the urban poor and their support organizations are partners in the city's development. It provided many opportunities for them to participate in local decision making through representation in technical working groups and multisectoral bodies and allowing more room for effecting change in local policies. The scale and scope of housing delivery, upgrading, postdisaster assistance, and other basic services were much increased because of the resource sharing from the partnership.

Local government extended facilities/equipment and personnel (site engineer, surveyors, mappers) to provide technical assistance to the Federation on housing and disaster rehabilitation measures, and these also lowered the cost of projects. A portion of the relocation site was allocated to the construction of temporary housing units and communal facilities for families affected by Typhoon Frank. Being a member of the Resettlement and Monitoring Task Force, the Federation assisted in social preparations and other resettlement-related activities conducted by the local government. These include an Information Dissemination Campaign among communities living in danger zones (along riverbanks or shorelines, and those directly affected by the city's infrastructure projects) that will be transferred to government relocation sites.

The city government, through the Iloilo City Urban Poor Affairs Office, assisted in the federation's social mobilization, which included mapping of high-risk/disaster-affected communities, and identification and prioritization of communities to be given postdisaster assistance (temporary houses and material loan assistance for housing repair).

Source: N. Carcellar, J. Christopher, R. Co, and Z. O. Hipolito, "Addressing Vulnerabilities through Support Mechanisms: HPFPI's Ground Experience in Enabling the Poor to Implement Community-Rooted Interventions on Disaster Response and Risk Reduction," *Environment and Urbanization,* 23, no. 2 (2011).

In addition to the shared methodologies outlined earlier, such as public–private partnerships and grassroots mobilization, the federations that are members of SDI share a commitment to keep down costs and recover them when possible, so they can support other federation initiatives. The federations know that external (international) funding is limited and difficult to get, so it tends to be used for initiatives to show local (and national) governments the capacity of the federations. This will often include a demonstration that they can build houses or public toilets that are both of better quality and cheaper than the contractors used by local governments. When combined with attention to keeping down unit costs, this means that the federations with large-scale initiatives are mostly or entirely funded by their own (local and national) governments—as in India, Thailand, South Africa, and Namibia. The settlement profiles, community-driven enumerations, and mapping that most of the federations have done serve as the information base for designing and implementing improvements and are also far cheaper than if these were contracted out to companies. They also produce a level of detail and community verification that external agencies cannot accomplish. In addition, many important development activities that are performed by federation members have little or no cost to governments. For instance, in India, the management of community toilets by federation members provides cost-effective maintenance and repair and sets up the systems to generate finance from affordable user fees. The partnerships between community organizations and the police in providing policing in informal settlements mentioned earlier also require little or no new funding.

All of the processes described earlier have the goal of making local governments—and, where relevant, agencies from higher levels of government—valued partners in addressing and meeting their responsibilities. The federations know that increasing the scale and the scope of what they can do depends on government support.

THE IMPORTANCE OF CHANNELLING AID TO THE GRASSROOTS ORGANIZATIONS AND FEDERATIONS FORMED BY THE POOR

Although some international funding agencies do provide support for some of these federations and a few have supported these federations' own Urban Poor Fund International (described later), the proportion of development funding that goes to grassroots organizations formed by the urban poor is extremely small. The social policies that dramatically reduced poverty in high-income nations were strongly influenced by the demands of those suffering from poverty and their organizations, and by the democratic structures and processes that they pressed for and worked through. If we consider aid to be in part an international social policy, there are no comparable channels of influence or accountability for the urban or rural poor in Africa, Asia, or Latin America to influence aid agencies and development banks.[62]

There are two international funds that have sought to make aid accountable to and influenced by the urban poor: the Urban Poor Fund International and the Asian Coalition for Community Action managed by the Asian Coalition for Housing Rights. Short descriptions of how these work are given, before drawing some conclusions about equity challenges.

Starting in 2001, the Urban Poor Fund provided funding for initiatives costing between £10,000 and £50,000 to members of Slum/Shack Dwellers International chosen by the federations themselves. These initiatives sought to meet their needs and show local government what they were capable of; they also acted as demonstrations to other savings groups of what is possible within their own nation and other nations. Between 2001 and 2008, funding was provided to a wide range of environmental and development community initiatives, including land for housing in Cambodia, Kenya, India, Malawi, Colombia, Nepal, the Philippines, South Africa, and Zimbabwe; "slum"/ squatter upgrading and land tenure in Cambodia, India, and Brazil; bridge finance for initiatives in the Philippines, South Africa, and India (where promised government support was slow to come); improved water and sanitation in Uganda, Cambodia, Sri Lanka, and Zimbabwe (with improved land tenure); slum/shack enumerations to provide the information base for upgrading/new housing initiatives in Brazil, Namibia, Ghana, Sri Lanka, South Africa, and Zambia; exchange visits by federations to urban poor groups in East Timor, Mongolia, Angola, and Zambia; reconstruction after the 2004 tsunami in Sri Lanka and India; and supporting federation partnerships with local governments in housing initiatives in India, Malawi, South Africa, Zambia, and Zimbabwe.

These organizations addressed the priority needs of tens of thousands of low-income people in ways that were determined by the communities themselves. The projects implemented helped set new precedents that changed the urban poor's relations with local governments, by showing what the urban poor were capable of, what resources they could mobilize, and how far they could make funding go. These projects also showed the elements that had to be changed to support larger scale initiatives, such as inappropriate building codes and land subdivision regulations.

Around US$7 million was channelled through the Urban Poor Fund from 2001 to 2008. The initiatives supported involved over 150,000 people.[63] In addition, this funding leveraged far more than the Fund's contributions locally since the projects also drew support from government and brought in contributions from federation members.

Since 2008, the scale of this fund has increased with around $4 million a year available to SDI, allowing it to support larger scale initiatives.[64] The Urban

Poor Fund International has established its own international board of governors that includes housing ministers from several nations. The fact that this Fund has operated for 10 years shows the feasibility of a funding model that allows representative organizations of the urban poor real influence in how funding is used. The Fund's experience combined with the experience of National Urban Poor Funds that many of the federations have set up, show that far more external funding can be channelled through institutions providing direct support to grassroots organizations formed by slum/shack dwellers. Channelling external funding through these institutions would make it accountable to the urban poor *and* accountable to external funders.

Another example of funding available to the community organizations set up by low-income urban dwellers is the Coalition for Community Action Programme (ACCA).[65] This is a new fund to catalyze and support city-wide upgrading and partnerships between community organizations and local governments, set up and managed by the Asian Coalition for Housing Rights. In its first year of operation, it provided support to a range of different environmental and development initiatives in 64 cities, including paved roads and walkways, drains and bridges, water supply improvements, electricity and street lighting, solid waste management, and community centers. The ACCA sets very low budget ceilings for the funding it provides and leaves decisions on how best to use it and raise other funding in the hands of the implementing communities. The ACCA explains the principle of "insufficiency" as resulting from a lack of development funding to fund "sufficiently" all that needs to be done to meet the needs of all informal settlements. As the report on its first year of operation explained:

> The $3,000 for small upgrading projects and the $40,000 for big housing projects which the ACCA Program offers community groups is pretty small money but it is available money, it comes with very few strings attached, and it's big enough to make it possible for communities to think big and to start doing something actual: the drainage line, the paved walkway, the first 50 new houses. It will not be sufficient to resolve all the needs or to reach everyone. But the idea isn't for communities to be too content with that small walkway they've just built, even though it may be a very big improvement. Even after the new walkway, the people in that community will still be living in conditions that are filled with all kinds of "insufficiencies"—insufficient basic services, insufficient houses, insufficient land tenure security and insufficient money…the ACCA money is small but it goes to as many cities and groups as possible, where it generates more possibilities, builds more partnerships, unlocks more local resources and creates a much larger field of learning and a much larger pool of new strategies and unexpected outcomes.[66]

One important issue in regard to cost-effectiveness for both the Urban Poor Fund International and the ACCA program is the extent to which the funding these provide stimulates other support and helps build partnerships with local governments whose support can greatly increase the scale and scope of what is done. For instance, between 2008 and 2011, projects funded by the Urban Poor Fund International secured 443 plots of land free of charge from the state and an additional US$7.6 million worth of support from local and national governments.[67] As noted earlier, within the ACCA program, the small grants catalyze community contributions and partnerships with local governments, unlocking more local resources. This suggests the need for assessments of cost-effectiveness to include the value of local (monetary and nonmonetary) resources that were catalyzed and the value of benefits achieved through the policy changes stimulated or supported. It is difficult to put an economic value on key policy changes such as the success of many federations of slum/shack dwellers in getting acceptance by city and/or national government of in situ upgrading for their informal settlements. But these changes can bring very large and valuable health and environmental benefits for a very large proportion of low-income urban households, including the costs and impoverishments avoided as in situ upgrading replaces the previous lack of public provision in informal settlements and stops evictions and inappropriate resettlement programmes.

CONCLUSIONS

One important reason for widening the measurement of inequality beyond income or assets is that governments and international agencies have far more scope to reduce other inequalities, for instance, inequalities in the quality of housing, the extent of secure tenure and the quality of provision for water, sanitation, drainage, health care, schools, emergency services, and electricity. Cities that have a very unequal income distribution may not have very unequal health outcomes between income groups because differentials in other key health determinants have been addressed, for instance, when even low-income households have good quality water piped to their home, sewer connections, electricity, solid waste collection, and access to health care services. City and municipal governments that can work with the representative organizations of urban poor groups in their city can reduce many of these inequalities while also addressing the profound inequalities in who within the city has voice and influence. This has important implications for how development is monitored; at present, the reliance of international agencies on household surveys for representative samples of national populations means there are no detailed data on the inequalities within urban (and rural) populations and within cities.

The Millennium Development Goals can be seen as an initiative to help address inequalities—both in health outcomes (for instance, reducing infant, child, and maternal mortality rates) and in provisions that contribute to better health (for instance, in improving provision for water and sanitation). There is now a growing worry that many of the Millennium Development Goals will not be met in many nations by 2015, even though the targets for many such goals were fairly modest. There is also the worry that inappropriate indicators will be used; for instance, the use of the dollar-a-day poverty line enormously understates the scale and depth of urban poverty because the costs of food and nonfood needs are so much higher than this in many cities.[68] As noted earlier, there are significant limitations in measurements for who has "improved" water and sanitation, yet these are the official indicators being used to monitor provision for water and sanitation. It is also important to consider how many nations actually had a lower proportion of their urban population with water piped to their premises in 2010 compared to 1990.

Current discussions within aid agencies about aid effectiveness give too little attention to what actually reduces inequalities. These discussions focus on so-called efficiencies (for instance, lowering staff costs), "value for money," or the simplistic search for quick wins and silver bullets. Where is the discussion around making decisions about aid allocations more accountable to and influenced by "the poor" by having the aid-funded institutions who work on the ground be accountable to the representative organizations of the urban (and rural) poor and involving them in their decision making? Meeting the equivalent of the Millennium Development Goals in what are today high-income nations depended on the political influence on government by those whose needs were not being met.

International agencies need to rethink what role they should have in encouraging and supporting local processes that reduce urban poverty. This includes supporting solutions that low-income groups and their organizations develop themselves and what they prioritize and negotiate with local government and other agencies. As this chapter has shown, external funding can achieve high "value for money" when it catalyzes, supports, or even helps leverage local contributions from households, community organizations, and local governments and supports urban poor groups to negotiate policy change. This means international agencies will have to rethink how they will support this engagement on the ground; this can be helped by the fact that most of the urban poor federations have set up their own National Urban Poor Funds, which they manage but which are also accountable and transparent to any external funders.[69,70] It does not mean only support for local action; obviously national and international issues need addressing, too, as Figure 2.1 makes clear. But if only 1 percent of aid supported representative organizations of the urban poor (in ways that were determined by them and accountable to them), the effectiveness of urban poverty reduction would be much increased in many nations.

NOTES

1. J. E. Hardoy, D. Mitlin, and D. Satterthwaite, *Environmental Problems in an Urbanizing World: Finding Solutions for Cities in Africa, Asia and Latin America* (London, England: Earthscan Publications, 2001).

2. A. Sverdlik, "Ill-health and poverty: a literature review on health in informal settlements," *Environment and Urbanization* 23, (2011): 1123–56.

3. World Health Organization, "Creating Healthy Cities in the 21st Century," chap. 6 in *The Earthscan Reader on Sustainable Cities*, ed. D. Satterthwaite (London, England: Earthscan Publications, 1999), 137–72.

4. I try to avoid using the term "slum" because of its derogatory connotations. Classify a settlement as a slum and it helps legitimate the eviction of its inhabitants. In addition, the term is often used as a general term for a range of different kinds of housing or settlements, many of which provide valuable accommodation for low-income groups and that do not need replacement but provision for infrastructure and services. But it is difficult to avoid the term slum for at least two reasons. The first is that some urban poor groups have organized themselves as slum dweller organizations or federations as described later. In some Asian nations, there are advantages for residents of informal settlements in being recognized officially as a "slum"; indeed, the residents of such settlements may even lobby to become a "notified slum." The second is that the only global estimates for deficiencies in housing collected by the United Nations are for "slums."

5. S. Agarwal, "Health and Inequality in Urban Populations in India," *Environment and Urbanization* 23, no.1 (2011): 13–28.

6. S.T Lama-Rewal, "Urban Governance and Healthcare Provision in Delhi," *Environment and Urbanization* 23, no.2 (2011): 563–81.

7. UN-Habitat, *Water and Sanitation in the World's Cities; Local Action for Global Goals* (London, England: Earthscan Publications, 2003).

8. For instance Embakasi in Nairobi. See African Population and Health Research Center, *Population and Health Dynamics in Nairobi's Informal Settlements* (Nairobi, Kenya: APHRC, 2002).

9. UN Habitat, *Water and Sanitation* ...

10. J. Thompson et al., "Waiting at the Tap: Changes in Urban Water Use in East Africa Over Three Decades," *Environment and Urbanization* 12, no. 2 (2000): 37–52.

11. APHRC, *Population and Health Dynamics* ...

12. Hardoy, Mitlin, and Satterthwaite, *Environmental Problems...*

13. UN Habitat, *Water and Sanitation...*

14. World Health Organization and UNICEF, *Progress on Sanitation and Drinking Water: 2010 Update* (Geneva, Switzerland: WHO/UNICEF Joint Monitoring Programme for Water Supply and Sanitation, 2011).

15. S. Arrossi, "Inequality and Health in Metropolitan Buenos Aires," *Environment and Urbanization* 8, no. 2 (1996): 43–70.

16. Global Research Network on Urban Health Equity, *Improving Urban Health Equity through Action on the Social and Environmental Determinants of Health*, (London, England: GRNUHE, University College London and the Rockefeller Institute, 2010).

17. C. J. L. Murray et al., "Eight Americas: Investigating Mortality Disparities across Races, Counties, and Race-Counties in the United States," *PLoS Medicine* 3, no. 9 (2006). doi:10.1371/journal.pmed.0030260.

18. Commission on Social Determinants of Health, *Closing the Gap in a Generation: Health Equity through Action on the Social Determinants of Health.* Final Report, (Geneva, Switzerland: World Health Organization, 2008).
19. Hardoy, Mitlin, and Satterthwaite, *Environmental Problems...*
20. UN Habitat, *Water and Sanitation ...*
21. Hardoy, Mitlin, and Satterthwaite, *Environmental Problems...*
22. D. Satterthwaite, "Cities' Contribution to Global Warming; Notes on the Allocation of Greenhouse Gas Emissions," *Environment and Urbanization* 20, no. 2 (2008): 539–50.
23. D. Satterthwaite, "Cities' Contribution ..."
24. See also G. Haughton, "Environmental Justice and the Sustainable City," *Journal of Planning Education and Research* 18, no. 3 (1999): 233–43 for another way of considering environmental inequities.
25. D. Satterthwaite, *The Scale and Nature of International Donor Assistance to Housing, Basic Services and Other Human Settlements Related Projects*, Helsinki, Finland: WIDER, 1997)
26. D. Satterthwaite, "Reducing Urban Poverty: Constraints on the Effectiveness of Aid Agencies and Development Banks and Some Suggestions for Change," *Environment and Urbanization* 13, no. 1 (2001): 137–57.
27. O. Fergutz, S. Dias, and D. Mitlin, "Developing Urban Waste Management in Brazil with Waste Picker Organizations," *Environment and Urbanization* 23, no. 2 (2011): 597–608.
28. J. Arputham, "Developing New Approaches for People-Centred Development," *Environment and Urbanization* 20, no. 2 (2008): 319–37.
29. J. Arputham, "How Community-Based Enumerations Started and Developed in India," *Environment and Urbanization* 24, no. 1 (2012): 27–30.
30. S. Boonyabancha, "Mankong: Going to Scale with 'Slum' and Squatter Upgrading in Thailand," *Environment and Urbanization* 17, no. 1 (2005): 21–46.
31. S. Boonyabancha, "Land for Housing the Poor by the Poor: Experiences from the Baan Mankong Nationwide Slum Upgrading Programme in Thailand," *Environment and Urbanization* 21, no. 2 (2009): 309–30.
32. J. Bolnick, "The People's Dialogue on Land and Shelter: Community Driven Networking in South Africa's Informal Settlements," *Environment and Urbanization* 5, no. 1 (1993): 91–110.
33. J. Bolnick, "uTshani Buyakhuluma (The Grass Speaks): People's Dialogue and the South African Homeless People's Federation, 1993–1996," *Environment and Urbanization* 8, no. 2 (1996): 153–70.
34. See for instance S. Patel, "Tools and Methods for Empowerment Developed by Slum and Pavement Dwellers' Federations in India," *Participatory Learning and Action* 50 (2004): 118–9.
35. S. Patel and A. Jockin, "An Offer of Partnership or a Promise of Conflict in Dharavi, Mumbai?" *Environment and Urbanization* 19, no. 2 (2007): 501–8.
36. S. Patel and J. Arputham, "Plans for Dharavi: Negotiating a Reconciliation Between a State-Driven Market Redevelopment and Residents' Aspirations," *Environment and Urbanization* 20, no.1 (2008): 243–54.
37. Community Organisation Research Center, *Profiles of Informal Settlements within the Johannesburg Metropole* (Cape Town, South Africa: CORC, 2005).
38. Community Organisation Research Center, *Profiles of the Informal Settlements within Cape Town Metropole* (Cape Town, South Africa: CORC, 2006).
39. J. Weru, "Community Federations and City Upgrading: The Work of Pamoja Trust and Muungano in Kenya," *Environment and Urbanization* 16, no. 1 (2004): 47–62.

40. Pamoja Trust and Shack/Slum Dwellers International, *Nairobi Slum Inventory*, (Nairobi, Kenya: Pamoja Trust, Urban Poor Fund International, and Shack/Slum Dwellers International, 2008).
41. I. Karanja, "An Enumeration and Mapping of Informal Settlements in Kisumu, Kenya, Implemented by Their Inhabitants," *Environment and Urbanization* 22, no.1 (2010): 217–39.
42. A. Muller and E. Mbanga "Participatory Enumerations at the National Level in Namibia: The Community Land Information Program," *Environment and Urbanization* 24, no. 1 (2012): 67–75.
43. B. Chitekwe-Biti et al., "Developing an Informal Settlement Upgrading Protocol in Zimbabwe—the Epworth Story," *Environment and Urbanization* 24, no. 1 (2012): 131–48.
44. B. R. Farouk and M. Owusu, "If in Doubt, Count: The Role of Community-Driven Enumerations in Blocking Eviction in Old Fadama, Accra," *Environment and Urbanization* 24 (2012):147–57.
45. A. Livengood and K. Kunte, "Participatory Settlement Mapping by Mahila Milan," *Environment and Urbanization* 24, no. 1 (2012): 77–97.
46. Arputham, "How Community-Based Enumerations ..."
47. D. Mitlin, "With and Beyond the State: Co-Production as a Route to Political Influence, Power and Transformation for Grassroots Organizations," *Environment and Urbanization* 20, no. 2 (2008): 339–60.
48. B. Chitekwe-Biti, "Struggles for Urban Land by the Zimbabwe Homeless People's Federation," *Environment and Urbanization* 21, no. 2 (2009): 347–66.
49. M. A. Z. Manda, "Mchenga—Urban Poor Housing Fund in Malawi," *Environment and Urbanization* 19, no. 2 (2007): 337–59.
50. D. Mitlin and A. Muller, "Windhoek, Namibia: Towards Progressive Urban Land Policies in Southern Africa," *International Development Planning Review* 26, no. 2 (2004): 167–86.
51. S. Patel and D. Mitlin, "Grassroots-Driven Development: The Alliance of SPARC, the National Slum Dwellers Federation and Mahila Milan," in *Empowering Squatter Citizen: Local Government, Civil Society and Urban Poverty Reduction*, eds. D. Mitlin and D. Satterthwaite (London, England: Earthscan Publications, 2004), 216–41.
52. Boonyabancha, "Mankong: Going to Scale ..."; Boonyabancha, "Land for Housing the Poor ..."
53. S. Boonyabancha, "The Urban Community Development Office: Increasing Community Options through a National Government Development Programme in Thailand" in *Empowering Squatter Citizen; Local Government, Civil Society and Urban Poverty Reduction*, ed. D. Mitlin and D. Satterthwaite (London, England: Earthscan Publications, 2004), 25–53.
54. Boonyabancha, "Mankong: Going to Scale ..."; Boonyabancha, "Land for Housing the Poor ..."
55. S. Burra, S. Patel, and T. Kerr, "Community-Designed, Built and Managed Toilet Blocks in Indian Cities," *Environment and Urbanization* 15, no. 2 (2003): 11–32.
56. SPARC-NSDF-Mahila Milan, *Citywatch India*, Mumbai: 6, (June 2010).
57. Patel, "Tools and Methods ..."
58. Burra, Patel, and Kerr, "Community-Designed ..."
59. SPARC-NSDF-Mahila Milan, *Citywatch ...*
60. A. N. Roy, A. Jockin, and A. Javed, "Community Police Stations in Mumbai's Slums," *Environment and Urbanization* 16, no. 2 (2004): 135–8.

61. J. C. Rayos Co., *Community-Driven Disaster Intervention: The Experience of the Homeless Peoples Federation Philippines,* (working paper IIED/ACHR/SDI, London, England, 2010).
62. Satterthwaite, "Reducing Urban Poverty ..."
63. D. Mitlin, D. Satterthwaite, and S. Bartlett, *Capital, Capacities and Collaboration; the Multiple Roles of Community Savings in Addressing Urban Poverty* (working paper IIED/Human Settlements Group, London, England, 2011).
64. Ibid.
65. Asian Coalition for Housing Rights, *64 Cities in Asia; First Year Report of the Asian Coalition for Community Action Programme* (Bangkok, Thailand: ACHR, 2010).
66. Ibid., 9.
67. Mitlin, Satterthwaite and Bartlett, *Capital, Capacities ...*
68. D. Satterthwaite, "The Millennium Development Goals and Urban Poverty Reduction: Great Expectations and Nonsense Statistics," *Environment and Urbanization*, 15, no. 2 (2003): 181–90.
69. D. Mitlin, *Urban Poor Funds: Development by the People for the People* (working paper, Poverty Reduction in Urban Areas Working Paper, London, England, 2008).
70. S. Phonphakdee, S. Visal, and G. Sauter, "The Urban Poor Development Fund in Cambodia: Supporting Local and Citywide Development." *Environment and Urbanization* 21, no. 2 (2009): 569–86.

CHAPTER 3

Achieving Environmental Equity

Race, Place, and the Movement to Build Healthy
Communities in the United States

ANGELA GLOVER BLACKWELL

Local environments either nourish or undermine the well-being of individuals, families, communities, and society, and it is well known which way this cuts in low-income communities and communities of color in the United States. Years of research have shown that these communities have the highest pollution levels; the most limited access to fresh foods, park space, and other resources for health; the most entrenched barriers to economic opportunities; and the fewest social supports to overcome these obstacles. Stark, racially based environmental inequities lie at the root of poverty, rising inequality, and glaring health disparities.

The community factors that influence well-being can be categorized into four broad environments: economic, social, physical, and service. These environments have been shaped and distorted by a long history of inequitable policies and investments that have isolated low-income communities, particularly poor communities of color, from opportunity. Alleviating poverty and building healthier, sustainable communities for all require long-term investments in policies and strategies that strengthen the environments of distressed communities while empowering the people who live there. These approaches must intentionally respond to changing demographics, and they must forcefully address the vestiges of racism, which remains the most intractable barrier to equitable opportunity in the United States. This chapter presents a framework for transforming vulnerable communities with an emphasis on policy change focused on equitable results.

Americans cherish the idea of our nation as a land of equal opportunity. Yet the economic isolation and environmental degradation of low-income communities in the United States—and particularly of low-income communities of color—parallel conditions in poor communities in developing countries. Scores of rural communities from Central California to the Mexican border, from Arizona to North Carolina, lack such basics as clean drinking water and sewer systems. Nor are isolation and policy neglect limited to invisible rural outposts. New Orleans, one of the most storied, beloved cities in the United States, became a symbol of raw poverty, racial exclusion, environmental injustice, and government disregard during the catastrophic flooding after Hurricane Katrina in 2005.

The growing understanding of the connections between health and place—that is, the links between the physical, economic, and social well-being of people and the physical, economic, and social conditions in which they live, work, study, and play—has propelled a broad-based movement in the United States to transform ailing, disinvested neighborhoods into healthy communities.[1] Animating this movement is a commitment to equity: just and fair inclusion in a society rich with opportunities for all to reach their full potential. The goal of equity is to create conditions that allow all to participate and prosper. In short, equity creates a path from hope to change.

The actions of the movement range in scale from city block to rural county to metropolitan region. For example, in Lanare, California, a very low-income, predominantly African American and Latino community in the Central Valley, one of the richest agricultural regions in the nation, residents, many of them migrant workers, have organized to demand government funds to fix their contaminated and at times dysfunctional water system.[2] In Baldwin Hills, the historic African American heart of Los Angeles, community groups worked for years to create a park and have waged one battle after another to protect it, first from the construction of a power plant, then from development of a garbage dump, and recently from expansion of oil drilling in adjacent fields.[3]

Recognizing the complex interconnection among issues confronting vulnerable communities, advocates and experts in land use, transportation, environmental justice, workforce development, and housing are formulating equity-focused planning agendas for their cities and counties—blueprints that look beyond traditional brick-and-mortar community development to integrate health, environmental quality, job training, and economic vitality. Grassroots advocates also have forged partnerships with unions, faith organizations, and business groups, among others, to eliminate long-standing environmental barriers to health—in particular, by improving access to healthy food and by reducing pollution from the ports, freeways, and refineries that often scar the landscape of poor communities of color.

Although poverty is largely absent in current political discourse, amid the clamor over taxes and the deficit, the Obama Administration recognizes that a nation where approximately one in four African Americans, Latinos, and noncitizens are poor, and where people of color soon will represent the majority, is squandering its human capital and jeopardizing its future. The Administration has launched collaborative, comprehensive, place-based initiatives to improve the lives of low-income people.[4] To cite just two examples: the Partnership for Sustainable Communities, a joint effort of the US Department of Housing and Urban Development, the Department of Transportation, and the Environmental Protection Agency, is working with urban, suburban, and rural communities to expand transportation choices, promote affordable housing and energy efficiency, enhance economic competitiveness, and strengthen neighborhoods. The federal Promise Neighborhoods program, inspired by the successful Harlem Children's Zone, is supporting community-based efforts to provide children and families with high-quality, coordinated health, social, community, and educational support services from cradle to college to career, with the goal of improving student outcomes. Innovations such as these offer the best opportunities in years to bring to national scale local wisdom and promising equity-driven models for community revitalization.

THE EQUITY IMPERATIVE

Catalytic changes can provoke groundswells of social and political action. The New Deal, born of the Great Depression, revolutionized the role of the government and paved the way for Social Security, Medicare, and other safety nets. The rejection of second-class citizenship by African American soldiers returning from World War II, followed by African independence movements, set the stage for the civil rights protests of the 1950s and 1960s. The publication of Rachel Carson's *Silent Spring* aroused concern for natural resources and inspired the modern environmental movement.

The movement to build healthy communities has caught fire at a pivotal moment. The United States continues to struggle to recover from the worst financial collapse since the Depression. And it does so in a global economy that, even before the Great Recession, had devastated the economies of whole cities and regions. Across the country, the education system and public infrastructure are crumbling, the middle class is disintegrating, and the social safety net is unraveling. Against this backdrop three forces of change—increasing inequality, a health crisis that threatens the nation's future productivity, and shifting demographics—have converged, demanding new thinking and innovative approaches in every field, from community development to public health to environmental justice to economic recovery.

Inequality

After steadily worsening for decades, inequities in income, wealth, and opportunity have reached unprecedented levels; the United States has the third worst income inequality among advanced industrialized nations.[5,6] Since 1976, the share of income going to the top 1 percent has more than doubled, and this upper echelon of earners now receives more than one-fifth of the nation's economic pie.[7] Of all wealth generated between 1983 and 2009, 82 percent went to the richest 5 percent of households, while the typical household's wealth actually declined. The median wealth of white households is now 20 times that of black households and 18 times that of Latino households—the largest disparities since the federal government began tracking these data 25 years ago.[8] A key cause is the mortgage foreclosure crisis, which has disproportionately stripped African American and Latino families of their biggest—often, their only—asset: their home.

Even before the housing and financial collapse, deindustrialization and the loss of union jobs had taken a huge economic and social toll, particularly in older cities in the Northeast and Midwest. From 1990 to 2010, low-wage jobs grew by 31 percent, high-wage jobs by 20 percent, and middle-wage jobs by just 3 percent.[9]

Persistent residential segregation by race and income, coupled with the inequitable distribution of opportunity structures (i.e., the concentration of high-quality schools, good jobs, and social services in wealthier communities), deepens and cements the economic divide. It isolates low-income people and people of color from the resources, institutions, and social networks that enable Americans to get ahead. Limited economic mobility perpetuates poverty and disadvantages people of color from generation to generation.

A study by the Economic Mobility Project, a nonpartisan collaborative effort of The Pew Charitable Trusts, found that two-thirds of black children live in high-poverty communities, compared with 6 percent of white children.[10] These statistics have not changed in 30 years. In addition, American children have less relative mobility than their counterparts in northern Europe. One study found that 42 percent of US children born to low-income families (the bottom 20 percent) will remain there, and another 42 percent will make it out just barely.[11] Race is a determinant of mobility: more than half of black children born to parents whose incomes are in the bottom fifth remain there as adults, compared with 30 percent of white children. And the specter of downward mobility is more prevalent for African Americans: 45 percent of middle-class African American children end up poor, compared with 16 percent of middle-class white children.[12]

Economic inequality has always been the target of antipoverty advocacy. But the new extremes, combined with the geography of poverty, call for comprehensive approaches to create pathways for upward mobility and access to the opportunities of the future.

Health Crisis

By almost every measure, the health status of people of color is a national disgrace. Compared with white babies, African American babies are 2.4 times as likely to die at birth and four times as likely to die of complications related to low birthweight.[13] Lung disease, hypertension, hepatitis B, AIDS, and certain cancers are among the debilitating conditions that are far more prevalent, and deadly, among African Americans, Latinos, and to a lesser degree Asian American and Pacific Islanders.[14]

Racial health disparities have been evident for years, but the obesity epidemic has propelled the issue to the policy forefront. Obesity rates have nearly doubled among US adults and more than tripled among children in the past four decades,[15,16] with negative consequences for the prevalence and severity of chronic illnesses, quality of life, productivity, and health care costs.[17] While the epidemic cuts across lines of race, class, and geography, it disproportionately affects low-income communities and communities of color. Nearly 43 percent of Mexican American children ages 6 to 11 years, and nearly 37 percent of African American children in that age group, are overweight or obese, compared with 32 percent of white children.[18] Without concerted efforts to reverse obesity trends, today's generation of young people may be the first in modern US history to live sicker and die younger than their parents.[19]

Obesity and related illnesses such as heart disease and Type 2 diabetes are often viewed as "lifestyle" conditions attributable to an individual's behavior. In reality, they are the consequences of inequitable policies and investments that have shaped the built environment, land use patterns, economic development, and transportation plans. It is virtually impossible for residents of many distressed communities to follow official guidelines for diet and physical activity because of limited or no access to the requisite resources. More than 23.5 million people in low-income communities have no supermarket or large grocery store within a mile of their homes,[20] and the problem is most acute in communities of color. In California, lower income communities have 20 percent fewer healthy food sources than higher income communities.[21] In Albany, New York, 80 percent of nonwhite residents live in neighborhoods where one cannot find low-fat milk or high-fiber bread, a staple in any middle-class American community.[22] High-poverty communities and predominantly black neighborhoods also have fewer athletic venues, parks, bike trails, pools, and recreation facilities that provide practical, safe opportunities for active play, walking, and exercising.

In short, address has become a determinant of health and a proxy for opportunity. No doctor can undo the deleterious effects of living in a place without affordable fresh foods, green spaces, clean air, or safe, walkable streets. No medication can reverse the damaging consequences of living in a place with sweeping, systemic obstacles to wellness, including joblessness, dilapidated housing, abysmal schools, crime, and violence. While better access to health care is critical, broad environmental changes are needed to address the urgent health needs of communities of color.

Demographics

Equitable policies and investments are not simply the right thing to do; they are an economic imperative as well. If people of color do not thrive—if the wealth and health gaps persist and widen—the United States will not thrive. The 2010 US Census shows the nation's demographics changing faster than projected: in less than a generation, the majority of Americans will be people of color. They already represent the majority in California, Texas, New Mexico, and Hawaii. Nationwide, 46 percent of people under 18 years are children of color, and they will tip to become the majority by 2015.[23] There is a growing generation gap between the increasingly diverse youth population and primarily white seniors (not to mention the political establishment).

The changing face of America demands efforts to include people of color in the economy and in social and political life. Organizing efforts must address demographic changes in communities, engage all groups represented in a neighborhood or a region in planning and decision making, and find ways to work through the complexities of race dynamics and the cultural and language barriers in increasingly diverse neighborhoods.

A FRAMEWORK FOR COMMUNITY TRANSFORMATION

When the Health Department in Alameda County, California, asked its staff, area residents, youth, advocates, and local leaders what makes a community healthy, they answered with remarkable consistency: having access to good jobs, healthy foods, decent housing, and home ownership; living in an environment with clean air, clean water, and places to safely walk and play; enjoying trust among neighbors, good relations with police, safety from violence and crime, and an atmosphere free of prejudice and discrimination.[24]

In essence, the movement to build healthy communities is a push to improve conditions in the economic, social, physical, and service environments of a place. While this chapter discusses these environments one by one, they do not exist or affect people's lives in isolation. Rather, they blend into, respond to, and influence one another. The most effective organizing strategies and the most durable solutions reflect this melding.

Economic Environment

A thriving local economy—the presence of diverse businesses such as grocery stores, banks, restaurants; opportunities to own homes and build wealth; and pathways to jobs and entrepreneurship—is a requisite for healthy communities and the people who live and work there.[25] Conversely, well-being suffers when a moribund local economy leaves residents to cope with joblessness, the threat of homelessness, and the violence and alienation that can be fueled by dim prospects.[26] Transformative investments that revitalize the economies of disinvested inner cities, aging and increasingly impoverished suburbs, and isolated rural communities are critical.

Retail is an important piece of this equation. The vibrancy of a commercial district is a leading indicator of, and a major contributor to, community vitality. Robust neighborhood businesses draw foot and car traffic, create local jobs, and stimulate more commerce. When local businesses wither, communities tend to spiral downward: The tax base shrinks, resulting in public disinvestment. Streets are not swept, and trash piles up. Residents must shop outside their neighborhood, and without a critical mass of customers, new businesses do not locate there. The result is an image of decay that contributes to the overall negative perception of communities of color and depresses property values, which makes it difficult or impossible for homeowners to accumulate wealth.

The food retail environment is especially salient. Not only do grocery stores provide the benefits of any other robust business—foot traffic, commerce, jobs, many of them unionized—but they also foster better eating.[27]

People of color know they are being disrespected in their neighborhood when they cannot find a place to buy groceries. Unfortunately, this is all too common, and it is symptomatic of broader retail patterns. Communities of color have less access to essential commercial and financial services. For example, a 2009 national survey by the Federal Deposit Insurance Corporation found that 21.7 percent of black households, 19.3 percent of Hispanic households, and 15.6 percent of Native American households have no checking or savings account, compared with 3.3 percent of white households.[28] At the same time, research has shown that communities of color, particularly African American, have higher densities of liquor stores and bars, which are associated with more injury, drunken driving arrests, cirrhosis deaths, and violent crimes.[29] In a study of the cities of Contra Costa County, California, for example, researchers found that San Pablo, where 84 percent of residents are people of color, had 12.6 liquor stores per 10,000 residents, and Richmond, where 79 percent of the population are people of color, had 6.5 liquor stores per 10,000 residents. In contrast, neighboring, affluent Orinda and Lafayette—where people of color represent 16 percent of the population—had 1.7 and 3.3 liquor stores for every 10,000 residents, respectively. Together, San Pablo and Richmond were home to 25 percent of the county's liquor stores but only 14 percent of its population.[30] These trends are evident nationwide. In a study of 9,361 urban zip codes, RAND researchers found that the concentration of liquor stores and bars was consistently higher in black communities, and highest of all in low-income black neighborhoods—a disparity the researchers called "an environmental injustice for minorities and lower-income persons."[31]

This disparate economic landscape did not arise from blind market forces. From the post–World War II period through the 1960s, federal and state policies provided powerful incentives for homeownership, which promoted white flight first from inner cities and then to the ever-distant suburban edge.[32] Many businesses, including supermarkets, left the inner city, taking with them their jobs and tax revenues. Chain stores became oriented to the new suburban locations, with their abundant, inexpensive land and customers who owned cars. Many large chains did not regard urban locations, especially low-income ones, as viable.

Recent studies demonstrate how the marketing analyses that influence retailers' location decisions systematically undervalue inner-city neighborhoods.[33,34] Marketing firms often rely on national data sources such as the US Census, which tend to undercount low-income people and people of color— for several reasons. According to an analysis by the Leadership Council on Civil and Human Rights, low-income communities have lower response rates for mail and door-to-door collection methods. People with lower education levels, lower literacy, and limited English may have difficulty understanding the census. Furthermore, people may fear that immigration or law enforcement officials may use census responses to deport or incarcerate family members.[35] Market studies also tend to look at average household income rather than at total area income, a measure that more accurately captures the density of an urban neighborhood and therefore its purchasing power.

Some marketing firms use distorted generalizations and even gross stereotypes to assess investment potential. For example, one firm described the residents of predominantly African American neighborhoods in Milwaukee as "very low-income families [who] buy video games, dine at fast food chicken restaurants, use nonprescription cough syrup, and use laundries and Laundromats." The company described the residents of a suburban community as "interested in civic activities, volunteer work, contributions, and travel."[36] Setting aside the ethical and moral issues with these stereotypes, such assessments can steer companies away from investing in underserved communities that may very well offer good opportunities.

While advocates have worked for decades to reverse the grocery store exodus and establish supermarkets and other healthy fresh food outlets in underserved communities, the effort has gained traction in the face of the obesity epidemic. Research by PolicyLink, the Center for Public Health Policy, and the University of California, Los Angeles, has revealed that people who live in neighborhoods where fast food restaurants far outnumber fresh food stores are at significantly higher risk for obesity and Type 2 diabetes.[37] Conversely, numerous studies show that greater access to supermarkets corresponds with healthier eating.

Pennsylvania Fresh Food Financing Initiative, a public–private partnership, has emerged as a model for the nation in solving the problem of healthy food access while creating jobs and stimulating neighborhood economies.[38] The initiative has broken through a barrier that had long bedeviled food access advocates: money. The work dates back to 2001, when The Food Trust, a nonprofit organization in Philadelphia, documented the connection between lack of supermarkets and deaths from diet-related disease in the city. The findings sparked hearings in Philadelphia—Pennsylvania's most populous city, with 1.5 million residents—and the creation of a task force composed of a diverse group of local leaders charged with recommending solutions.

Financing was identified as the single greatest obstacle to stimulating grocery retailing in underserved communities. To overcome this hurdle, the task force recommended the creation of a statewide fund to support fresh food retail development. Pennsylvania subsequently appropriated $30 million over 3 years to create the Fresh Food Financing Initiative (FFFI).

Since it began in 2004, the initiative has led to the creation of 88 supermarkets, grocery stores, farmers markets, and co-ops—1.7 million square feet of retail space, all in underserved areas. The initiative has also created or protected more than 5,000 jobs, and the new supermarkets are helping to revitalize neighborhoods. With just $30 million from the state government for one-time grants and loans, the program has garnered $190 million in investment and improved healthy food access for almost half a million people.

The Obama Administration has created the Healthy Food Financing Initiative (HFFI), based on the Pennsylvania program, to encourage supermarkets, farmers markets, and other healthy food outlets to locate in underserved areas.[39] The federal initiative, which would include $330 million in loans, grants, and tax credits, has the potential to bring benefits to communities across the country.

A strong local retail environment means more than a grocery store, of course. And the retail environment is only one aspect of community economic development. Investments and policies must address all the factors that contribute to a strong local economy, including housing, employment, job training, noncommercial development, and local public finance.

Social Environment

We all need a strong social fabric to thrive. This matters at an individual level: people who are socially isolated are at higher risk for a variety of illnesses, accidents, homicide, suicide, drug abuse, and premature death.[40] This also matters at the level of community. When people are connected to those around them, and when they trust their neighbors, their local shopkeepers, their community leaders, and the teachers in their children's schools, they feel greater attachment to and investment in the place they live.

Research suggests that weak social networks, less cohesive neighborhoods, and environments marked by social conflict are associated with poor health outcomes and higher mortality. A study of urban teens found that weak social bonds are a strong predictor of the rates of four common sexually transmitted diseases: gonorrhea, Chlamydia, syphilis, and AIDS.[41] One of the most revealing studies on the impact of social bonds—because it looked at an actual event rather than a survey of a sample population—comes from an analysis of deaths during a Chicago heat wave in 1995. A neighborhood with relatively weak social bonds and cohesion had a mortality rate 10 times higher than the rate in a neighborhood of similar income but with stronger relationships.[42] Conversely, studies also show that more social connections and higher community cohesion are associated with greater well-being. For example, a study of Filipino Americans found that learning about one's cultural heritage, participating in cultural practices, and experiencing a sense of pride and ethnic connection buffer the emotional stress of perceived discrimination and are strongly associated with fewer symptoms of depression.[43]

The concept of social capital is key to understanding the intersection between the social environment and community well-being. The lack of resources and opportunity structures in many poor communities and communities of color—parks, thriving commercial districts, good schools with well-funded athletic teams and fields, indeed, the factors in all four environments of this framework—strips neighborhoods of the amenities and gathering spaces that knit people together and inspire community service and action. The inequities can feed on themselves. Weak community networks make it difficult for residents to organize and advocate for the very services, investments, and policies that would strengthen civic cohesion, build pride and a sense of ownership, and improve prospects for a healthy, sustainable future. For example, research has found that neighborhoods experiencing ethnic and racial changes were more likely to have toxic waste dumps located within their boundaries.[44]

Mentoring, supportive relationships, and social networks can teach, model, and reinforce virtually all the behaviors and activities that help people and places thrive: from healthy eating to civic engagement to leadership. And when diverse people come together for a common goal, they not only increase their potential to achieve it, but they discover opportunities for bridging differences as well. For example, Barrios Unidos in Santa Cruz, California, is working with former gang members, other out-of-school youth, and young prisoners to strengthen their self-esteem, cultural pride, and other life-affirming qualities as an alternative to violence.[45] Building black-brown alliances is emphasized, even in the tough terrain of the prison system. As for the young members, who are largely Latino, Barrios Unidos helps them rediscover their drive to succeed by reconnecting them with their culture, often through the practice of indigenous spiritual traditions.

More grocery stores, cleaner air, safer streets, better housing—indeed, all the positive factors in the four environments presented here—are possible with strong organizing, mobilization, and staying power. When neighbors know one another, when they feel invested in the betterment of their community, and when they feel empowered to raise their voices, they create ways to join together and fight for changes that improve the lives of everyone.

Physical Environment

Clean water and air; well-maintained sidewalks and parks; structurally sound and attractive housing; clean, safe school buildings—good physical conditions are bedrocks of a thriving neighborhood.[46] Conversely, inadequate and dilapidated public facilities and infrastructure discourage economic investment and commerce, they limit opportunities for physical activity and social engagement, and they expose residents to toxins and other hazards. Unfortunately, poor physical conditions are all too common in underinvested communities of color.

The history of metropolitan sprawl and inner-city disinvestment created and perpetuates these problems. The pattern described in the economic environment section is etched in concrete in the physical environment of low-income urban communities: the exodus to the suburbs of jobs, businesses, tax base, and white residents; and the isolation of people of color in neglected, underinvested neighborhoods.[47,48,49] Many older urban neighborhoods may have been built to the standards of earlier eras as compact communities with public gathering spaces and commercial districts. But after decades of economic isolation, sidewalks are often poorly lit and maintained; streets roar with traffic; and parks are often unsafe, unkempt, and much too small for the current population, if they exist at all.

Bus depots and facilities that spew pollutants are disproportionately located in low-income communities of color, highways often run through them, and ports and airports frequently abut them.[50] These foul the air of already vulnerable neighborhoods. In 2005, the California Air Resources Board found that the ports and movement of goods throughout the state caused more than 2,400 premature deaths annually, mostly related to particulate pollution, and was responsible for 2,000 hospital admissions because of respiratory problems.[51] The predominantly black community of West Oakland sits against a busy freeway, a major port, and an airport. A 2003 study found the air inside some homes in this area was five times more toxic than in other parts of the city.[52]

Truck and ship fumes, of course, are far from the only environmental hazard in low-income communities. Substandard housing construction and rundown apartments are sources of pollutants and allergens in low-income communities of color.[53,54] Peeling paint may contain lead, which causes mental and physical developmental delays in fetuses, infants, and children.[55,56,57] Deficient housing is associated with higher rates of injuries and higher health care costs, and it exacts an emotional toll.[58,59,60] A study in Detroit found that people living in neighborhoods with a greater number of buildings in poor condition suffered increased stress levels and more symptoms of depression.[61]

Deplorable school facilities continue to be a problem in underfunded, overcrowded districts. They pose the same health risks as substandard housing, compounding the dangers for children, particularly those with asthma and other respiratory conditions, who get no respite either at home or school.

Spending on the "built" environment—school buildings, roads, parks, transportation systems, and other essential infrastructure—is among the largest investments made by governments and the private sector. Planning and decision making must be done with the explicit goal of promoting health, sustainability, and equity. Local residents must be engaged at every step, particularly people of color, who have been left out of these conversations for too long.

Thanks in large part to grassroots advocacy, a growing number of municipalities are recognizing the connections between health and community design and are integrating health concerns into zoning and planning decisions. In San Francisco, for instance, the Healthy Development Measurement Tool, designed by the Department of Public Health in conjunction with leaders of several diverse low- and moderate-income neighborhoods, is used to forecast the health consequences of redevelopment proposals.[62] By holding projects accountable for long-overlooked outcomes, including sustainable transportation, healthy housing, access to goods and services, and resident participation, tools like this mark a striking departure from traditional approaches to urban planning.

For decades, environmental justice activists have called attention to the connections between pollution, illness, land use planning, and public policy. They also have documented their heavy burden on communities of color, and they have challenged the mainstream environmental movement's disregard of these issues. By revealing insights into the juncture of social inequity and public health, environmental justice activism laid important groundwork for advocacy on health and place. The history of the environmental justice movement also offers a cautionary lesson: unless a social change movement intentionally focuses on equity and engages communities of color in crafting policies and programs that benefit everyone, solutions to broad societal problems are likely to overlook the most vulnerable people and may harm them even further.

Service Environment

The inequitable distribution of public services—hospitals, clinics, good schools, sanitation, and police and fire protection—is a long-standing issue in inner cities and many smaller communities. Local governments raise revenues and allocate resources in patterns that systemically reproduce inequities by race and income, resulting in community infrastructure and a range of social, educational, and protective services that vary tremendously in quality and effectiveness. Services that would enhance community health and the prevention of chronic diseases are poorly supported, while ineffectual and counterproductive criminal justice systems consume an ever-larger share of local budgets. These inequities and skewed priorities have dire consequences for residents from birth, or even earlier: As discussed earlier, African Americans are more likely to lack access to health care, prenatal care included. Black babies are more likely to be born preterm (18 percent in 2009, compared with 12 percent for Hispanic babies and 10.9 percent for white babies) and are nearly twice as likely as white infants to be born at low birthweight.[63] The effects of underinvestment spiral from there. Not until 2005 did the percentage of black children attending preschool, the foundation for academic success, equal that of white children at nearly 70 percent. Latino children still lag behind, with only 48 percent attending preschool. African American children begin elementary school about 1 year behind white children in vocabulary knowledge—and that gap widens to 4 years by the end of high school.[64] Racial gaps also persist in math and reading scores,[65] and in high school graduation rates. In 2009, according to the most recent federal data available, the high school dropout rate among 16- through 24-year-olds was 17.6 percent for Hispanics, 9.3 percent for African Americans, and 5.2 percent for whites.[66] The reasons for these disparities are complex, but certainly inequities in education resources play a significant role: schools attended predominantly by students of color are more likely to have inexperienced teachers, inadequate materials, less demanding curricula, and overcrowded, outdated, facilities.

The education gap is becoming a crisis, as the job market offers fewer and fewer opportunities for less-educated workers. The unemployment rate for African American men ages 16 to 19 years was 33 percent in 2009, a higher rate than the United States suffered during the Great Depression.[67]

A gaping racial divide also characterizes the law enforcement and the criminal justice systems. Police, rather than offer protection that is culturally sensitive and responsive to the needs of low-income communities of color, are often quick to detain residents, especially men. And the criminal justice system is far more willing to incarcerate these men than to reintegrate them into society after their release. African Americans are imprisoned at nearly six times the rate of whites, and Latinos at nearly double the rate of whites.[68] Traditional rehabilitation and reentry approaches are failing, draining limited resources that might otherwise be available for education, health services, and social welfare programs that could keep people out of the criminal justice system and launch them on the road to success. In California, for example, more than 60 percent of formerly incarcerated men return to prison within 3 years.[69] US incarceration rates, by far the highest in the world, harm the life chances not only of those who wind up behind bars. When so many men are marginalized economically and socially, in prison and after their release, their families and communities also suffer.[70] And when so many children of color find themselves in a cradle-to-prison pipeline, hope becomes elusive.

A growing number of advocates are focusing on service improvements for the population most vulnerable to violence and its health effects—and disproportionately punished by get-tough policies: boys and men of color. The San Francisco–based W. Haywood Burns Institute for Juvenile Justice Fairness and Equity, for example, has piloted restorative justice projects that have proven to be effective alternatives to punitive school policies—dramatically reducing the number of African American youth detained for aggravated battery (the legal term for school fights).[71] The institute has also collaborated with probation departments, courts, schools, child welfare agencies, and local groups around the nation to change policy and provide alternatives to youth detention.

Prison rehabilitation and reentry programs must offer people who have been incarcerated a real chance for a productive life. Healthy, equitable communities require the full range of health and human resources, including well-funded programs, innovative and responsive leadership, and effective services that protect, assist, and empower all people to reach their full potential.

Underinvestment and government neglect have a different cast in rural America—no less dire than in cities, but far less visible. Thousands of poor, unincorporated communities lack the basics that mainstream America takes for granted. California's San Joaquin Valley, for example, is one of the most agriculturally rich regions in the United States, yet it is home to some of the nation's most isolated, distressed communities. A PolicyLink analysis of 2010 Census data found that across the region's eight counties, poverty rates ranged from 18 percent to 27 percent. Many of these communities lack safe tap water; one study found that 92 water systems in the region had a well with nitrate levels above the legal limit, potentially affecting the water supply of 1.3 million residents.[72] Many residents also live without other features of a healthy environment, including sewer systems, safe housing, sidewalks, and access to healthy foods, due to decades of neglect and exclusion from formal decision making by city, county, and state governments.

To respond to these problems, the Community Equity Initiative (CEI) was established in 2007 as a partnership of California Rural Legal Assistance, Inc., California Rural Legal Assistance Foundation, and PolicyLink.[73]

The initiative convened San Joaquin Valley residents, policy and legal advocates, and researchers to identify the root causes of the service and infrastructure deficit and to develop solutions. Participants agreed that achieving service and infrastructure equity would require at least four primary strategies: support and education for resident participation and leadership in governance and decision making; reform of local and state policies; legal representation; and research.

CEI is working directly with residents and local leaders throughout the San Joaquin Valley, developing capacity to participate meaningfully in critical decisions shaping their communities and their region. Residents are organizing and learning how to become effective members of the boards of agencies that control water and local services.

CEI has achieved concrete changes in law and policy locally and statewide. Perhaps most notably, CEI developed a focused strategy to make sure that sustainable growth planning grants provided by a state law are distributed equitably, and that funds are set aside for communities in desperate need. In the unincorporated community of Matheny Tract, just south of the city of Tulare, CEI worked with residents to achieve an unprecedented planning decision by the local land commission, which secured safe drinking water, facilitated the development of a sewer system, and institutionalized fair planning processes. CEI is now representing a coalition of 17 communities in a lawsuit against the State of California for its failure to prepare a mandated Drinking Water Plan, a blueprint to ensure that every community in the state has safe potable water. With respect to the long-term plans for the region, CEI is training local leaders to influence the state and federally funded planning grants intended to spur more sustainable growth. Sustainability means not simply less sprawl, but a coherent strategy to address the service and housing needs of the region's lower income communities of color.

Applied research is the underpinning of all CEI strategies. The most basic approaches include mapping and identifying the communities, often for the first time, surveying residents about local conditions, and analyzing the effects of prospective policies. These activities, undertaken with the full engagement of residents, build the case for positive change and create a collective understanding of the breadth and scale of service and infrastructure deficits and governance issues. Many unincorporated areas are not defined as distinct neighborhoods by the US Census or county planning agencies. As a result, their needs are often unaccounted for, they are not acknowledged in planning processes, and they cannot compete for government investments. When communities are invisible, they stand little chance of being well represented or well served, which makes mapping analyses especially important in identifying the many rural outposts that low-income families and people of color call home. Being seen is a first step toward being heard.

GUIDEPOSTS FOR ACTION

Building healthy, opportunity-rich communities demands comprehensive approaches and multidisciplinary strategies grounded in four principles of equity. These have relevance not only in the United States but also in a global context.

1. *Integrate "people" strategies and "place" strategies.* Fair, sustainable development—in rural communities, urban neighborhoods, recently disinvested suburbs, or metropolitan regions overall—requires a dual focus: on people-oriented strategies that support residents (for instance, job training, child care, and workforce development); and on place-oriented strategies that stabilize and improve local environments (for instance, supermarket development, affordable housing, and infrastructure investment).

2. *Reduce local, regional, and national disparities.* Policies at all levels of government must focus on improving outcomes for low-income communities and communities of color while building strong regional and national economies. A growing body of research, most of it based on developing countries, suggests that inequality is harmful to economic growth.[74,75,76,77,78] A smaller, growing body of literature focusing on the United States has reached the same conclusion. For example, an analysis of the growth of 74 metropolitan regions in the 1980s found that greater equality within regions (measured by poverty reductions in central cities) corresponded with stronger regional economic growth (measured by increases in per capita income).[79] Regions and nations that systematically address both economic growth and economic distress set themselves up to compete more effectively in the global marketplace.

3. *Promote "triple bottom-line" investments* that deliver fair returns for investors, benefits for the community, and positive impacts on the environment. This means investing in sustainable public transportation; in modern, energy-efficient affordable housing; in jobs and workforce development in the growth industries of the future, including the "green" sector; and in small business and local entrepreneurship opportunities. It also means that private investments, when guided, complemented and provided incentives by public policies and spending, can and should be structured to return benefits to the local community. Financial institutions, private developers, and large corporations must collaborate with policy makers, local leaders, grassroots advocates, and community residents to ensure that investments are equitable and catalytic.

4. *Ensure meaningful community participation, leadership, and ownership.* Civic engagement lies at the heart of equitable policy making, and it is a pillar of a thriving community. Government officials and well-meaning experts must move beyond top-down decisions and actively listen to community voices and local wisdom. Residents must have full access to the tools, skills, knowledge,

and resources that allow authentic participation at every stage of the planning and decision making that will shape the future of the place they call home.

Environmental awareness and advocacy has always been rooted in, and motivated by, an appreciation for the interrelatedness of all spheres of human and natural activity. The movement to build healthy communities embodies a similar integrated perspective and builds on insights into the connections between the health of the environment and the life prospects of the people who live in that environment. Our collective future—as a nation and as a planet—depends on our ability to create community environments that afford all people meaningful opportunities to participate and prosper. An explicit, unwavering commitment to equity is essential to ensure that the environmental and societal changes we are fighting for do not simply benefit a privileged few, but improve the lives of people who have been left behind for too long.

NOTES

1. J. Bell and M. Lee, *Why Place and Race Matter* (Oakland, CA: PolicyLink, 2011), accessed June 20, 2011, http://www.policylink.org/site/c.lkIXLbMNJrE/b.6728307/k.58F8/Why_Place___Race_Matter.htm
2. Ibid.
3. The City Project, accessed May 2, 2013, http://www.cityprojectca.org/ourwork/baldwinhills.html
4. R. Fox and S. Treuhaft, *The President's 2011 Budget: Creating Communities of Opportunity.* (Oakland, CA: PolicyLink, 2011), accessed June 20, 2011, http://www.policylink.org/atf/cf/%7B97c6d565-bb43-406d-a6d5-eca3bbf35af0%7D/FINAL_2011BUDGET_FINAL.PDF?tr=y&auid=6436296
5. A. Gilbert, "Inequality and Why it Matters," *Geography Compass* 1, no. 3 (2007): 422.
6. B. Einhorn, "Countries with the Biggest Gaps Between Rich and Poor," *Business Week*, October 16, 2009, accessed June 20, 2011 http://finance.yahoo.com/news/pf_article_107980.html
7. T. Piketty and E. Saez, *Striking it Richer: The Evolution of Top Incomes in the United States* (Updated with 2008 Estimates), accessed July 17, 2010, http://elsa.berkeley.edu/~saez/saez-UStopincomes-2008.pdf
8. Pew Research Center, *Wealth Gaps Rise to Record Highs Between Whites, Blacks, and Hispanics*, accessed November 14, 2011, http://pewresearch.org/pubs/2069/housing-bubble-subprime-mortgages-hispanics-blacks-household-wealth-disparity
9. S. Treuhaft, A. G. Blackwell, and M. Pastor, "*America's Tomorrow: Equity is the Superior Growth Model,*" PolicyLink and USC Program for Environmental and Regional Equity, accessed November 1, 2011, http://www.policylink.org/site/c.lkIXLbMNJrE/b.7843037/k.1048/Americas_Tomorrow_Equity_is_the_Superior_Growth_Model.htm
10. P. Sharkey, "Neighborhoods and the Black-White Mobility Gap." Pew Charitable Trusts Economic Mobility Project. 2009, accessed May 26, 2013,

http://www.pewtrusts.org/uploadedFiles/wwwpewtrustsorg/Reports/
Economic_Mobility/PEW_SHARKEY_v12.pdf

11. J. B. Isaacs, "Economic Mobility of Families Across Generations," in *Getting Ahead of Losing Ground: Economic Mobility in America*. (Washington, DC: Brookings Institution, 2008) ed. Ron Haskins, Julia B. Isaacs and Isabel V. Sawhill, accessed June 20, 2011, http://www.brookings.edu/~/media/Files/rc/reports/2008/02_economic_mobility_sawhill/02_economic_mobility_sawhill_ch1.pdf

12. Ibid.

13. *Infant Mortality and African Americans*, U.S. Department of Health and Human Services, Office of Minority Health, accessed June 20, 2011, http://minority-health.hhs.gov/templates/content.aspx?ID=3021

14. Data/Statistics from U.S. Department of Health and Human Services, Office of Minority Health, accessed June 20, 2011, http://minorityhealth.hhs.gov/templates/browse.aspx?lvl=1&lvlID=2

15. K. M. Flegal et al., "Prevalence and Trends in Obesity Among US Adults 1999–2008," *Journal of the American Medical Association* 303, no. 3 (2010): 235–41.

16. C. L. Ogden and M. D. Carroll, *Prevalence of Obesity Among Children and Adolescents: United States Trends, 1963-1965 Through 2007-2008*, Centers for Disease Control and Prevention, accessed June 20, 2011, http://www.cdc.gov/nchs/data/hestat/obesity_child_07_08/obesity_child_07_08.htm

17. National Heart, Lung, and Blood Institute. *Clinical Guidelines on the Identification, Evaluation, and Treatment of Overweight and Obesity in Adults (US): The Evidence Report* (NIH publication no. 98–4083, Bethesda, MD: Washington, NHLBI, 1998).

18. C. L. Ogden, M. D. Carroll, and K. M. Flegal. "High Body Mass Index for Age Among US Children and Adolescents 2003–2006." *Journal of the American Medical Association* 299, no. 20 (2008): 2401–5.

19. S. Jay Olshansky et al., A Potential Decline in Life Expectancy in the United States in the 21st Century. *New England Journal of Medicine* 352, no. 11 (2005): 1138–45.

20. USDA Economic Research Service, *Access to Affordable and Nutritious Food: Measuring and Understanding Food Deserts and Their Consequences. Report to Congress* (Washington, DC: U.S. Department of Agriculture, 2009).

21. California Center for Public Health Advocacy, PolicyLink, and the UCLA Center for Health Policy Research, *Designed for Disease: The Link Between Local Food Environments and Obesity and Diabetes* (Oakland, CA: PolicyLink, 2008).

22. A. S. Hosler et al., "Low-Fat Milk and High-Fiber Bread Availability in Food Stores in Urban and Rural Communities," *Journal of Public Health Management Practice* 12 (2006): 556–62.

23. *Population Projections*, U.S. Census Bureau, accessed May 26, 2013, http://www.census.gov/population/projections/data/national/2008.html
PolicyLink analysis of U.S. Census data available at http://www.censusscope.org/

24. M. Beyers et al., *Life and Death from Unnatural Causes: Health and Social Inequity in Alameda County* (Oakland, CA: Alameda County Public Health Department, 2008).

25. J. R. Kahn and E. M. Fazio, "Economic Status Over the Life Course and Racial Disparities in Health," *Journals of Gerontology Series B: Psychological Sciences and Social Sciences*, Special Issue 2 60 (2005): S76–S84.

26. A. J. Schulz et al., "Social and Physical Environments and Disparities in Risk for Cardiovascular Disease: The Healthy Environments Partnership Conceptual Model," *Environmental Health Perspectives* 113, no. 12 (2005): 1817–25.

27. T. Giang et al., "Closing the Grocery Gap in Underserved Communities: The Creation of the Pennsylvania Fresh Food Financing Initiative," *Journal of Public Health Management and Practice* 14, no. 3 (2008): 272–9.

28. *National Survey of Unbanked and Underbanked Households*, FDIC, accessed May 26, 2013, http://www.fdic.gov/householdsurvey/2009/full_report.pdf

29. J. Romley et al., "Alcohol and Environmental Justice: The Density of Liquor Stores and Bars in Urban Neighborhoods in the United States," *Journal of Studies on Alcohol and Drugs* 68, no. 1 (2007): 48–55.

30. Pacific Institute, "Liquor Stores and Community Health," in *Measuring What Matters: Neighborhood Research for Economic and Environmental Health and Justice in Richmond, North Richmond, and San Pablo*, 2009, accessed November 14, 2011, http://www.pacinst.org/reports/measuring_what_matters/issues/liquor_store.pdf

31. J. Romley et al., "Alcohol and Environmental Justice: The Density of Liquor Stores and Bars in Urban Neighborhoods in the United States," *Journal of Studies on Alcohol and Drugs* 68, no. 1 (2007): 48–55.

32. M. Seitles, "The Perpetuation of Residential Racial Segregation in America: Historical Discrimination, Modern Forms of Exclusion, and Inclusionary Remedies," *Journal of Land Use and Environmental Law*, accessed June 20, 2011, http://www.law.fsu.edu/journals/landuse/Vol141/seit.htm

33. J. Pawasarat and L. Quinn, *Exposing Urban Legends: The Real Purchasing Power of Central City Neighborhoods* (Washington, DC: Brookings Institution Press, 2001).

34. The Boston Consulting Group and The Initiative for a Competitive Inner City, *The Business Case for Pursuing Retail Opportunities in the Inner City*, accessed May 26, 2013, http://imaps.indygov.org/ed_portal/studies/bcg_inner_city_retail.pdf

35. The Leadership Conference, *Reasons Behind Inaccuracy in the Census*, accessed May 2, 2013, http://www.civilrights.org/census/accurate-count/inaccuracies.html

36. Pawasarat and Quinn, *Exposing Urban Legends...*

37. California Center for Public Health Advocacy et al., *Designed for Disease...*

38. The Food Trust, accessed May 26, 2013, http://thefoodtrust.org/

39. *Healthy Food Financing Initiative*, U.S. Department of Health and Human Services, Office of Community Services, accessed May 2, 2013, http://www.acf.hhs.gov/programs/ocs/ocs_food.html.

40. Centers for Disease Control and Prevention, *Report of the National Expert Panel on Social Determinants of Health Equity: Recommendations for Advancing Efforts to Achieve Health Equity*, (Atlanta, GA: Centers for Disease Control and Prevention, 2009).

41. D. R. Holtgrave and R. A. Crosby, "Social Capital, Poverty, and Income Inequality as Predictors of Gonorrhea, Syphilis, Chlamydia, and AIDS Case Rates in the United States," *Sexually Transmitted Infection* 79 (2003): 62–4.

42. E. Klinenberg, *Heat Wave: A Social Autopsy of Disaster in Chicago* (Chicago, IL: University of Chicago Press, 2002).

43. K. N. Mossakowski, "Coping with Perceived Discrimination: Does Ethnic Identity Protect Mental Health?" in "Race, Ethnicity, and Mental Health," special issue, *Journal of Health and Social Behavior* 44, no. 3 (2003): 318–31.

44. R. Morello-Frosch et al., "Environmental Justice and Regional Inequality in Southern California: Implications for Future Research," *Environmental Health Perspectives* 110, supp. 2 (2002): 149–54.

45. Barrios Unidos, official website, accessed May 2, 2013, http://www.barriosunidos.net/

46. H. Frumkin, "Healthy Places: Exploring the Evidence," *American Journal of Public Health* 93, no. 9 (2003): 1451–6.

47. D. Acevedo-Garcia and K. Lochner, "Residential Segregation and Health," in I. Kawachi and L. Berkman, eds., *Neighborhoods and Health* (Oxford, England: Oxford University Press, 2001), 264–87.

48. J. A. Powell, "Race and Space," *Brookings Review*, Fall (1998). accessed May 26, 2013, http://www.brookings.edu/research/articles/1998/09/fall-politics-powell

49. M. Orfield, *American Metropolitics: The New Suburban Reality* (Washington, DC: Brookings Institution Press, 2002).

50. C. Lee, "Environmental Justice: Building a Unified Vision of Health and the Environment," *Environmental Health Perspectives* 110, supp. 2 (2002): 141–4.

51. California Environmental Protection Agency, *Emission Reduction Plan for Ports and Goods Movement in California: Update on Implementation*, (Air Resources Board Meeting. Oakland, California. April 24, 2008), accessed June 20, 2011, http://www.arb.ca.gov/bonds/gmbond/docs/slides_only_for_apr2008_gmerp_board_update.pdf

52. H. K. Lee. "Diesel Exhaust Poses Health Risk in West Oakland, Study Finds," *San Francisco Chronicle*, November 16, 2003, accessed, http://www.sfgate.com/cgi-bin/article.cgi?f=/c/a/2003/11/16/BAGQE334JL1.DTL

53. J. Krieger and D. L. Higgins, "Housing and Health: Time Again for Public Health Action," *American Journal of Public Health* 92(5):758–68 (2002).

54. R. D. Cohn et al., "National Prevalence and Exposure Risk for Cockroach Allergen in U.S. Households," *Environmental Health Perspectives* 114, no. 4 (2006): 522–6.

55. D. Bellinger et al., "Low Level Lead Exposure and Infant Development in the First Year," *Neurobehavioral Toxicology and Teratology* 8 (1986):151–61.

56. Committee on Environmental Health, "Lead Exposure in Children: Prevention, Detection, and Management," *Pediatrics* 116, no. 4 (2005): 1036–46.

57. H. L. Needleman et al., "The Long-Term Effects of Exposure to Low Doses of Lead in Childhood: An 11-Year Follow-up Report," *New England Journal of Medicine* 322, no. 2 (1990): 83–8.

58. G. R. Istre et al., "Deaths and Injuries from House Fires," *New England Journal of Medicine* 344, no. 25 (2001): 1911–6.

59. M. Sandel and J. Sharfstein, *Not Safe at Home: How America's Housing Crisis Threatens the Health of Its Children* (Boston, MA: Children's Hospital Medical Center, The Doc4Kids Project, 1998).

60. D. Chenoweth, *The Economic Cost of Substandard Housing Conditions Among North Carolina Children*, (report, North Carolina Housing Coalition, Raleigh, NC, 2007).

61. *Annual Report 2004–2005*, Healthy Environments Partnership, accessed May 26, 2013, http://www.hepdetroit.org/en/our-documents/hep-reports

62. The Healthy Development Measurement Tool, accessed May 26, 2013, http://www.thehdmt.com/

63. Forum on Child and Family Statistics, accessed May 26, 2013, http://childstats.gov/americaschildren/health.asp

64. G. Farkas, *Racial Disparities and Discrimination in Education: What Do We Know, How Do We Know It, and What Do We Need to Know?*, accessed May 26, 2013, http://www.hrpujc.org/documents/TCRecordFarkas.pdf

65. R. G. Fryer and S. D. Levitt, "Understanding the Black-White Test Score Gap in the First Years of School," *The Review of Economics and Statistics* 86, no. 2 (2004): 447–64.

66. *Fast Facts*, National Center for Education Statistics, accessed May 2, 2013, http://nces.ed.gov/fastfacts/display.asp?id=16

67. S. Wessler, *Race and Recession: How Inequity Rigged the Economy and How to Change the Rules* (New York, NY: Applied Research Center, 2009).

68. M. Mauer and R. S. King, *Uneven Justice: State Rates of Incarceration by Rates and Ethnicity* (Washington, DC: The Sentencing Project, 2007), accessed June 20, 2011, http://www.sentencingproject.org/doc/publications/rd_stateratesofincbyraceandethnicity.pdf.

69. California Department of Corrections and Rehabilitation, *Recidivism Rate: Three Year Follow-up Period by Commitment Offense*, (Sacramento, CA: Adult Research Branch, California Department of Corrections and Rehabilitation, 2009).

70. J. B. Hyman, *Men and Communities: African American Males and the Well-Being of Children, Families, and Neighborhoods* (background paper, Joint Center for Political and Economic Studies, Washington, DC, 2006), accessed May 2, 2013, http://www.jamesbhyman.com/Publications/Men%20and%20Communities.pdf

71. W. Haywood Burns Institute, official website, accessed http://www.burnsinstitute.org.

72. E. Moore and E. Matalon, *The Human Costs of Nitrate-contaminated Drinking Water in the San Joaquin Valley* (Oakland, CA: Pacific Institute, 2011), accessed November 20, 2011, http://www.pacinst.org/reports/nitrate_contamination/nitrate_contamination.pdf.

73. *Achieving Policy Impact: Unincorporated Communities: The Community Equity Initiative*, PolicyLink, accessed May 2, 2013, http://www.policylink.org/site/c.lkIXLbMNJrE/b.5160111/k.8DA6/Unincorporated_Communities.htm

74. A. B. Atkinson, "Is the Welfare State Necessarily an Obstacle to Economic Growth?" *European Economic Review* 39 (1995): 723–30.

75. J. Pontusson, *Inequality and Prosperity: Social Europe vs. Liberal America* (Ithaca, NY: Cornell University Press, 2005).

76. W. Korpi, "Economic Growth and the Welfare State: Leaky Bucket or Irrigation System?" *European Sociological Review* 1, no. 2 (1985): 97–118.

77. P. Aghion, E. Caroli, and C. Garcia-Penalosa, "Inequality and Economic Growth: The Perspective of the New Growth Theories," *Journal of Economic Literature* 37, no. 4 (1999): 1615–60.

78. W. Easterly, "The Middle Class Consensus and Economic Development," *Journal of Economic Growth* 6, no. 4 (2001): 317–35.

79. M. Pastor Jr. et al., *Regions That Work: How Cities and Suburbs Can Grow Together* (Minneapolis, MN: University of Minnesota Press, 2000).

CHAPTER 4

Building Income and Social Equity through Urban Sustainability

Lessons from Vancouver's Downtown Eastside

MITRA THOMPSON

Locally based, income-generating initiatives have an extremely important role to play in fostering healthy communities. Poor and marginalized communities are increasingly turning to the social economy as a means of revitalizing impoverished neighborhoods. Increasingly, these socially motivated enterprises are simultaneously addressing environmental challenges. Recent Canadian scholarship on the social economy suggests that promoting sustainable urban development and other "green" goals should also be seen as social goals in and of themselves. One argument put forward is that environmental goals form an intrinsic part of a social enterprise's social mission, as they represent the goals of people living within society "and therefore one form of social objective."[1] For United We Can, a Vancouver-based social enterprise, this combined approach to social and environmental goals involves linking job creation for low-income urban residents with a mandate of creating "economic opportunities for people with multiple barriers living in the Downtown Eastside, through environmental initiatives."[2] United We Can is located in Vancouver's Downtown Eastside, a neighborhood sometimes referred to as Canada's poorest postal code, where community members face high incidences of social and health inequalities, including poverty, drug addiction, and mental health issues.

In 1995, after 5 years of campaigning and organizing, Ken Lyotier founded a nonprofit social enterprise that would become the main source of legal work and income for some of the poorest and most vulnerable people in the city of Vancouver. United We Can has harnessed the economic potential of a previously untapped area of Vancouver's informal economy—binning—and made huge strides toward legitimizing it as a type of employment. Binning is the practice of retrieving large quantities of cans and bottles from dumpsters, to be redeemed against their designated value. In the 1980s, Lyotier himself spent several years working as a binner as he struggled with addiction and homelessness while living in Vancouver's Downtown Eastside.

At United We Can, local people are hired regardless of addiction, mental health issues, or other barriers to employment, and they earn an hourly wage to run a bottle depot that processes the bottles and cans brought in by binners, before sending them off for recycling. The bottle depot guarantees payment in full to all binners for as many beverage containers as they can collect, providing them with a legal source of daily income.

When United We Can was created, most nonprofit organizations in the Downtown Eastside (DTES) were either local political activist groups or traditional charities. Amid a throng of highly vocal community advocacy groups and social service providers with distinct clientele pools in line with funder preferences,[3] United We Can set itself apart early on by calling for change without taking political sides, and by actively building relationships with local business in addition to trade union and government representatives to advance its work. Today, it provides mostly recycling-based jobs with flexible work hours and an understanding that, for DTES residents who live with multiple barriers to full-time employment, time off will be granted on an as-needed basis.

This chapter examines the impact United We Can has had on a community of highly marginalized, largely unemployed people living in the most expensive city in Canada. First, it sets the scene for United We Can by providing social context about the Downtown Eastside and the challenges faced by its resident community. Then, it goes on to analyze the role of United We Can in terms of social equity outcomes and explores their link to environmental sustainability. Finally, it weaves together this analysis with the challenges faced by United We Can, offering lessons to other social enterprises focused on job creation in marginalized communities.

METHODOLOGY

United We Can was selected as a case study for its success in building social equity and improving environmental sustainability within a local urban context. Fieldwork was conducted from May 17 to July 9, 2010 in Vancouver, British Columbia, Canada. A total of 44 United We Can employees, management, binners, city councillors, municipal workers, community stakeholders, and academics were interviewed during the case study. Participants were selected primarily through snowball sampling, and particular effort was made to ensure that the managers, supervisors, and as many employees as possible from each of the four United We Can projects targeted were involved. Present throughout the participant selection process was the need to balance the overall sample as much as possible between representatives of United We Can and other community stakeholders not affiliated with the organization. In the end, 27 of the 44 interviewed participants worked for or were in some way linked to United We Can. Gender representation among this sample of 27 is somewhat skewed, with only three female interviewees. It should be recognized, however, that the ratio of men to women among United We Can staff is heavily weighted in favor of the former, owing largely to the heavy physical nature of the work but also reflecting a male bias in the local population[4]: according to United We Can's executive director, female employees make up just 15–20 percent of all staff at any given time.

CANADA'S POOREST POSTAL CODE

Canada's third largest city is known for its stunning ocean and mountain views, its West Coast coffee-and-yoga lifestyle, its thriving Asian food scene... and the soaring prices of its forest of gleaming new condominiums. In 2011, it was estimated that more than one in five Vancouver houses sold for over C$1 million, and the average house cost more than 11 times a typical family income.[5] Affordable housing and the cost of living in general is a source of concern for many Vancouverites, and the nature of the city's housing market means that many people who would be able to buy their first house elsewhere often end up renting, creating downward pressure on the rental market that ends in demand for social housing that outstrips supply. Nowhere is the struggle for housing more starkly depicted than in the Downtown Eastside.

The Downtown Eastside is the oldest part of Vancouver and forms its historic core. Situated in east-central Vancouver, it had a total population of more than 16,500 in 2001.[6] Historically, the area has always been working class, and since the early 20th century it has been dotted with single-room occupancy hotels (commonly referred to as SROs) that were originally used to house the casual laborers of BC's construction and natural resource industries during the off-season. Today, privately owned SROs are the second biggest source of low-income housing in the Downtown Eastside in terms of overall room numbers, after nonmarket (subsidized) housing.[7]

A variety of factors contributed to the protracted economic downturn and social issues that have impacted the Downtown Eastside since the early 1980s. The downturn of BC's resource-based industries such as fishing and logging left behind a depressed local economy and a large pool of unemployed laborers for whom the most affordable housing option was to take up permanent residence in cheap city lodgings. A generation of low-income SRO residents were evicted in the early 1980s when a number of hotel landlords opted to rebrand their buildings as tourist hotels for Vancouver's hosting of the 1986 World's Fair.[8] Homelessness grew in tandem with rising housing costs and the declining availability of affordable housing throughout the city. In 2010, Vancouver's homeless count stood at 1,715 people,[9] some 9 percent more than 2008 and up 25.7 percent from 2005.[10]

Poverty levels in the Downtown Eastside have also been exacerbated by cutbacks to social assistance coverage by the provincial government since the early 1990s, when the province of British Columbia saw its social assistance funding capped by the federal government. Cutbacks on social assistance measures have placed low-income Downtown Eastside residents in the unenviable situation of having the lowest minimum wage of any Canadian province[11] and low-income assistance rates while residing in the most expensive city in the country in terms of living costs.

Evidence of hard drug addiction—the Downtown Eastside's most visible social issue—can be traced back to at least the 1960s. Poorly conceived government efforts to clamp down on drug use have had disastrous public health effects; the incidence of HIV linked to intravenous drug use saw a massive spike in the early 1990s, for reasons that remain hotly contested. While sharing syringes was recognized as the most direct cause of HIV transmission among local intravenous drug users, research suggests this was compounded by several factors: a shift in local drug-use patterns from heroin to cocaine injection that dramatically increased the number of daily injections, limited access to sterile needles, the temporary suspension of Vancouver's mobile needle exchange program, a concentration of low-income housing within a very limited area of the city, and a policy to charge re-entry fees to SRO residents who left their residences at night, resulting in many choosing not to venture out to the needle exchange center.[12]

The deinstitutionalization of BC's psychiatric patients in 1992—and Vancouver's unpreparedness to implement the much-touted "care in the community" alternative to institutionalized treatment—meant the arrival of a significant cohort of new residents with mental illnesses in the DTES. These people were quickly exposed to a black market of prescription drugs and narcotics sold on the street.[13]

Despite these troubling realities, efforts are being made at a variety of levels in the public, private, and voluntary sectors to improve conditions for Downtown Eastside residents, mostly aimed at providing affordable housing for low-income and homeless people. On the employment front, a wave of new business investment over the past 10 years has meant fewer boarded-up storefronts in the neighbourhood. The employment this generates does not always benefit local residents, many of whom face a variety of barriers—whether physical, mental, or the negative perception of their work abilities by employers unfamiliar with the community—that prevent them from finding and maintaining regular employment. In 2001, unemployment in the Downtown Eastside stood at 22 percent compared with 8 percent for

Vancouver as a whole, but it had declined from 28 percent and 11 percent, respectively, a decade before.[14]

The popularity of binning as an alternative income-generating activity can be explained in part by the comparative laxity of municipal regulations on business recycling. The City of Vancouver "does not provide recycling [...] collection services to small businesses at this time," and businesses looking to recycle their beverage containers in particular are advised but not legally obliged to "find a Return-It recycling depot."[15] The many containers not returned to depots, but disposed of instead in dumpsters or garbage cans, provide rich pickings for binners, who use commercial dumpsters as their main source for the cans and bottles they bring to stores and bottle depots, including United We Can.

Social Marginalization of the Binning Community

In the early 1990s, when United We Can was founded, binners faced institutional as well as social marginalization due to their perceived association with the drug scene. The end result was that binners had no guarantees they would receive the full deposit value of the beverage containers they returned to the store. People binning in Vancouver in the early 1990s recall that store owners were reluctant to refund the large quantities of containers brought in by binners, and that some businesses would even reimburse binners with nonmonetary goods:

> In those days a lot of the retailers really didn't want to serve us. We were dirty, and our stuff was dirty, and they were trying to sell food out of their stores, and they didn't have the storage space, and they didn't want to part with their money, and there was a whole bunch of issues. [...] I can remember one woman who got more actively involved [with United We Can], and she said what really makes her mad is that when she took her cans and bottles to the store, the store keeper would only pay her in chewing gum. Like, he wouldn't give her the cash, right? And for me it was just such a classic example of how, when you're poor and powerless, you have a very limited voice to try and address problems that you face on a daily basis.[16]

Binners today are also marginalized in more obvious ways, having extremely low-income, low-quality housing or no permanent housing at all, being politically powerless and largely dependent on food and services provided by charitable organizations, as well as social assistance funding.[17] Long-term dependence on state welfare or disability payments, and the inability to work at a regular paying job for too many hours per month for fear of losing crucial health care coverage included in these payments, is a condition that differentiates the binners from wider society and contributes to their social exclusion by people who do not view binning as a legitimate form of employment.

CREATING ENVIRONMENTAL, ECONOMIC, AND SOCIAL CHANGE

Environmentalism arguably comes second to United We Can's main objective of job creation for local residents, although recycling and sustainability are central to all of its social enterprise projects. In 2007, United We Can recycled 16 million beverage containers, thus preventing them from ending up in the landfill. United We Can's executive director says this figure has grown significantly since then, and today stands closer to 30 million containers annually. The organization also refunded $2.7 million to one of the most marginalized groups in Vancouver—the binning community—and created 22 full-time and 127 part-time jobs for residents of the Downtown Eastside. United We Can has been recognized both locally and nationally for the successful impact of its social enterprise model; the efforts of its founder have been repaid with an Arthur Kroeger College Award from Carleton University and a Meritorious Service Medal from Canada's Governor General in 2005, while the City of Vancouver proclaimed February 24, 2005, "United We Can Day" in recognition of the organization's work toward community development.

United We Can's original mission was to improve working conditions for binners by ensuring they received the full deposit on all their bottles and cans and had access to a working environment into which they would be welcomed. A simultaneous goal was to provide validation for binning not only as a legitimate means of income generation but as a valuable way of reducing the number of beverage containers sent to the landfill. Today, the largest of seven social enterprise projects hosted by United We Can is a bottle depot staffed entirely by Downtown Eastside residents, where binners can return the containers they collect. All seven projects are based on the idea of creating "green-collar" jobs and helping local people alleviate the burden of poverty. The organization employs roughly 150 people in a mix of part-time and full-time jobs, and sees as many as 700–800 binners a day pass through the bottle depot.

United We Can's social enterprise projects aim "to support environmental, social, and economic improvement in the inner city of Vancouver," particularly for Downtown Eastside residents.[18] Accurately measuring United We Can's impact in these areas is challenging and would require much more in-depth research than the scope of this case study permits. The organization itself does not have the capacity to conduct follow-up assessments of the people it hires, nor is it required to provide this type of data to funders. As such, no statistics exist on the number of former employees who have gone on to find work elsewhere, who have managed to leave the welfare system, or who have transitioned from unstable to more stable housing situations as a result of working at United We Can. This section therefore represents a rare attempt to qualitatively assess the organization's impact in terms of environmental and social equity outcomes. It examines the effects of four of the organization's seven social enterprise projects: the Bottle Depot, the Lanes Cleaning Project, the Urban Binning Unit, and the SOLEfood Urban Farm.

There is no shortage of current employees with positive things to say about what the organization has brought to their lives. Most display a genuine sense of pride in their work. There is widespread staff recognition that United We Can has made the surrounding area cleaner and safer, while offering a space for local people to interact and escape the isolation of unemployment. At the same time, living in a neighborhood where drug addiction is a significant issue means that many employees have limited trust in the people around them, which hampers efforts at building community. Staff members welcome the income they receive from United We Can as an important supplement that makes monthly expenses easier to bear, but most continue to rely on various forms of income assistance. A majority of employees gain years of work experience at United We Can, but many choose to stay at the organization rather than seek work elsewhere. Business owners, municipal government, and other local stakeholders are also positive about United We Can's impact on the surrounding community, although wider political tensions can sometimes taint the group's public perception.

Grassroots Approach to Community Empowerment and Engagement

United We Can's connections to the binning community are deep seated and reach as far as the organization's founder, who has himself overcome addiction and homelessness and had been earning a living as a binner for several years before founding United We Can. This firsthand knowledge of the challenges faced by binners and the wider Downtown Eastside community was essential in defining goals for the fledgling organization that were not only practical and achievable but that would resonate strongly with those it was trying to help. In describing the issues that motivated the group's creation, the founder clearly views himself as part of the same group of people the organization was trying to help:

> We had three or four objectives. The first one was that we wanted to have an ability to take in all the cans and bottles that we were able to scavenge, and get refunds on them. The second was that we wanted all beverage containers to be included within the refund deposit system. A third one was that some of the people [involved] wanted to see an increase in the deposit amount, so that theoretically we would get more of a return when we collected and took the bottles and cans in. There was a debate around that inasmuch as some people said that wouldn't be a good idea, because if you made the deposit rate higher, people would take the cans and bottles in themselves, and that way we would lose out on the pickings. As a kind of a codicil to that group of objectives, there was an evolving objective of doing it ourselves, that we could operate a better system ourselves than what was being offered to the retail stores.[19]

Representatives from the City of Vancouver, the beverage industry, and labor unions were consulted regularly as the organization grew. From the start, however, United We Can's core development took place at a very grassroots level: binners were invited to share their ideas for change and have them taken seriously at a series of open community meetings, where those who wanted to participate in forming the organization could do so.

Basing United We Can around an economic activity that was already taking place in the community created a degree of ownership of its structure and vision that binners would likely not have had in an organization centered on a completely unknown trade, or indeed a provider of social services to a targeted client population. United We Can engaged the local community from the start and paved the way for binners to organize themselves politically as and when necessary.

IMPACT

Environmental Sustainability

United We Can's bottle depot saves an average of 16–20 million beverage containers from the landfill each year. The Urban Binning Unit hires people to pick up empties from local businesses and bring them back to the depot by bicycle, using a specially adapted cart that attaches to the back wheel. The Lanes Cleaning Project removes litter—including hazardous waste such as used needles and condoms—from streets and laneways within a 40-block radius of United We Can. The SOLEfood Urban Farm, which had only just begun operating at the time that fieldwork for this case study was being conducted, converted an abandoned parking lot into a green space to grow organic produce for sale. It is expected to enhance the biodiversity of the surrounding area and, in the long term, improve food security for local residents. Community groups with which United We Can has partnered are quick to recognize the organization's role in raising awareness of local environmental sustainability:

> They [United We Can] were some of the leaders in terms of the local environmental movement and in terms of getting recyclables out of the landfill and that kind of stuff, so there is an environmental benefit for sure.[20]

Others credit United We Can's championing of the binners with bringing home the importance of recycling to the city in general, even influencing municipal policy. Since 2005, over 900 garbage cans across Vancouver have featured built-in recycling racks for beverage containers.[21] The racks have the dual purpose of making it safer for binners to retrieve the cans and encouraging people to recycle rather than simply discard their empty drink containers.

There remains a distinct lack of statistical evidence of United We Can's impact on environmental sustainability, which can perhaps be ascribed to the secondary nature of environmentalism to job and income creation within the organization's mission. In the absence of solid data, the group's founder speculates that its environmental impact is likely to be quite small, despite the large volume of bottles and cans that it helps recycle each year:

> Let's see, we've been at it for 15 years. Let's say for the first three, even five years, I'd say on average it was 5 million containers a year [that we saved from the landfill]. By year six, it was around 15 million. Today, [in an] average year, it's about 20 million containers that go through there. So what that has in relation to the region's environmental circumstances in terms of solid waste: beverage containers represent about 5 percent, I think, of the solid waste, and our piece of that would be way, way less, like maybe 0.1 percent of the total solid waste in the system in the province. So it's not significant.[22]

United We Can uses its mandate of green job creation to develop social enterprises dedicated to improving the local environment in different ways, whether through recycling beverage containers, removing litter from the surrounding urban environment, or promoting biodiversity and food security. As new jobs have been created, the scope of each social enterprise has grown, as has its capacity for cleaning up the local environment. However, urban environmental outcomes are not the only indicator of United We Can's commitment to sustainability.

As businesses, United We Can's social enterprise projects have always strived to develop sustainably. Dedicated sustainability manager and coordinator roles have meant that the management of each social enterprise consistently seeks new ways to make operations as environmentally friendly as possible within their allocated budget. Examples range from finding ways to reduce United We Can's carbon footprint to avoiding the use of pesticides or chemical fertilizers on the crops at the SOLEfood Urban Farm. There is a recognition by United We Can of further potential for fostering sustainable development, taking inspiration from similar groups elsewhere. Some of this has already been harnessed through the development of new projects such as SOLEfood:

> I'd already had ideas about what we could accomplish here, just taking the mission and using that as a guide. Because although we are directly dealing with binners and that's kind of what our main focus is, there's this underlying mission that was maybe not so front and center in the things [United We Can's founder] did, or wasn't being communicated. So I tried to figure out where the opportunities were. And I thought there were a lot of synergies going on with what we were doing and what was going on at least in North America, with a lot of other communities that were focused on the same kind of things United We Can was focused on.[23]

The organization can also be said to have indirectly influenced policy that will impact on future environmental sustainability, namely through succeeding in their campaign to alter provincial law on refund deposits, which now insists on higher levels of corporate product stewardship. At the time of the case study, United We Can's founder and executive director both sat on the Advisory Committee of Encorp Pacific, British Columbia's beverage container stewardship group, pushing for environmental reforms in the sector from the inside.

Employee Development

Economic Development

Employment is the basic mechanism for United We Can to stabilize local residents' long-term economic circumstances, and training new employees in a way that builds their self-confidence is the first step. Job training at most United We Can projects is informal in nature, but it is an effective method of preparing employees to perform well in their jobs. Just as important, it is flexible enough to allow different employees to progress at their own pace without the threat of losing their job if a certain level of achievement is not quickly reached. Job training at United We Can acclimatizes employees—some of whom have not worked for many years—to continuous employment in a busy working environment. Time management, worker interaction, and income management are essential skills that help prepare employees for a longer life in the workforce.

Many of the casual (part-time) workers at United We Can tend to work for a period of weeks or months before leaving for a variety of personal reasons, often related to addiction issues or mental health. When they are ready to return, United We Can is usually willing to let them pick up their job where they left off. One employee describes how he went through a similar experience:

> I started partying for a little while. Fell off the wagon, I guess. I went missing for about two weeks. Yesterday was my first shift back in the bottle depot in about two weeks. I had to go talk to [the Executive Director], and [he] said they liked the way I worked, they didn't want to lose me, and just said 'Nice to have you back.[24]

Paradoxically, this rapid turnover creates more opportunities for hiring new staff. On the basis of this high volume of job creation, United We Can describes itself as the biggest employer in the Downtown Eastside. Of the 19 nonmanagerial[25] staff members interviewed, 14 (nearly 74 percent) were unemployed immediately before joining United We Can. A further three (15.8 percent) had been working in the construction business, one had recently left a long-term job at a DTES community center, and another had joined from a rival bottle depot.

One reason why some staff members treat these jobs as short-term employment is that they see only limited prospects for career advancement within United We Can. As a former bottle depot worker explains:

> I know the people that are there in the top management positions. They're probably going to be there for awhile. So there's advancement to a certain point, but only to that point. And like, some of those guys, [the bottle depot Supervisor] and some of the other people, they've been there for a long period of time. There's not going to be much advancement past them. [...] I'm 52 years old, [the Supervisor] is maybe in his early 40s. I mean, am I going to get [his] job? Not likely. [...] And some of the other assistant managers that work there, you know, there's not much space for those guys either.[26]

Despite the flexible ties between United We Can and its casual workers, management considers a large proportion of the staff base to be long-term employees:

> About 50 percent of our staff are five years and up. There's not a big turnover. Turnover usually comes when an addiction issue has got the better of somebody, and they're left on their own or been terminated for one reason or another. The termination is only a last resort, and it's when people's safety or our ability to do our business are, you know, grossly affected.[27]

A brief survey of nonmanagerial staff suggests that this estimate is accurate. Of the 19 interviewees listed earlier and one binner who has been redeeming cans at United We Can since 2006, only three are permanent payroll staff, but 25 percent have worked for 2.5–5 years and a further 25 percent have worked for 6–10 years. The remaining 50 percent are split equally between staff who have been at United We Can for 1–2 years and those who have been with the organization for less than 12 months. In considering their future options, 68 percent of interviewed nonmanagerial staff who were formally employed by United We Can said they hoped to keep working for United We Can into the long term. Approximately 26 percent felt United We Can was more of a stop-gap for them before moving onto other things, while one interviewee was undecided.

Part-time staff at United We Can are hired at a starting wage of $8 per hour,[28] while supervisors can make anywhere from $12 to $20 an hour depending on seniority. Only payroll staff (full-time) receive a biweekly paycheck. All part-time staff at United We Can are paid in cash at the end of each day's work. This can make saving difficult, a fact that is recognized by management:

> A lot of them don't make a lot of money. You know, for their money to last to the end of the month is almost impossible. Some of them have pets, and they need pet food, and some of them smoke and they need cigarettes, and whatever else.[29]

Despite this inherent challenge, daily cash wage payment is locally accepted as the best known solution for people coping with addiction or mental health issues (including fetal alcohol syndrome) while on a very tight budget to manage their money on a daily basis.

> If they did not do it that way, I don't believe [United We Can] would have the amount of employees they have now. I believe that if everybody went onto the payroll, the majority of the people there would not do it. I think a lot of them would leave. They'd lose employees left, right, and center. 'Cause a lot of them are basing their week on the fact that if they're working three shifts, that they're gonna get 32 dollars this day, a day off, then they get 32 dollars the next day that they're on. To buy whatever they're buying.[30]

> So when I'm talking to friends in the street who are fetal-alcohol, they've all got this extreme work ethic; they really, really, really want to work. But they really can't understand how if you work today, you get paid in two weeks, and then that's all gone in a day anyway, and you've still got to work another two weeks to get more money. This is not how that brain tracks it, right? And what we need is to have these [low-barrier, daily-pay] jobs, because they can figure it out on a daily basis. But they can't figure it out over time.[31]

The majority of people hired by United We Can receive some form of income assistance—typically welfare or disability support—and are consequently limited in the amount of money they can earn and legally declare per month. This is one of the biggest practical hurdles to United We Can's mission to help people escape poverty. Only two people interviewed for this case study confirmed that they had been able to stop receiving welfare as a result of working for United We Can, although this does not mean that others have not managed to do the same. Increases in the minimum wage can also have the inverse effect of limiting employees' ability to earn money at United We Can, as earning too much per month would disqualify them from the income assistance benefits they receive, such as prescription drug coverage. As such, people within and outside the organization recognize that the income it provides helps to ease the burden of poverty rather than escape it completely:

> What kind of poverty are we escaping? Are we escaping the poverty where we don't eat for half of the month? [...] Are we escaping the poverty where we can't go to a greasy spoon and get something that looks like a normal meal once a day? That's escapable. To be in a position of saving money to buy a condo in Vancouver? No. To be in a position of moving up to a supervisory level in the bureaucracy? Not gonna happen.[32]

> Most of the people that we've got working with us are not able to work full time, based on the barriers that they have. So we're never going to be able to take

them completely out of poverty because there's always going be a certain reliance on the system to help them, whether it's through mental health or through welfare or through disabilities. There's always going to be a connection to the system as a whole, but this [United We Can] helps them with some of the little things, and most of them are on programs that allow them to make a certain amount of money every month. We help them do that.[33]

Personal and Social Development

In a neighbourhood where 61 percent of all residents live in "non-family" housing and more than half of non-family dwellers live alone,[34] social isolation is a serious issue, particularly for the unemployed and those living with addiction issues. A critical component of United We Can's mission to build community, therefore, is to build up the confidence necessary for individuals to interact with the community around them. A significant number of United We Can staff interviewed said that their self-confidence had improved as a result of their job. One employee said that working there after several years of unemployment had strengthened her personality:

I'd say I talk more now. I used to be very quiet, I never used to speak up. But since I've been here I've been more assertive. Yeah. Ever since that. 'Cause before it was just that people would step all over me. Totally, just step on me, so I wouldn't say a word. Now I speak up. I've learned how to do that here, thanks to the people, you know. They're very supportive. I like that part.[35]

There is no official strategy for fostering self-esteem, but a positive impact is achieved through a policy of actively recruiting people with barriers to traditional employment and then finding ways around these barriers to allow them to participate in the work in any way that they can. After years of unemployment and a succession of personal traumas, this brings a level of personal validation that cannot be found while living on income assistance alone.

Regardless of their chosen level of interaction, staff at United We Can work in open, communal areas, surrounded by a large group of coworkers who reflect the diversity of the neighborhood. For people used to feeling upset or ashamed by the barriers they live with, seeing other people with similar issues succeeding at holding down jobs at United We Can may reinforce their own sense of self-confidence and capability. This sense of belonging is familiar to many who live in the area:

I'll tell you the truth: until I moved into this neighbourhood, I was never happy. Down here, there's all kinds of other people like me. Yes, I have issues, but I'm fairly high-functioning, because I'm willing to look at my problems and deal with my problems. [...] Moving into this neighborhood, where a lot of other people have issues, and most of them wear them right out on their sleeve, I felt normal for the first time in my life. And all the staff that work here [at United We Can], you know, it employs them, makes them feel better about themselves. So yeah, definite impact on the neighborhood.[36]

A third way in which United We Can helps local people increase their self-esteem is by providing them with a means of earning a living. Employees take pride in the fact that they *earn* the money they receive from United We Can and are not given it out of charity. A majority of nonmanagerial staff receive long-term income assistance, and employment at United We Can reduces their sense of dependence on welfare or disability cheques. This resonates with the original commitment of United We Can's founder to changing the discourse around unemployed Downtown Eastside residents to one focusing on how to provide jobs for the many local people who desperately want to work but cannot get hired. One employee explains how her job has changed her sense of self:

> One of the main things it does is it gives me my self-esteem and self-respect back. Even by working the little bit that I do, it's being paid for what I do. It's like, when I get my pension cheque, I haven't done anything for it; I'm just receiving it. [With] this, I'm doing something. It just gives me that sense of confidence and self-respect back. And I see that with people that come in and work for a time, or whatever. It gives them their self-respect back. And that's what's really neat.[37]

A significant number of interviewees said that they enjoyed working at United We Can because they liked interacting with the other staff members. A number of employees show up at United We Can up to an hour before their shift, or even on days when they are not scheduled to work, simply to chat with friends over coffee and a cigarette. This phenomenon must be seen in the context of the SRO hotels that house the majority of employees; SRO occupants live alone and are often prohibited from bringing guests to their rooms, reinforcing their sense of social exclusion. United We Can therefore acts as a balance to this and helps to engage otherwise isolated residents in the community around them. One bottle depot employee said that working there had not only reduced the isolation he felt while unemployed but had given him the opportunity to make new friends that could be relied on in an emergency, underscoring an important beneficial impact of social inclusion:

> *It's a thing that makes me feel like I'm doing something. I'm not sitting at home in my bachelor apartment flipping through 500 channels of nothing. [...] I've made a few friends. I'm not completely alone, and I know if something happens that probably people here will do something to help me. Like when I was in the hospital, you know, they were hanging out, they were able to help me.*[38]

Another employee agrees that support from coworkers and management makes working at United We Can an enjoyable experience that has helped him come out of his shell. Reacclimatizing people to socializing with others is an essential building block of community development but also improves job performance and, potentially, future employability:

> The social environment is really nice. I'm kind of a loner, and the [jobs that I do here] are both loner jobs. But you know, I'm interacting with people all the time, but it's just quick interactions. It's just, okay, here's your order, thank you, on your way. You know, I smile at people and I say good morning and that kind of thing, but I'm just focused on my task. And on the floor [in the bottle depot], people are yelling and screaming at each other, and joking, and talking about all kinds of things, hockey games, stuff that I don't know anything about! But they're all very supportive of each other, and I've felt supported.[39]

Supporting the Binning Community

Depending on the number of containers they collect, binners can make anywhere from $10 to $50 from a day's work by redeeming their product at United We Can. Since United We Can runs the largest bottle depot in the Downtown Eastside—and is the one most closely associated with the binning community—this daily economic support is depended on by a large group of people. This group received $2.7 million in cash payouts from United We Can in 2007 alone. For some, the independence and freedom of binning make it a more attractive—and potentially more lucrative—way of making money than working fixed hours at United We Can. One binner, who had found an abandoned bicycle he was planning to sell on the street shortly after being interviewed, explains:

> I'm sort of at that balancing act where, let's say my [binning] route, if I go for 2 hours, let's say I make $8 [an hour]. So [with another] $20 on the bike out there, so I'd probably make 40 bucks today, in 2 ½ hours. Working indoors [for 4 hours at United We Can] for 8 bucks an hour with no deductions is 32. So I have issues with my own self right now, in pulling myself off my route that I do, that makes me a good chunk of change in a shorter period of time.[40]

Community Development

Beyond encouraging community building among its own employees, United We Can also contributes to the community around it. The object of this section is not to demonstrate a direct link between the organization's presence and changes to different aspects of Downtown Eastside community life—too many independent variables exist to make this a valid causal relationship—but rather to show that United We Can has its place in the mix of forces bringing change to the Downtown Eastside.

All interviewees agreed that retail business was beginning to return to the Downtown Eastside after years of empty, boarded-up storefronts. Two coordinated government policies—the Great Beginnings project and the Vancouver Agreement—are in place to bring economic revitalization to the area. While this cannot be attributed to United We Can, the impact of the Lanes Cleaning Project and other United We Can programs in keeping the areas around local businesses clean and recycling their beverage containers has been recognized by community stakeholders as contributing to making the Downtown Eastside more attractive for prospective business investors:

> The lane cleaning aspect of it helps our business. If you live and work in an area that's tidy and people have pride in it, then the whole neighborhood has pride.[41]

Another way that United We Can impacts local business development is by reinforcing links between different business stakeholders. United We Can's reputation for effective street cleaning and job creation for local people has won them the admiration of many local businesses, which tend to have the organization in mind when they hear of another business looking to partner with a social enterprise from the community:

> When I was talking to [a local business looking to donate to a social enterprise] and I suggested strongly United We Can, I said [it's] because you're not only helping an organization that's doing well, you're giving a job to people. And it's making a difference in our neighbourhood because they're cleaning it up. So I just see it as a win-win, and certainly our lanes have been an awful lot better.[42]

LESSONS LEARNED

Financial Survival Takes Planning

While United We Can has grown steadily in terms of revenue and as a business since its creation in 1995, the last 2 years have seen the organization's finances suffer somewhat. This is largely due to a decision made 3 years ago under a previous executive director to install a benefit plan and increase wages across the board—a decision that was ethically the "right" thing to do but that created a large dent in the group's finances. While United We Can's Board Chairman is committed to keeping the benefit plan in place, the lost capital still needs to be rebuilt. This, in addition to guarding against seasonal lulls in trade, finding ways to compensate for anticipated large cutbacks from the City of Vancouver contract for the Lanes Cleaning Project, and heavy start-up costs for the SOLEfood Urban Farm all present serious challenges to ensuring the long-term survival of United We Can's social enterprise projects.

The issue of financial sustainability has been raised with the Board, and at the time of fieldwork for this case study, the executive director had agreed that it was necessary to develop a strategic plan to develop and grow the business in such a way that there are sufficient profitable enterprises to supplement those that are loss making. The plan will represent something of a departure for United We Can, which has only had one major external review of its operations in the past. The nature of working at the organization is such that managers are constantly "putting out fires" in terms of dealing with staff issues as and when they arise, leaving little time to look at the bigger picture of the organization as a whole.

Build and Maintain Relationships

A 2009 investigation by *The Province* newspaper found there to be over 170 different social service providers of various sizes based in the Downtown Eastside.[43] United We Can is therefore one of many nonprofit organizations jockeying for grant money from the City of Vancouver and other sources, both public and private. This is a challenge that is set to persist and unavoidably politicizes the relationships between nonprofit groups serving the same community. Research from elsewhere in Canada suggests that "as community groups compete for limited funding, they are potentially pitted one against another, or divided between those who participate and support the federal government's agenda and those that do not, taking to the level of community notions of 'deserving' and 'undeserving' that have long been identified in social welfare programs."[44] The point is equally valid in situations where the funding comes from other levels of government, such as provincial or municipal.

Since its inception, United We Can's approach has been to ensure that communication channels with government and business are kept open at all times. It is a method that has served the organization well and looks set to remain the approach of choice for the foreseeable future. Referring to Ken Lyotier, United We Can's founder, the group's executive director says:

> Ken always walked that middle line, you know, he's always got friends on both sides of the fence, if you will, whether it's political or whether it's economic. He's built allegiances throughout the community by taking that high ground. And I made it my mission to sort of continue on that route, and I know it's something that the Board certainly supports.[45]

United We Can's nonconfrontational and collaborative approach to the political and business communities is well recognized by community stakeholders, who concur that it has given it an advantage over several other groups. In the words of one of the group's funders:

> The thing I think that's really important to know about United We Can is how successful they have been at fostering relationships with all sorts of different groups within the city. And that's important, because those groups not only bring the connections and the money that can help carry the group on, but they bring a lot of skills that help govern and manage the United We Can organization. That's very important. And I don't see that to nearly the same extent with other good social organizations.[46]

Challenge Not-in-My-Backyard Attitudes

Public support for United We Can is high (the City of Vancouver is a firm backer of the organization), but the perception that the bottle depot is inadvertently "funding" the local drug trade remains persistent among some sections of the community. The perception is reinforced in the public consciousness through the visible concentration of drug dealers who congregate daily on the sidewalk directly outside United We Can's premises. Binners who bring their beverage containers to United We Can are forced to share the stretch of sidewalk outside with the drug dealers, who are fully aware that binners will be leaving the bottle depot with disposable cash. While drug use is banned outright at United We Can, its workforce and customers do include people who use drugs. The negative public perception of this state of affairs can be found in many parts of the community, and even resonates with employees themselves. One worker recounts:

> It supports their habits. That's all people use it for. It supports their addictions. I've even had friends tell me that. Like I said, when the Playoffs were on, like, [the] World Cup's coming up—it's gonna be beer money.[47]

A plan to move United We Can's operations to new premises some years ago was effectively blocked by a residents' association near the proposed site, owing to fears that the organization's funding to buy the new building had come from the drug trade:

> The owner of the property we made an offer on—a good friend of mine is a friend of his—and he told my good friend that it was, you know, drug money. That he didn't want to sell it to us because it was all drug money. So they've never ever had a problem [at] United We Can, ever, with drugs or police or whatever.

But the broader community went absolutely crazy and shrieked and said, not in my backyard. So we had to retrench back into our little hole in the Downtown Eastside, which was very disappointing for a lot of people.[48]

This not-in-my-backyard attitude could easily jeopardize future attempts at expansion into areas outside the Hastings Corridor. Indeed, expanding operations to include a second bottle depot in central or West-End Vancouver, where many binners operate, has been ruled out by United We Can's executive for, among other reasons, the fact that recycling operations are not a "good fit" in more prosperous and well-developed areas of the city. United We Can is fully aware of this obstacle to its future development. At the same time, it has learned with time to make the best of it and to keep making efforts at fostering new community links, including with apparent naysayers. A perfect illustration of this is the apartment blocks represented by the residents' association that blocked United We Can's move—today, they are a regular client of the Urban Binning Unit program, meaning that United We Can employees are paid to routinely visit the apartment block to collect empty bottles and cans. Challenging not-in-my-backyard attitudes by working around them has helped develop important links between a very marginalized community of people and the city that surrounds them.

Integrate Workforce Issues into the Business Model

Addiction and mental health issues mean that there can be gaps in task completion within each of United We Can's social enterprise projects when people suddenly stop showing up. Work absences that are drug related can be a cyclical issue, with fewer binners bringing in beverage containers and sometimes fewer employees working at United We Can on days when monthly welfare cheques are deposited. It is also understood and accepted that employees typically need to take time off several times per month to attend to medical needs or deal with housing, legal, or other personal issues.

There have been instances in the past of bottle depot employees stealing money from the cash; hiring trustworthy cashiers who stay on for longer than a few months remains one of the biggest challenges faced by the depot. The cumulative effect reduces workplace efficiency and could—in the case of key jobs such as cashiers—potentially lead to monetary loss. This is also a concern for the SOLEfood Urban Farm, where hiring people willing to work early-morning shifts at minimum wage is proving difficult; staff shortages can equate with irregular maintenance and harvesting of crops, again at significant monetary loss.

United We Can recognizes and accepts these challenges as intrinsic to the nature of the work that it does—job creation and training for local people who have extremely limited employment options elsewhere will always take precedence over profit at United We Can—but there are some subtle signs that the organization is trying to guard against the worst effects. Examples include promoting existing staff internally instead of always hiring people from outside United We Can to fill new positions, and the recent shift from the "binners' meeting" model of job interviews—where anyone could show up and be considered for hiring on the spot—to a more traditional approach of submitting an application form.

Redefine Poverty

United We Can uses green jobs as a tool to reduce poverty by going out of its way to ensure that these jobs are suited to the abilities of the people it hires, who in a majority of cases are unable to find work elsewhere. The division of labor is such that a variety of tasks are available to suit different employee strengths, abilities, and temperaments. Complemented by a managerial commitment to flexibility and tolerance toward short-notice work absences, this low-barrier approach to job creation provides an informal but routine and legal way for local residents to supplement their income.

Economic outcomes for United We Can staff do change upon employment, typically shifting from financial uncertainty to a higher degree of financial stabilization, albeit on a monthly income that remains extremely low when compared to the average cost of living in Vancouver. Improvements to living standards as a result of stabilized finances are small but important for those they benefit and can include money for food, clothing, public transit, and personal entertainment. The ability to cover these basic items is not guaranteed for those who spend a large proportion of their income assistance money on monthly rent, and as such, United We Can provides a lifeline to these people.

At the same time, the vast majority of nonmanagerial staff—particularly those who work part-time—remain on welfare or disability allowance while working for United We Can. For those earning minimum wage for their shift work, the income provided is simply not sufficient to survive on without the additional support of a government check. Conversely, those receiving state benefits are unable to work more than a set number of hours per month at United We Can without seeing their income assistance cut dollar for dollar. This is something of a catch-22 situation for employees, who remain caught between the need to survive financially and the systemic restrictions imposed on the poorest members of society. Viewed this way, United We Can eases the economic situation of people who have been let down by inefficiencies within the broader social policy framework. While this is undeniably a critical and much-needed public service for residents of the Downtown Eastside, some wonder whether the organization's successes in the local community may be providing an excuse for policy makers to delay important antipoverty reforms.

While escaping poverty remains at the heart of United We Can's mission, the concept of poverty itself needs to be readjusted in relation to the context of policies and other factors impacting life in the Downtown Eastside. A more meaningful definition of poverty would be one that is broadened in scope to include nonmaterial indicators such as self-worth, social inclusion, and community engagement. In many Canadian provinces, and indeed elsewhere, poverty as a concept is defined as deprivation not only from money, food, lodging, and other material goods but also from culture, education, and social interaction. This last element is particularly absent in the lives of Downtown Eastside residents, many of whom spend long hours of unemployment in SRO rooms, estranged from their families and with few friends in the neighborhood whom they can rely on. In provinces such as Quebec, government antipoverty strategies emphasize reducing social exclusion as a crucial way to alleviate the worst ravages of poverty. Such legislation has yet to be passed in British Columbia.

NOTES

1. J. Quarter, L. Mook, and A. Armstrong, *Understanding the Social Economy: A Canadian Perspective* (Toronto, ON: University of Toronto Press, 2009), 4.
2. United We Can, "About Us" http://www.unitedwecan.ca/about-us. Accessed May 23, 2013.
3. G. W. Roe, "Fixed in Place: Vancouver's Downtown Eastside and the Community of Clients," *BC Studies: The British Columbian Quarterly* 164 (2010): 75–101.
4. In 2006, the gender split among DTES residents was 62 percent male, 38 percent female, compared with roughly 49 percent male, 51 percent female for Vancouver as a whole. City of Vancouver, *2005/06 Downtown Eastside Community Monitoring Report.* (Vancouver, BC: City of Vancouver, 2006), 8.
5. S. Ladurantaye, "What's Driving Vancouver's House Prices?" *The Globe and Mail*, June 23 2011.
6. City of Vancouver, *2005/06 Downtown...*, 6.
7. Ibid., 15.
8. H. A. Smith, "Planning, Policy and Polarization in Vancouver's Downtown Eastside," *Tijdschrift voor economische en sociale geografie* 94, no. 4 (2003): 496–509.
9. This figure includes people staying in shelters and with friends. Vancouver's Zero Homelessness by 2015 policy is credited for contributing to a nearly 70 percent increase from 2008 to 2010 in the number of homeless people living in shelters as opposed to on the streets. D. Kraus et al., *Vancouver Homeless Count 2010: Off the Street and into Shelters* (Vancouver, BC: Eberle Planning and Research, 2010), 10.
10. Ibid.
11. Government of British Columbia, *Minimum Wage*, ed. Employment Standards Branch, (Victoria, BC: Government of British Columbia, 2011).

12. M. V. O'Shaughnessy et al, "Deadly Public Policy: What the Future Could Hold for the HIV Epidemic among Injection Drug Users in Vancouver," *Current HIV/AIDS Reports* 9 (4; 2010): 394–400 et al.,

13. G. W. Roe, 2010, 85.

14. City of Vancouver, *2005/06 Downtown...*, 12.

15. City of Vancouver, "Is it Really Garbage?" Accessed May 23, 2013: http://vancouver.ca/home-property-development/dispose-of-other-items.aspx http://vancouver.ca/doing-business/waste-collection-for-businesses.aspx

16. Ken Lyotier, (Founder and former Executive Director, United We Can), interview July 8, 2010.

17. A reliable estimate of how many binners receive income assistance is difficult to provide: since declaring the income earned from binning could entail the same amount being cut from their monthly cheques, most binners that do receive income assistance do not declare this meagre extra income.

18. United We Can, *About Us*. Accessed May 23, 2013: http://www.unitedwecan.ca/about-us

19. Ken Lyotier, (Founder and former Executive Director, United We Can). Interview July 8, 2010.

20. Anonymous, 29, (Business and Social Enterprise Developer, Building Opportunities with Business), interview June 23, 2010.

21. City of Vancouver. *City of Vancouver—2005 Annual Report* (Vancouver, BC: City of Vancouver, 2005), p 9.

22. Ken Lyotier, interview.

23. Manager of Sustainability, United We Can, interview May 21, 2010.

24. me], (SOLEfood Urban Farm worker, United We Can), interview July 9, 2010.

25. This figure includes one current managerial-level employee who was initially employed in the bottle depot.

26. Interview with binner and former United We Can bottle depot worker, June 8, 2010.

27. (Executive Director, United We Can), interview May 17, 2010.

28. The official minimum wage in British Columbia at the time of interviews was $8 per hour. Hourly pay at United We Can has since risen in accordance with minimum wage increases for British Columbia in 2011 and 2012.

29. Lanes Cleaning Project Manager, United We Can, interview May 19, 2010.

30. Interview with bottle depot worker, June 11, 2010.

31. Social Housing Coordinator, City of Vancouver, interview June 29, 2010.

32. Ibid.

33. Executive Director, United We Can, interview July 8, 2010.

34. City of Vancouver, *2005/06 Downtown...*, 9.

35. Interview with bottle depot worker, United We Can, June 11, 2010.

36. Interview with bottle depot worker, June 22, 2010.

37. Office Administrator, United We Can, interview June 9, 2010.

38. Interview with bottle depot worker, June 11, 2010.

39. Interview with bottle depot cashier and Bintek assistant, June 2, 2010.

40. Interview with binner and former bottle depot worker, June 8, 2010.

41. Manager, Donnelly Fund; Donnelly Hospitality Management), interview June 3, 2010.

42. Executive Director, Gastown Business Improvement Society, interview June 17, 2010.

43. D. Carrigg, "Downtown Eastside Costs $1 Million a Day," *The Province*, February 16, 2009.

44. Murray, Karen Bridget. "Do Not Disturb: 'Vulnerable Populations' in Federal Government Policy Discourses and Practices." *Canadian Journal of Urban Research* 13, no. 2 (2004), 63.
45. Executive Director, United We Can, interview July 8, 2010.
46. Director of Development, Vancity, interview June 9, 2010.
47. Interview with SOLEfood Urban Farm worker, July 9, 2010.
48. Chairman of the Board, United We Can, interview June 7, 2010.

CHAPTER 5

New Skills for the Green Economy

Two Training Programs for Job Seekers in the

United States

COSMIN PADURARU AND KARA QUENNELL

If we are to have any hope of mitigating the effects of climate change and depletion of natural resources, many of our industries and the jobs they provide must change to employ sustainable and environmentally friendly practices. In addition to being important for environmental sustainability, a greener economy can have an important role to play in improving economic, environmental, and health inequalities. Other chapters examine how low-income populations persistently experience greater environmental burdens along with reduced access to employment opportunities, which ultimately lead to inequalities in health and well-being. Studies have shown that participation in the formal economy resulting in a steady living wage has positive impacts on health, quality of life, social development, and psychological well-being for individuals and their families.[1,2] In light of these facts, environmentally focused education and green job training can simultaneously address issues of poverty while promoting environmental sustainability. This notion is the basis for the existence of programs such as Casa Verde Builders (CVB) and Sustainable South Bronx's (SSBx) BEST academy.

CVB, located in Austin, Texas, focuses on a combination of high school level education and hands-on green construction training. The program is targeted at disadvantaged youth, typically low-income high school dropouts, who are often burdened with additional challenges such as homelessness or criminal records. The program's main goals are to have the students graduate and be placed in jobs or higher education (not necessarily in green sectors, although they do emphasize sustainable practices in their education).

BEST Academy is a green job training program run by Sustainable South Bronx, an organization that works toward environmental sustainability in conjunction with social and economic equity in the South Bronx of New York City. The program is targeted at those who are un- or underemployed and living in communities that bear disproportionately high environmental burdens. BEST is an individual-focused program that empowers its participants by giving them the skills needed to get and retain a job within the green economy, encouraging the development of self-reflection and self-knowledge, and offering them the chance to make positive and tangible changes in their communities through environmentally sustainable practices.

CVB and the BEST academy work with individuals who experience barriers to employment and who have thus far had little success getting and retaining jobs. Both programs work toward creating and supporting the movement toward a greener economy while simultaneously effectively addressing the problems of chronic un- and underemployment through education.

CONTEXT AND RAISON D' ÊTRE FOR THE TWO PROGRAMS

Greenhouse gas emissions and average temperatures have both been increasing since the industrial revolution. Current projections warn of catastrophic climate change unless significant emission cuts are achieved. Such a change will require substantial changes to many industries and that more jobs become "green," that is, mindful of environmental aspects. In particular, both CVB and BEST focus an important part of their training on energy-efficient construction, which could lead to significant emission reductions: in the United States, which was responsible of 19 percent of global CO_2 emissions in 2007,[3] the residential sector was responsible for close to 22 percent of total greenhouse gas emissions in 2011.[4] Green jobs are a particularly attractive opportunity for those who wish to use job training as a means to increase social equity. This is in large part because green jobs are perceived as a niche and growing market for which few training programs exist. This means that, in theory, participants are being trained to get newly created jobs—not simply take jobs from others. Moreover, green jobs are often labor intensive yet require specified knowledge, which makes them an ideal target for this type of training program.

While environmental impacts pose a rising concern, poverty and inequalities remain a central challenge in urban centers. It is well known that an increased level of education correlates strongly with earnings potential. In the second quarter of 2010, the median weekly wage in the United States was $440 for people without a high school degree, versus $629 for people with a high school degree and $774 over the entire US population.[5] CVB and BEST operate in (and get most of their incoming students from) poor urban areas. In the target area for CVB, which can be roughly described as South East Austin, the poverty rate is 42 percent, dropout rate is 69 percent, and unemployment rate is 21.7 percent,[6] compared to figures of 15.3 percent, 3.5 percent, and 3.5 percent, respectively, in the City of Austin as a whole. The South Bronx is historically known for underdevelopment, high rates of un- and underemployment, and crime. It is located in the United States' poorest congressional district and has an estimated unemployment rate of 24 percent. Although many industries do operate out of the Hunts Point and South Bronx area, this high level of industrialisation has not led to high levels of local employment. Instead, it has led to high levels of air pollution and a lack of accessible public space. Consequently there is a sense that residents of these neighborhoods have the worst of both worlds: they are subjected to the health, safety, and environmental concerns that accompany industrial production without benefitting from the employment opportunities generated by this proximity.

In addition, the people joining the programs are often at a disadvantage even with respect to their neighbors. All incoming CVB students have dropped out of school, and, as with BEST students, some of the other major challenges they face are poverty and homelessness, former criminal justice involvement, drug abuse and dependency issues, the absence of a supporting family or entourage, and a lack of essential soft skills such as team work or communication. Many of the participants come to the program after receiving some form of government financial assistance such as welfare.

METHODOLOGY

These programs were selected for their focus on offering pathways out of poverty through education with a strong emphasis on energy efficiency and environmental sustainability as a means of working toward social and economic equity. During the research process a total of 69 interviews were conducted with individuals connected to CVB and SSBx. Interviews took place during May and June of 2010. Interviewees were selected primarily through snowball sampling, and they included present and past program participants, community members, senior program management, teachers, trainers, representatives of funding agencies and local governments, and potential or current employers of program graduates. These interviews followed a general script but were left open ended in order to allow for a wide range of perspectives and new ideas, as well as to understand what participants themselves would consider important topics and issues. Informed consent was obtained from the participants prior to the interviews. Program participants and graduates were also informed that their name or other personal information would not appear in the case study.

In addition to the interviews, information was gathered through observing meetings and classes, visiting construction sites, speaking informally with program participants, conversations with staff members, e-mail communication with program staff and government officials, and attending staff meetings and community events. Documentation reviewed includes internal documents such as budgets or policies and procedures, program brochures, Web sites, curricula, grant applications, and external evaluations. Efforts were made to seek multiple sources of evidence for the claims made in this study, including interviews with a variety of individuals, external and internal documentation, and participant observation.

PROGRAMS: HISTORY AND MISSION

Casa Verde Builders

American YouthWorks is dedicated to transforming the lives of at-risk youth through education, service, and green jobs training.

    official mission of American YouthWorks, Casa Verde's parent organization

Casa Verde Builders (CVB), created in 1994, is one of several subprograms of the American YouthWorks (AYW) charter school. Throughout its history, CVB has worked toward simultaneously addressing social and environmental goals. They use hands-on training in energy-efficient construction as a way to prepare disadvantaged youth for the job market and sell the houses built in the process to low-income residents at affordable prices. Incoming students must be between the ages of 17 and 24 years. At least 75 percent must be high school dropouts and meet specific income or disadvantage criteria.[7] Up to 25 percent do not have to meet these conditions as long as they are basic skills deficient.[8] Students stay in the program for 6 months to 2 years. CVB currently serves around 70 students per year.

Currently, CVB is divided into a classroom-based academic component and an on-site construction training component. The academic component consists of either General Education Development[9] (GED) preparation or high school classes. Since most CVB students are in the GED part of the program, the academic component consists in most cases of writing practice tests under the supervision of an instructor. Classes are made up of 10–15 students, and the instructors are able to provide individualized feedback and assistance.

The on-site component provides hands-on training via the construction of energy-efficient housing. All the house components, except for the foundation and the electrical part, are built by the students themselves. In addition, CVB instructors use the different stages of the construction process to relate mathematical concepts learned in class to applied situations. For instance, students learn how to use fractions to evenly space windows, or how to use the Pythagorean theorem in order to create a right angle. Relating abstract mathematical concepts to practical work in this fashion is viewed by the staff as an effective way of enhancing academic learning, particularly for the types of students they serve. Students receive a stipend of $7.25/hour (minimum wage at the time of the study) for the time they spend on site.

The on-site training component is designed with sustainable building practices in mind. In particular, many relatively simple and inexpensive design techniques that can significantly reduce energy consumption are used in the construction process. Orienting the house for good air circulation, building the roof at an angle that lets the sun in during the winter but keeps it out during the summer, allowing heat to escape through holes on top of the roof, or placing the water boiler in the middle of the house are all part of the repertoire of simple yet effective energy-reduction techniques that CVB students learn. These techniques are complemented by the use of more advanced (yet still rather inexpensive) construction materials, with an emphasis on the use of recycled materials. According to CVB staff, the energy efficiency techniques they use do not add more than a few thousand dollars to the house's cost. In some instances, solar panels (often donated) are also installed on the rooftops.

Through their training, CVB students have the opportunity to obtain a range of certificates, such as safety certificates from the Occupational Health and Safety Administration (OSHA), National Center for Construction Education and Research (NCCER) certifications, and a preapprenticeship construction training certificate from CVB. Supplemental programs offer students a range of extracurricular activities, covering mostly soft skills training (from interview preparation to nutrition to personal finance) and environmental awareness.

BEST ACADEMY

The goal of the BEST program is to give [participants] employable skills and be able to couple the trades that they are receiving with the soft skills to make them more employable than the average person in that job market.
SSBx staff member

In 2003, SSBx started its first job training program, the Bronx Environmental Stewardship Training (BEST) program. The problem of unemployment had come up repeatedly during the community visioning meetings held around SSBx's other projects, and it was concluded that a green job training program could both complement existing endeavors and help create positive change in the lives of disenfranchised individuals. The BEST program is seen as offering "pathways out of poverty" for those who live in neighborhoods with few employment opportunities. It seeks to provide participants with a steady living wage job along with a renewed sense of self-worth. Participants in the program tend to be from Hunts Point and the South Bronx, as SSBx recruits many through word of mouth and other community-based organizations. Participants must have their GED and pass basic math and reading tests along with an interview and a 2–3 day tryout before they are admitted. Participants tend to be in their late twenties or early thirties and unemployed. While participating in BEST, participants are provided with an unlimited metro card and $5 a day to purchase their lunch, and they can also continue to receive any government transfer money they were receiving previously. Participants are trained to build and maintain green infrastructure by learning skills such as river restoration, brownfield remediation, greenroof construction and maintenance, and horticultural skills. To complement these skills, participants receive several widely recognized certifications, including HAZWOPER,[10] OSHA Confined Space, and OSHA construction safety[11] and first aid-CPR C,[12] as well as some more specific certifications such as Trees New York Citizen Pruner and Pervious Pavement Technician. In addition to practical, hands-on skills, the BEST program teaches soft skills that enhance the social capital of participants by helping them learn how to conduct themselves professionally, communicate effectively, and manage interpersonal conflict. In the training they practice resume writing, team building, and interview skills. They also do daily physical fitness training. This training lasts between 17 and 19 weeks and seeks to make participants as employable as possible. Once the training is complete, SSBx's job developers help them find and maintain jobs. These jobs are in various types of work and tend to be entry level, paying $12–$14 an hour.

In 2009, SSBx expanded the BEST program to include a new type of training, BEST 4 Buildings (B4B). This training focuses on the skills needed to work in green construction. Participants learn basic carpentry and plumbing skills, to build green roofs, retrofit buildings for increased energy efficiency, and do energy efficiency audits. Like BEST ECO, B4B participants gain several certifications, including HAZWOPER, OSHA Construction Safety, NYC and NYS Asbestos Handler, Building Performance Institute Building Analyst, First Aid and CPR-C, and AEA Energy Efficient Tech. In 2011 they planned to run three cycles of each program with 20–25 participants in each, training about 120 people per year.

TEACHING ENVIRONMENTALLY FRIENDLY SKILLS
AND RAISING AWARENESS

CVB teaches green building techniques and builds houses that are significantly more energy efficient than average newly built homes and that use as few new materials as possible. All of the houses that CVB built in the last 3 years received a five-star energy efficiency rating from Austin Energy. In addition, one of the CVB homeowners interviewed, who also happens to be an energy auditor, confirmed that CVB-built homes use significantly less energy than typical new houses, explaining that he never had an electricity bill over $8, whereas for similarly sized homes he estimated that "the average electricity usage would probably be between $80 and $150."[13] Recently, CVB students have built about two new houses each year.

The graduates of the BEST 4 Buildings programs also learn green building techniques and have recently taken on initiatives such as offering local energy audits to allow low-income residents of the South Bronx to reduce their energy consumption and costs, as well as building green roofs, which help trap storm water, increase biodiversity, and decrease heating and cooling needs and costs. Many BEST ECO graduates go on to build or maintain the green infrastructure of New York. The Bronx River alliance employs BEST graduates and has been an important part of transforming the Bronx River from an unpleasant and polluted waterway to an accessible public space. BEST graduates also work maintaining the street trees of the million-tree initiative and are expected to be instrumental in both building and maintaining the city's greenways. Thus, the environmental benefits can be broadly understood as improving the maintenance and encouraging the construction of green infrastructure.

In addition to teaching green construction and maintenance techniques, these programs raise awareness of the impact of environmental issues. Because so much of what CVB students learn on-site is geared toward minimizing energy consumption, waste, and the need for new materials, it seems natural that these concepts will remain ingrained in the students' minds even after the training is over. Students had a generally heightened level of environmental awareness because of being in the program. For one, being on the site made them more aware of energy efficiency. Students expressed how they had become more knowledgeable when it came to energy efficiency from a construction standpoint—"let's say I was building my house [...] I know what is the green elements, and everything like that"[14] as well as in terms of reducing consumption. This increased knowledge could lead to direct financial benefits from the savings in energy use, as one student explained, "I learned so much that me and my sister's light bill is not even as high as it used to be."[15] In addition, extracurricular activities also made them more aware of a range of environmental issues. Students spoke about local issues like water management, explaining how "if we just stop using cements for ground and start using the pavers so that the water can go through to the aquifer, it would make a big difference in our water systems."[16] They also expressed concerns over global issues such as climate change.

These benefits are more prominent in the BEST program in that encouraging an awareness of one's ability to create environmental change is understood both by staff as one of the program goals and by the students as one of the major things they have learned and take away from their time with BEST. The environmental aspect of the program is a key part of the program's goal of self-empowerment, and participants leave the program really valuing what they have learned about the environment and feeling proud that they will be working in a field that makes a positive difference in communities. This is often a new experience for participants who grew up in urban communities with little green space. As one participant explained,

I understand more clearly about the surface that I am standing on, you know, I understand the ground, the soil. I just recently started digging the soil for the first time in my life. Growing up, I mean after growing up in the city, just in buildings, I mean not really aware of gardens and stuff like that …this is a big change, it is a big improvement on a whole different scale.[17]

The focus on the environment was a significant motivator for students, for whom it provides a sense of pride and belief that they are engaging in a practice that will benefit their communities. A graduate from the BEST program who now works in the greenway project explained how he saw the greenway impacting community members: "It is good because it is going to have a lot of trees and benches so that they can come out of their house. Some of them are like locked in their house because they don't have nowhere to go. Maybe now they will coming out because of trees and benches they can associate with other people, with their community."[18]

FOSTERING SOCIAL AND ECONOMIC DEVELOPMENT

Both BEST and CVB play positive roles in the lives of the young men and women that they serve, helping them obtain and keep jobs and promoting personal and social development.

The YouthBuild federal program, which is responsible for a large part of CVB's funding, requires all grant recipients to submit data about member outcomes.[19] The numbers in Table 5.1 indicate that CVB is performing above average among programs with similar funding and objectives.

CVB has seen 87.5 percent of its graduates go on to higher education or employment, compared to a 41.4 percent aggregate rate for similar programs. CVB has also stood out in achieving high rates of job retention for its graduates. YouthBuild, a network of 273 training programs in 45 states, awarded CVB the Outcome Award for Highest Retention in 2010.

Table 5.1. OUTCOME DATA FOR CVB GRADUATES
TRAINED UNDER
THE 2007 DOL GRANT

	Aggregate	Casa Verde Builders
Placement in employment or higher education	41.44 percent	87.50 percent
Attainment of a degree or certificate	58.08 percent	67.65 percent
Literacy/numeracy gains	48.02 percent	58.62 percent

Students and graduates of CVB were eloquent about the impact the program had on their lives. When asked what they thought they would be doing if it was not for CVB, many participants said that they would not have a job or have a low-paying job that would barely allow them to make ends meet. In addition, some of the students said that they would probably be in jail or involved in criminal activities. The following quote is typical of how interviewed students viewed the impact that CVB was having on their lives:

> They helped me get my schooling, they paying me to work, they're gonna help me find another job. Before I found this program I wasn't doing nothing. I was in the streets and now I found something positive in my life to keep going.[20]

In addition, during the course of the program many CVB students discover ways in which they can have career aspirations that they had never thought possible as the staff actively work on changing participants' perceptions of what they can achieve. Student interviews illustrated this perception of increased opportunities and potential:

> Before CVB I never thought it would be possible for me to ever go to college and now that I can graduate and go, it's just so many doors that have been opened.[21]

> And it just showed me that I can do anything, like, I'm building a house and I never thought "me, hammer?" It's just like giving you, making you believe you can do just like so much better. You got these people motivating you, telling you you could do better.[22]

> Casa Verde, it feels like they trying to help us, they don't want us to stay at that one point our whole life. They want us to move on and mature. But like other schools they are just, they'll let you sit there.[23]

CVB students also noted the importance of having a positive, stable period in their otherwise troubled lives. One student who talked of many personal issues said that "as soon as I started this program everything kind of went alright, I mean it helped a lot."[24] Another appreciated the fact that he got "6 months of positive, good quality, work experience" and that he has "learned how to talk to people and work in a positive environment."[25] Confirming the positive role of the CVB environment, another student noted that "I done seen some people come here and they're like they act all crazy and young and then a week being on site, they all grown up."[26]

The BEST program also has high level of job placement (approximately 80 percent) and, more important, job retention (approximately two-thirds hold their first job for more than a year.) At the time of this research 14 of the 20 most recent graduates were employed. This level of success is considered especially impressive given that the population they target often faces social and personal obstacles in entering the workforce. In comparison, the Parks Opportunity Program, a job training welfare-to-work program administered by the city of New York had a job placement rate of less than 64 percent in 2007. As an employee for the city of New York explained, "the [BEST] job training is really special. I think it is very difficult to have the placement rate that it does and it is very difficult to motivate people to change their lives whether it is leaving public assistance or not re-offending if they just got out of jail."[27] Participants in the training program were confident that it would lead to better employment opportunities, as stated by a recent BEST graduate: "I believe that it will change my situation a lot because a lot of these opportunities are being afforded to us now that other people might not be able to do in their lifetime so basically that is why I wanted to get involved with the program."[28]

BEST targets a mixture of individuals but about two-thirds enter the program after receiving some sort of government transfer (this may include food stamps, Medicare, housing allowances, or cash aid) for an extended period of time (of the 279 that had graduated by the summer of 2010, 185 had been supporting themselves through welfare or welfare-to-work programs.) BEST is also one of the few job training programs that accepts ex-felons into their program (employment rates for ex-felons tend to be about 6 percent lower than those of individuals with comparable demographic backgrounds who have not been incarcerated).[29] This brings with it additional challenges, both in terms of the end goal of finding those individuals employment and in terms of addressing some of the psychological issues that accompany serving extended prison time. Ex-offenders must readjust to function outside of the daily structure of prison and reestablish social relationships within a context where many of their old friends and relationships were built around illegal activity. This, along with employer reluctance to hire ex-offenders, makes it extremely difficult to find gainful employment and contributes to the high rates of recidivism experienced in neighborhoods with chronic unemployment and underemployment. As a former BEST staff member explained, "even if someone [comes] out of jail wanting to change their life, there really is very limited opportunity for them to do that because it is very difficult to get work as a convicted felon."[30]

Enabling individuals to make changes in their lives and thinking is considered one of the primary strengths and goals of BEST. Within the teachings and discourse of the program there is a strong promotion of the idea that the program's success stems from the success of each individual participant in transforming his or her life. While discussing the program's success, one staff member explained:

> I think it is about quality, not too much about our quantity. We are small in number, we train, not 500 people a year, but our training has so much quality. It has so much intent and concern about the person, not the dollar, not the amount or whatever; it is about the person and them building their self up to become the person they need to be.[31]

Participants are encouraged to view the program as an opportunity to learn about themselves and grow. BEST staff explain the program as "[avenue] for these individuals to better their lives and make something of themselves."[32] This imparts both agency and autonomy to participants who are given the responsibility for ensuring that they make use of this opportunity. This rhetoric of self-determination is paired with an emphasis on self-reflection. Along with an intense focus on life skills, the curriculum is designed to engender self-awareness and self-appreciation. Participants are encouraged to recognize their own good and bad qualities, to understand what they find aggravating in others, and why and how they can move past that within themselves. Overcoming insecurities and expectations of failure is considered to be an important element of this; as one staff member explained, this portion of the curriculum "becomes where they really learn to love themselves, like who they are so they are able to deal with people in the outside world."[33]

MERGING SOCIAL AND ENVIRONMENTAL GOALS

CVB and BEST have as their main goal to improve the lives of those in need through education and job training. Both see green jobs as a potential way of achieving this goal, and both see environmental sustainability as a goal in itself. On the other hand, environmental aspects appear to have a more prominent role for BEST than for CVB, both in terms of program philosophy and of day-to-day activities.

The official mission of American YouthWorks (AYW), CVB's parent organization, is "transforming the lives of at-risk youth through education, service, and green job training"—a mission statement that emphasizes the social goals of CVB more than environmental objectives. Interviews with staff members underlined this emphasis even more, as most interviewees mentioned only their social goals when asked about the program's mission.

In this context, CVB's focus on environmental sustainability is seen primarily by staff as an effective means of achieving their social goals. The decision to focus on green jobs training was also motivated by greater opportunities for funding. Focusing on energy-efficient construction allowed the program to tap into a niche market and facilitated getting initial funding as well as playing a positive role in later funding applications. In addition, CVB's management believes that the green industry will continue to expand in the future, and they hope that the green building skills that their students acquire will give those students a better chance to succeed in the economy of the future. They also believe that green jobs will be good jobs, because they require more advanced skills and knowledge (compared to traditional construction, for instance). This view seems to be supported by an International Labor Office study that found that traditional construction jobs such as roofing or glazing will require increasingly advanced knowledge, in particular with respect to the insulating properties of materials and building geometry.[34] Finally, the science of green building allows program staff to teach theoretical concepts more effectively, by relating them to hands-on things that students can do.

Daily program operations reflect the vision that, while environmentally aware practices are important both as a means of achieving social goals and as a goal in themselves, the social aspects have primacy. For instance, students can (and are encouraged to) choose the career path that they find most appropriate after they graduate, rather than being geared specifically toward green jobs. GED preparation or regular high school classes, which make up about half of a normal school day, have very little to do with environmental sustainability. And the students also perceive that their development is the main goal of the program: none of the current members and program graduates interviewed mentioned joining the program because of its environmental focus. At the same time, green education is incorporated whenever possible—for instance, "Ed lab" activities include climate change education, organic gardening, or visiting waste treatment facilities.

While environmental sustainability may be a secondary or complementary concern at CVB, at BEST it is an ideological and foundational goal. SSBx sees environmental sustainability as inexorably intertwined with social and economic equity. Consequently BEST was conceived and is always understood within a framework that promotes environmental sustainability alongside social and economic equity.

Like CVB, SSBx also sees the economic practicality of training people for green jobs. SSBx expects the green economy to be an industry in which growth will occur despite the economic downturn in the United States, which will allow the BEST program to expand as well. This also provides a space for SSBx to push for policy measures (such as incentive programs and the creation of green space) that will grow this industry and provide jobs for their trainees. Much like at CVB, the green curriculum allows BEST to teach students through hands-on fieldwork, which can be more successful with a population that is not accustomed to a classroom. Finally, it allows the BEST program to attract funds from groups interested in addressing one of or both environmental issues and chronic unemployment and underemployment.

Despite both the ideological and practical motivations for BEST's green focus, staff members at the BEST academy, much like those at CVB, see getting people jobs as their top priority. But because everything that SSBx does operates within this environmentally sustainable ethic, the green aspect is built into every facet of the program. The ethic of environmental sustainability is pervasive throughout the BEST process. It is evident in more than just the skills they teach and informs everything from their selection process to their focus on individual self-reflection.

BEST's training is aimed entirely at working within the green economy. The original program, BEST ECO, focuses on the skills needed to create and maintain green infrastructure, including green roof installation and brownfield remediation, while the newer program, BEST 4 Buildings, focuses on green building and energy efficiency techniques. This curriculum looks at environmental sustainability as a source of individual and community empowerment, teaching participants that they can make positive and tangible change in their own lives and in their communities by using and promoting environmentally sustainable practices. Moreover, many BEST graduates do end up being placed and working in the green economy. In 2008, 90 percent of those graduates who were employed were employed in green jobs.[35] As a BEST graduate who was employed as an administrator at SSBx described, training in green jobs leads to multiple benefits: "If you train folks in that, then you are creating the jobs and if you are creating the jobs and now working on sustainability that means a better, helping the environment at the same time and when you help the environment you are helping health overall and a better quality of life for folks everywhere. So you are looking at, you solve issues like poverty, you solve issues of unemployment and you work on sustainability and at the same time you are helping our environment. What is better than that, I don't know."[36]

Part of the reason why CVB and BEST can use their green credentials to more effectively pursue their social goals is that both programs operate in areas of strong local environmental leadership. Having the support of local governments helps both programs in their funding and in the creation of a strong local green economy sector. Austin Energy, the publicly owned electrical utility in Austin, claims on its Web site to have developed the top performing renewable energy program in the United States, the first and largest green building program, and one of the most comprehensive residential and commercial energy efficiency programs. Travis County (where Austin is located) has a history of supporting workforce development programs based at least partly on environmental merits. The BEST program is greatly facilitated by the number of local partnerships that SSBx has forged. There is a great deal of environmental activism in Hunts Point and the South Bronx, and the city of New York's Bronx River Alliance is a major partner and employer of BEST graduates. The development of local greenways along with the Million Tree Initiative may also be indicators of the city's commitment to creating and maintaining greenspaces, which would provide jobs for BEST graduates who are trained in the creation and maintenance of green infrastructure.

LIMITATIONS

BEST and CVB are producing some real successes in both promoting environmental sustainability and social mobility. However, one needs to always keep in perspective the magnitude of the benefits that these programs are able to bring, compared to the magnitude of the needs. The jobs that participants are able to get through these programs tend to be physically demanding; some do not have standard hours, which can be difficult for participants who have families or other obligations, and their starting wages tend to be between $12 and $14 (US) per hour. In the case of the BEST program, some of the jobs that graduates end up getting are those that would otherwise be filled by those in city welfare-to-work programs (although BEST graduates do tend to be better qualified and more successful in these jobs).

One must also be mindful of the fact that success in training people for green jobs is inherently limited by the number of jobs that are available. Predicting exactly when these jobs will be created is much more difficult than predicting that they will eventually come. Job creation depends on a myriad of factors, such as the economic climate, government policy, resource constraints, and so on. In particular, there is evidence that the number of green jobs created in the United States is not living up to expectations, and in some areas the green industry has actually lost jobs in recent years. Consequently, having effective training programs is only one aspect of creating the desired social, economic, and environmental change. The success of green job training as a means of lifting people out of poverty is intrinsically tied to the state of the economy. If the green sector is booming, then this can greatly help programs that invest significant resources into green job training. On the other hand, a slumping green sector can mean that investment in green job training is not the most effective way to help program members succeed after graduation.

Finally, one must consider the extent to which the "green" in these green job training programs is crucial to their success. Once again, this is complicated by the difficulty of measuring overall environmental impacts and the intangibility of benefits such as instilling environmental awareness and appreciation in participants. In the case of BEST the green aspect is integral to the governing philosophy, informing both the overall conception and specific practices and constituting an important factor in the program's success. In the case of CVB this is less clear, and it may be the case that the green aspect only enhances an already strong program and facilitates the creation of partnerships and attracting funding. Factors such as a focus on soft and interpersonal communication skills, selective participant criteria, and a strong staff who believe in and are aware of their programs goals appear to be the main reason these two programs have such comparatively high hiring and retention rates.

KEYS TO SUCCESS: INTEGRATED FACTORS CONTRIBUTING TO PROGRAMS' OUTCOMES

While CVB and BEST focus their training on specific skills, aiming to prepare participants for jobs in the green economy, there are certain overarching factors that play a central role in the programs' effectiveness.

A Strong Focus on Soft Skills and Interpersonal Communication

People joining these programs typically lack a variety of what is called "soft skills." One of the teachers interviewed at CVB noted that some of the skills that members lack are to "show up on time, know what's work-appropriate behaviour, be able to be the kind of person that knows where to draw those boundaries, you know, 'maybe I shouldn't say that in front of her because she is my teacher or that person is my supervisor.'"[37] CVB staff tries to address these issues primarily through a lot of reasoning and communication. They also work on developing more specific soft skills by providing sessions on resume and interview preparedness or even on more basic topics such as proper nutrition and birth control.

BEST's curriculum likewise includes a great deal of emphasis on teaching soft skills and encouraging self-awareness, understanding, and self-esteem. Participants are encouraged to try and identify what aspects of their lives and behaviors they need to change in order to be successful in finding and keeping a job. A board member explained that SSBx attributes the unemployment and underemployment of many of the BEST program participants to the institutionalised racism those participants have experienced throughout their lives. For many this meant they received an inferior education, moved a lot as children, and consequently were not encouraged to become engaged or invested in their communities; they grew up conceiving of themselves within a society where unrewarding and unstable employment or the underground drug economy appeared to be the only viable vocational options. The soft and life skills aspects of the training attempt to make up for this disparity. The BEST program includes within its curriculum classic "soft skills" such as how to interview, financial management with a focus on debt management, saving and budgeting, and conflict management, particularly in terms of dealing with one's boss or fellow employees.[38]

These aspects are greatly appreciated by the participants. As a former BEST participant explained, the "life skills" aspect of the training "was very useful because a lot of us that grew up in this community, we need some type of training like that because a lot of us, we not aware of those [skills] and a lot of us take day by day, we don't even look as far as the future cause you know, our surroundings doesn't motivate us to have a future,...I mean the broad sense of what a success story is in a lot of these communities is crime."[39]

Strong Case Management before and after Graduation

Both programs believe that individual case management is crucial in order to get jobs for their students (particularly at a time where unemployment is high) and help them retain these jobs.

CVB has three people that are hired specifically for case management—a postsecondary placement specialist, a career placement specialist, and a counselor. Based on personal observation and interviews, they do a wide range of things—from more traditional counselling and career advice, to helping students with homework or housing issues. CVB trainers and teachers sometimes act as part-time case managers: they have strategies for motivating members (for instance, by showing them what they can achieve through hard work) and dealing with inappropriate behavior (e.g., pulling people to the side). The administrative staff takes part as well—for instance, the program director is also a counselor.

CVB does its best to keep in touch with program graduates, with Facebook being one of the most effective means for doing so. They track their outcomes and also help them with jobs or community college issues if need be. Some of their graduates continue with other AYW programs, either as administrative staff or become members in other service programs such as E-Corps.

BEST has dedicated two staff positions to job developers who actively seek out job possibilities for program participants. The job developers make connections with employers working in green industry or businesses in order to know what skills and qualifications they are looking for. The job developers keep track of job opportunities and help individual graduates find and prepare for interviews.

Once graduates have found a job, the staff at SSBx follow them for 3 years, ensuring that they are successful and satisfied with their employment. They offer themselves as a point of contact for an employer if there is an issue to be addressed. This provides those in the program a source of ongoing support and employers an additional assurance of stability. This ongoing support likely accounts for the high rates of retention as SSBx can act as a mediator to prevent small problems and miscommunications from escalating and ending in a graduate being fired or quitting.

A Thorough Participant Selection Process

As mentioned before, there are some important differences between the demographics of the incoming students for CVB and those for BEST (most important, young high school dropouts for CVB versus slightly more mature people who have at least a GED for BEST). This may allow BEST to be more ambitious in their goals, since the type of members in the program can have a significant effect on the program's success. CVB staff members in particular have given this issue a lot of thought, possibly due to the fact that in 2007–2008 they had a grant requiring them to only take on people from the criminal justice system, and this grant "almost killed Casa Verde."[40]

CVB has an interview process during which they look for "attitude, ability, and promptness"[41] and a 3-week voluntary orientation during which they can decide whether they officially enroll a student into the YouthBuild program. However, staff members claimed that new students often managed to stay on their best behavior during those 3 weeks but become significantly less interested and disciplined after they have officially joined the program.

The selectivity of the individuals admitted is probably a factor in BEST's impressive postprogram employment rate. The staff at SSBx is selective regarding who they admit into the program. Depending on the time of year, around 50–60 applicants apply each session and make it through the math and reading tests as well as a short interview. The 15–20 who are selected to go through the program are chosen through a 2– to 3-day training and tryout process comprised of teamwork exercises, mock interviews, and problem-solving activities. At the end of this session the BEST staff get together and discuss each participant and narrow down whom to accept. In doing so, they attempt to achieve a balance of those that they know will succeed with those that are not quite so stable. This is done with the understanding that they do not have the capacity to act as case workers, and so they do not take on participants who are struggling psychologically or have other major barriers that must be overcome (such as being in an unhealthy relationship or having addiction issues). In addition to a certain level of life stability, the main factors that BEST staff look for when choosing participants are drive and commitment. As one staff member explained, "We don't want everybody, we just want people who truly have a passion for this work because if they don't, they will not do well and they will not be successful." Consequently the staff look for participants who are interested, motivated to learn, and genuinely want to change their lives. They identify individuals who they believe are ready to commit the time and energy that the BEST program requires and who are "hungry for change for [themselves]." In their words,

> Most of the time the people that we get, we know that they are sick and tired of being sick and tired, and they want change. So we're able to you know, I really feel we've been very good at weaning away the bad seeds and making sure that people who are in this program are here for change for them, it's not about us, it's about you.[42]

Due to the rigor and length of the program as well as the significant investment of staff time and energy (and SSBx funds) into each individual, this selection process is very important. Like CVB, some of SSBx's recent grants for the BEST academy have had stipulations regarding the population it must serve (for example ex-convicts). At the time of this research it was not yet clear how or whether these restrictions on selectivity would affect hiring and retention rates, but given the clear importance of the selection process, it is doubtful that these limitations will be without consequences.

A Caring and Dedicated Staff

Having a caring staff that truly believe in the worth of the program has been crucial to the success of both programs. The high level of commitment and dedication of CVB staff was acknowledged by both students and outside observers, and it was identified by several interviewees as one of the key elements of their success. When asked what makes a YouthBuild program successful, the YouthBuild USA coach responded:

> I think having a committed staff, because I think it's really hard to run this type of program, and it means, again, kind of the extra hour, going the extra mile.[43]

And, according to one of the students:

> The difference between the other schools is like, you know you go to school and it's over. These people here man, it's like a family. You feel loved. They don't ever give up on you.[44]

The intensive development of each individual participant is made possible by BEST's passionate and engaged staff, who get to know each individual and are able to push and support them in this development. The individual class field managers are themselves graduates of the program, which gives them insight into what participants are experiencing. This also gives them a certain amount of legitimacy in the eyes of participants and to some extent prevents complex feelings regarding social issues such as class and race from becoming prominent in that encounter. Field managers know what they can reasonably expect from participants and explained that because they themselves had gone through the program and been in the position of those who are now their students, they were able to have more honest relationships with their trainees. These field managers were also able to act as role models for those in the program. As they are gainfully employed and respected, they serve as a model of the success that program participants seek to attain.

CONCLUSION

CVB and SSBx's BEST programs are able to take measurable steps toward simultaneously addressing environmental sustainability and providing opportunities for disadvantaged people through green job training. The programs' success can be measured both through indicators such as their high post-graduation placement rates, as well as through the way they manage to create positive change in the participants' mindsets. In particular, most participants become more aware of the environmental footprint of human activities and are able to learn about new ways to reduce this footprint.

The two programs are somewhat different in the extent of their focus on environmental aspects. While sustainability is a key part of both programs, CVB is more geared toward preparing their students for a variety of potential future careers, whereas BEST focuses entirely on green jobs. The successes that both programs have achieved despite these differences suggest that there is no single path toward lifting people out of poverty through green job training. In fact, a variety of approaches may be successful, as long as programs understand the population they are working with and the job market in the area where they function.

We have also identified several features that help programs with the difficult task of integrating a disadvantaged and undereducated population into the formal economy. We have seen evidence from both organizations concerning the positive effect of intensive case management, soft skills training, and having a staff that stays dedicated to the program's mission. We hope that the lessons drawn from this chapter will help guide similar programs toward successful paths, as well as inform policy makers about the nature and potential benefits of poverty alleviation through green job training.

NOTES

1. F. McKee-Ryan et al., "Psychological and Physical Well-Being During Unemployment: A Meta-Analytic Study," *Journal of Applied Psychology*, 10, no. 1 (2005): 53–76.
2. R. L. Jin, C. P. Shah, and T. J. Svoboda, "The Impact of Unemployment on Health: A Review of the Evidence," *Canadian Medical Association Journal* 153, no. 5 (1995): 1567–8.
3. U.S. Enviromental Protection Agency, accessed May 22, 2013, http://www.epa.gov/climatechange/ghgemissions/global.html
4. U.S. Environmental Protection Agency, "Inventory of U.S. Greenhouse Gases and Emissions and Sinks: 1990-2001", page ES-11, accessed May 22, 2013, http://www.epa.gov/climatechange/Downloads/ghgemissions/US-GHG-Inventory-2013-ES.pdf
5. Bureau of Labor Statistics, accessed May 22, 2013, http://www.bls.gov/news.release/archives/wkyeng_07202010.htm
6. Data compiled by CVB staff from the 2000 Census, Austin Independent School District, and the Intercultural Development Research Association; the target area for CVB is composed of Austin / Travis County census tracts 8.02, 9.01, 9.02, 10.0, 18.11, 18.12, 21.11, 22.02, 23.11, and 23.16.
7. They must be either from low-income families (80 percent of median), or in foster care, or a youth offender, or the child of an incarcerated parent, or a migrant youth, or have a disability.
8. This means less than ninth grade in any area according to the Test of Adult Basic Education (TABE) test.
9. In the United States and Canada, the General Educational Development (GED) tests are a group of five tests that, when passed, certify that the taker has high-school-level skills.

10. Hazardous Waste Operations and Emergency Response.
11. Occupational Safety and Health Administration.
12. Child and Adult CPR.
13. Interview with an owner of a CVB-built home, June 2010.
14. Interview with a CVB graduate, June 2010.
15. Interview with a CVB student, June 2010.
16. Interview with a CVB student, June 2010.
17. Interview with a BEST Eco Participant, June 2010.
18. Interview with SSBX's Greenway Steward, June 2010.
19. The most recent aggregate numbers for the 2007 grant cycle were obtained from DoL via email, and the CVB numbers were obtained from CVB staff. YouthBuild grantees all work with at-risk youth through a combination of classroom education and construction, but not all of them are focused on green building.
20. Interview with a CVB student, June 2010.
21. Interview with a CVB student, June 2010.
22. Interview with a CVB student, June 2010.
23. Interview with a CVB student, June 2010.
24. Interview with a CVB student, June 2010.
25. Interview with a CVB student, June 2010.
26. Interview with a CVB student, June 2010.
27. Interview with a former SSBx Staff member June 2010.
28. Interview with a recent BEST graduate, June 2010.
29. A. Geller, I. Garfinkel, and B. Western, "The Effects of Incarceration on Employment and Wages: An Analysis of the Fragile Families Survey," Center for Research on Child Wellbeing, accessed April 29, 2013, http://crcw.princeton.edu/workingpapers/WP06-01-FF.pdf
30. Interview with a former SSBx staff member, June 2010.
31. Interview with the Director of the BEST Academy, July 2010.
32. Interview with SSBx Job Developer, July 2010.
33. Interview with the Director of BEST Academy, July 2010.
34. *Skills and Occupational Needs in Green Building*, International Labor Office, accessed April 29, 2013, http://www.ilo.org/wcmsp5/groups/public/@ed_emp/@ifp_skills/documents/publication/wcms_166822.pdf.
35. M. Carter. "BEST Green Job Training Program," accessed April 29, 2013, http://www.majoracartergroup.com/services/case-histories/best-green-job-training-program/
36. Interview with BEST Academy Administrator, June 2010.
37. Bill Comeaux (CVB teacher), interview, June 2010.
38. This practice was evident in the interviews with participants done for this research in which many replied with full sentences, spoke with measure and included the question in their response to it.
39. Interview with BEST graduate, greenroof maintainer and installer, June 2010.
40. Chester Steinhauser (CVB Chief Operating Officer), personal communication, May 17, 2010.
41. J. Stuffel, "Addendum/Revision to Americorps Programs Recruitment Manual", internal AYW document redacted in the Fall of 2009.
42. Interview with BEST Academy Director, July 2010.
43. Leslie Newman, (YouthBuild coach working with CVB), interview July 2010.
44. Interview with a CVB student, June 2010

CHAPTER 6

Green Social Entrepreneurship as a Poverty-Reduction Strategy

TIDE India's Use of Technological Innovation

for Healthier and More Sustainable Communities

SHANNON LOCKHART

While all sectors of society are affected by increasing pressures on already-fragile ecosystems and overburdened natural resources, the poor bear a disproportionate share of the adverse consequences. As other chapters examine, the poor face worse environmental conditions, which have detrimental consequences on the health and development of low-income people and contribute to perpetuating the cycle of poverty. As environmental challenges continue to increase, the past few years have seen the detrimental impacts of the global financial crisis take a toll on the living standards and economic conditions of the vast majority of countries. Estimates from the World Bank suggested that the crisis left an additional 50 million people in extreme poverty by 2009 and some 64 million by the end of 2010 relative to a no-crisis scenario, principally in sub-Saharan Africa and Eastern and South-Eastern Asia.[1]

Traditionally, alleviating poverty has been seen as the responsibility of governments and charitable organizations. Social entrepreneurship instead attempts to harness the ingenuity and growth potential of the private sector to provide novel solutions for societal problems such as poverty, environmental degradation and gender inequality. Green social enterprises focus on solving the intertwined problems of environmental sustainability and poverty by finding ways to provide income-generating opportunities that simultaneously improve environmental conditions. Previous chapters examined initiatives to generate green enterprises in high-income countries; this chapter focuses on a green entrepreneurship program in India.

While robust economic growth has decreased poverty rates in India (the percentage of people living on less than $1 a day went from 49 percent in 1994 to 41 percent in 2004[2]) and propelled a substantial portion of the population into the middle class, poverty still remains a pressing concern, with almost 30 percent of the rural population living below the national poverty line. Rural areas continue to be home to the vast majority of India's population (72.18 percent)[3] but experience severe inequalities in terms of access to services and infrastructure as well as key human development indicators. Literacy rates in rural areas are 59 percent compared to 80 percent in urban areas[4]; access to infrastructure and health care is markedly lower in rural areas, with only 21 percent of the rural population having access to improved sanitation facilities compared to 54 percent of the urban population.[2] Gender inequalities are significantly more pronounced in rural areas. Literacy rates for men in rural areas are 70 percent compared to 46 percent for women, whereas in urban areas literacy rates are 86 percent for men and 72 percent for women.[4] Among the many health problems associated with rural poverty, one of the main aspects is indoor air pollution from the use of solid fuels, which is used by almost 90 percent of the rural population.[2] Indoor air pollution has been linked with increased child mortality from acute lower respiratory infections,[5] as well as an association of solid fuel with pneumonia mortality[6] and respiratory symptoms among children under age 5 years.[7] It is also directly linked to gender equity since it is women who are disproportionately exposed to indoor air pollution. Efforts to promote cleaner technology such as smokeless stoves are therefore an important element in combating the environmental and health consequences of rural poverty.

THE TIDE MODEL: COMBINING SOCIAL ENTREPRENEURSHIP WITH GREEN TECHNOLOGY

In Bangalore, India, nongovernmental organization (NGO) Technology Informatics Design Endeavour (TIDE) has been using a unique model to blend green technology design and social entrepreneurship to produce economic and environmental benefits for the rural poor. What is unique about their model is that TIDE neither creates the technology designs nor participates directly in entrepreneurship. Instead, TIDE turns green designs being produced by existing Indian research infrastructure into products that can be marketed and sold by entrepreneurs that TIDE incubates toward independence.

TIDE's model recognizes the necessity for environmental protection, the power of green technology to deliver that protection, and the ability of the social entrepreneurship model to deliver technology, knowledge, and economic opportunity to those that need it the most. TIDE's diffusion of green technology through its spin-off enterprises replaces energy-inefficient and polluting devices with new models that decrease both outdoor and indoor air pollution—providing direct benefits to the health of household members as well as long-term prevention of greenhouse gas emissions. In addition, a major part of TIDE's programs focus on educating entrepreneurs on how important environmental awareness and conservation are for both future generations and for the present marketing of their products.

TIDE's first green enterprise program began in 1998, funded by the India-Canada Environment Facility (ICEF), and focused on the diffusion of efficient biomass utilization technologies in nonformal industries in the southern Indian states of Karnataka and Kerala. The project concept was to decrease the amount of woody biomass burned for fuel in rural areas. High quantities of solid biomass, primarily wood, being burned in various processes contributes to deforestation in rural areas. By replacing conventional devices with newer, more energy-efficient models, biofuel requirements for activities conducted with traditional devices could be decreased.

TIDE chose a model of dissemination that spun off independent entrepreneurs who marketed and sold their devices. Although it is likely that the scale of dissemination of the devices TIDE has adapted could be increased through the use of a more centralized production and dissemination model, TIDE has consciously selected the green entrepreneurship model because of its potential to create economic opportunities, reduce poverty, and spread awareness in the project areas. TIDE's trainings go beyond technical training to address broader aspects of life, including personal development and environmental awareness. As such, their programs have been a catalyst for positive change for many of the participants.

When TIDE set out to channel technology design into marketable products for entrepreneurs, three guidelines for selecting the technologies were established:

1. Devices must have the potential to earn profits. The cost to build a device should not exceed the cost at which it could be sold.
2. Devices should be environmentally benign, meaning that they provide environmental benefits in the form of added efficiency relative to existing devices. Additionally, the devices should act as a medium for spreading awareness and educating people about environmental protection.
3. Device delivery should be socially and culturally acceptable.[8]

Since its inception, TIDE has tested over 54 types of technology from which it selects the most appropriate, efficient, and profitable to disseminate through TIDE-trained individual entrepreneurs and their companies. TIDE has tested designs in the areas of rainwater harvesting, agricultural greenhouses, waste management processes, silk processing, food drying, and Ayurvedic preparations, among others. This discussion will focus on the designs TIDE has adapted for entrepreneurial dissemination. Of the entrepreneurially disseminated products, there is a common focus on energy-efficient biomass-utilization technology for nonformal industries. The designs can mostly be fit into three categories: stoves, driers, and kilns. For their women's project, TIDE adapted three main types of technologies: a household cookstove (Sarala stove), a biomass drier, and a silk-reeling stove. Technologies were also customized to take advantage of the local resources in cluster areas in Karnataka, Kerala, Madhya Pradesh, and Tamil Nadu.

IMPROVING ENVIRONMENTAL HEALTH THROUGH THE DIFFUSION OF ENERGY-EFFICIENT TECHNOLOGIES

Improving the environment has been a fundamental goal of TIDE since its inception. With their unique model of spinning-off green enterprises to disseminate energy-efficient technologies, TIDE's program has created environmental benefits that include mitigating both outdoor and indoor air pollution, as well as spreading awareness and education about the importance of environmental sustainability to end users, typically the rural poor.

Outdoor Environmental Benefits

Because of the widespread existence of nonformal process industries in rural areas (silk-reeling, drying and selling of local food products, and tobacco curing), TIDE chose to focus on adapting energy-efficient technology into devices suitable to carrying out such processes. At the beginning of the project, TIDE conducted a survey of these industries and the technologies traditionally utilized as well as the biomass utilization of such technologies. During the survey period, TIDE staff "visited about 2,500 units of nonformal industries and analyzed the potential for biofuel savings in the industry."[9] TIDE chose sectors demonstrating the most potential for biofuel savings, availability of adaptable technologies, and profitability of the intervention for spin-off enterprises. For Karnataka state, TIDE identified jaggery making, brick kilns, tobacco curing, silk reeling, areca nut cooking, lime kilns, pottery kilns, cardamom drying, and arecanut drying as industries suitable for intervention. These industries combined utilized approximately 2,747,540 megatonnes (Mt) of biofuel annually, with per unit usage ranging from 1.8 Mt annually for arecanut drying to 156.7 Mt annually for brick kilns.[9] In Kerala state, TIDE selected the sectors of cardamom drying, rubber sheet smoking, hotels and restaurants, arecanut processing, Ayurvedic medicine preparation, coconut drying, cashew processing, and rubber band making. These industries combined for an annual biomass usage of 228,701 Mt. Within the identified Kerala state industries, per unit usage ranged from 7.9 to 165.6 Mt of biofuel per annum.[9]

Following this survey phase, TIDE tested different devices and adapted them for marketing and use by future enterprises they would spin off. The devices were different types of energy-efficient stoves, driers, and brick kilns, which provided higher energy conservation rates (e.g., 25 percent with the Sarala smokeless household cookstove). The dissemination phase, in which enterprises began to actively market and distribute the devices and/or their respective products began in 2001 and was tracked for 3 years. From 2001 to 2004 enterprises sold a total of 4,466 devices, which translates into a minimum decrease in biomass consumption of approximately 2,900 Mt per year.

Household Health Benefits

TIDE has since created another branch of the entrepreneurship program that focuses on women-led green enterprises in rural areas. Since women in rural India face large social constraints such as reduced autonomy, dominating domestic demands, and limited travel capacity, TIDE designed an independent program to address their specific needs.[11] Currently there are six women-run enterprises, of approximately five to eight members each, using driers to create products to market/sell and building Sarala smokeless household stoves.

The Sarala smokeless stove is a household cookstove TIDE has adapted that provides increased fuel efficiency and heat transfer, saving both fuel and time for its users, who are predominantly rural women. TIDE's design improves fuel efficiency by 25–30 percent while increasing the heat transfer to cooking vessels as well as increasing combustion chamber heat to enable multiple fuels, such as coconut husks and arecanut shells, to be used to replace wood.[12] While end users report appreciating these aspects of the device, the most important adaptation is that smoke emptied by traditional devices into the interior of the home is diverted by the Sarala stove outside of the kitchen, preventing residents of the home from inhaling harmful smoke whenever meals are prepared. One customer discussed how the stove had been so beneficial to her, in keeping her home, herself and her vessels clean, that she would like to begin stove building as way to make the lives of other women better.[13] Another conveyed her experience with the stoves:

> Because of building the stoves, there are many benefits. Especially for the women. And, these stoves are very safe and moreover, while washing the vessels, because the vessels would get blackened, all their hands would get blackened. And, moreover, when we blowed in the firewood stove, half the smoke would go into our stomach and most women would suffer from many diseases. But, with this stove, nothing like that happened.[14]

Grant officers at the Department of Science and Technology, New Delhi, discussed how the health benefits of diverting smoke outside of the home make this device one that could benefit every village household that does not currently possess it.[15]

Environmental Awareness and Education

TIDE's social enterprise model of dissemination has created a grassroots network of green enterprises committed to spreading environmental awareness and education along with their products. TIDE recognizes that the entrepreneurs they train are primarily interested in economic gains, but it instructs them on how environmental benefits such as increased fuel economy and heat transfer are marketable attributes of technologies that consumers will find appealing.[16] At the same time, TIDE emphasizes the broader importance of environmental awareness to its trainees. The energy-efficiency technology itself is what drew some participants to the program, with one participant leaving a career in agricultural research of tobacco product efficiency because he was interested in the environmental impacts of energy-efficient technologies specific to rural end users.[17] Another entrepreneur who is no longer working with TIDE discussed how TIDE's emphasis on the importance of environmental issues led him into the green energy sector and he has since established a rural hydroelectricity company that has received governmental recognition and support.[18] Another TIDE-affiliated entrepreneur has become the biomass fuels expert on a United Nations led Climate Change Community forum, focusing on how to decrease fuel consumption in India.[19]

For many of the female entrepreneurs, the future of their children is what makes environmental issues important to them. Women entrepreneurs conducting awareness programs for children and their mothers on environment conservation and management discussed their motivations: "Sometimes we feel more than for ourselves, [our work is] for our children's education."[20] These women also talked about the health of the village as being the motivator for their work, including preventing the spread of malaria and ensuring safe and adequate amounts of drinking water for the future:

> It helps the groundwater conservation and also the agriculture, as we consume more water, it will also help agriculture. Another reason is health because if we let water flow, and water stagnates then the mosquitos breed and it will lead to malaria, so we can also avoid that.[20]

CREATING ECONOMIC OPPORTUNITIES
IN RURAL COMMUNITIES

By selecting a model of dissemination for their devices that involves spinning off entrepreneurs and their microenterprises, TIDE's program has created income generation opportunities that have had direct economic impacts as well as indirect social benefits. TIDE entrepreneurs recognize and create their own economic opportunities, and as they leverage the extra income, they create promising opportunities in their families and communities.

Income Generation

TIDE's energy-efficient technology diffusion project began training entrepreneurs to disseminate the technologies in 1998. By the end of the first project, in 2004, TIDE had spun off 22 microenterprises[9] in various rural places in southern India. While reported earnings vary greatly among the men in this group, all men interviewed reported an increase in their annual income compared to before beginning TIDE's program. Direct income data were not collected during the project period because entrepreneurs were negotiating different prices for different devices in different areas. However, device dissemination was tracked, and between the 22 entrepreneurs, 5,170 devices were distributed during 2004 alone.[9]

Men in TIDE's entrepreneurship program typically take up fabrication and distribution of the energy-efficient technologies that TIDE provides as the activity of their enterprise. One man, Samson, began a career in Rain Water Harvesting technology installation through training and contracts that TIDE provided to him. Prior to his introduction to TIDE, Samson had been working as a laborer doing electrical wiring and plumbing work. TIDE taught him the technical aspects of the program, introduced him to the idea of systems and how to manage himself and others, and has set him up with clients who approach TIDE with interest in Rain Water Harvesting. Samson has been able to increase his monthly income by almost double, reporting an increase in earnings from 6,000 INR to approximately 10,000 INR these days. He has also been able to increase the size of his contracts since starting to work with TIDE, going from contracts worth between 15,000 and 50,000 INR to over 100,000 INR. Samson is now running a team of about 10 men, and he continues to conduct plumbing and electrical work in his downtime. He talked about how, "then even while he was working, for his kids' education he had to anyways borrow. But now, he is able to sustain his business, not borrow and he is able to take the money which he is getting, and also not being answerable to anybody because he is able to accomplish the work he is supposed to be [doing]."[21]

The first cohort of trainees consisted of only male participants. However, TIDE expressed the belief that money in the rural woman's hand might hold greater power to benefit her family and village,[22] so they began a program that would focus on recruiting and training female entrepreneurs in rural south India. In 2004, TIDE began a technical training for women to build and market household stoves, with the goal of supplementing the seasonal agricultural income that most rural women earned.[23] Data collected over the course of the women's project period, May 2004 to June 2006, show that 100 women (as well as 30 men who showed interest) were trained, 1,474 stoves were built in the three project districts, and 65,418 INR in revenue was earned from labor by the stove builders.[23] During the project, a high dropout rate was expected, as it was a pioneering effort in empowering women with alternate sources of income, against which there were known social and cultural pressures. Analysis of the reasons for dropout was undertaken, with family problems, poor health, and inability to travel being the main reasons women provided for not constructing stoves following the training.[23] In 2007, TIDE began another project that focused on energy-efficient biomass dryers for use by rural women running group food processing enterprises. Four groups of women were trained and it was discovered that stationary, group activities for women were much more accepted, successful, and sustainable than the independent and mobile stove-building activities. Today, TIDE works with six women working to market domestic energy-efficient lights, two to four women working on a greenhouse project, two women building smokeless stoves, and eight groups of six to ten women using biomass driers to market dried foods and goods.[24]

TIDE women participants talk freely about how the income-generation activities they have taken up through TIDE's green enterprise program have improved their economic situation. One of TIDE's most remarkable entrepreneurs, LalitaBai, is a woman who has taken up stove building to earn her livelihood. LalitaBai has received much publicity for the scale of her work, building over 10,000 stoves since starting her work with TIDE in 1992. She builds about 800 stoves per year with each stove bringing her approximately 80 INR in profit, for an annual, self-reported income of approximately 64,000 INR from stove building. LalitaBai's story has received a great deal of publicity in India. She is from the Lambani tribe, which is one of the lowest castes in India. She was the recipient of the Pan-India CII-Bharti Woman Exemplar Award of 100,000 INR, which "recognizes those [women] who have, against all odds, contributed in the fields of Education and Literacy, Health and Micro Enterprise,"[25] with which she was able to build a new home for her family, support her childrens' education, and pay for a medical procedure needed by her son. Prior to beginning TIDE's training program, LalitaBai had been working at a local NGO earning approximately 300 INR per month. She talks about how TIDE's program changed her life:

> After I joined TIDE, gradually my goals changed. My poverty reduced...I used to earn a meager salary of just 20 rupees [per week]. How would I buy ragi, rice or lentils? I have three kids and my husband would fall ill in those days...[The people at TIDE] have shown us the way to lead the life. And I think now it is our prerogative to stand on our own and lead the way.[26]

Shilpa is another TIDE entrepreneur, who works with a group of women in a coastal town of Kerala state in southern India, using TIDE's biomass drier to dry fish products and other local resources, market them, and sell them. The group started in 2005 and increased its earnings quickly, taking home 16,000 INR the first year, but increasing that to 144,000 INR in the last reported year (2009). Shilpa is happy with their success, which has enabled her to "build a house off that, and to get the land." The most recent goals of the group include expanding their business by increasing their number of biomass driers to keep up with the product demand as they expand their sales into international markets.[27]

Other women are not able or desire to commit full-time to the entrepreneurial activities that TIDE's technologies provide, but instead they use TIDE's trainings and technologies as a means of supplementing their incomes. To facilitate this, TIDE has selected technologies that can be produced and marketed with flexibility around the other domestic and labor duties of the entrepreneurs. Gita, a woman who markets solar products with a group of five other women, talks about how after she finishes her household duties, she takes about 2–3 hours to do work for her enterprise, and has the flexibility to choose which days she does this. Gita talked about how she is able to supplement her household income by about 3,000 INR per year without neglecting any of her familial responsibilities.[28]

Enterprising in New Markets

TIDE's training in entrepreneurial skills and microenterprise development encourages entrepreneurs to seek economic opportunity in new places as they see it arise, sometimes beyond TIDE-designed technologies. Ranveer is one such opportunity-seeking entrepreneur. Ranveer works in central Karnataka and began working as an entrepreneur after attending one of TIDE's trainings in 1997. He has since started his own spin-off enterprise, working in pico-hydroelectricity, where he installs units to generate hydro-electricity in off-the-grid locations in Karnataka state. Ranveer started this business in 2008 with the help of a subsidy from the government that he saw advertised in his local newspaper. Ranveer's business currently employs eight other people and he reports that he is currently earning 15 percent–20 percent profits each month so far. Ranveer talked about how, even though he is no longer using the technology that TIDE gave him, that he was able to get the start-up funding for his current business because lenders "trusted him based on the success of the TIDE project."[18]

Savir, another TIDE entrepreneur, has also expanded his business beyond TIDE technologies. Prior to working with TIDE in 2001, Savir inherited a company that cast spare automobile parts from iron and manufactured spinning wheels. After manufacturing and then testing some water heating devices for TIDE, Savir was convinced that these products were high-quality devices with significant improvements over traditional devices, and that there was a huge rural market for such energy-efficient devices. He began manufacturing and marketing TIDE's designs full time. Savir saw the opportunity for additional business and approached "five or six other organization which were doing similar things...[like] a cookstove, a charcoal stove and all that." He said, "So I contacted them and said, "Can we market and manufacture your stove?" They said [we] could market one and manufacture the other. So we started doing that. Then we contacted [another organization]."[19] But Savir didn't stop there. He got in touch with the Indian Institute of Science (IISc) and Indian Institute of Technology (IIT) to see if he could manufacture and market energy-efficient biomass designs to rural users for them. His company now distributes a line of about 20 different products for about 10 organizations.

He is also currently part of a United Nations-sponsored group talking about how to increase the use of green technologies in rural areas. He conveyed that the purpose of this group is to find ways to respond to the fact that "90 percent of the innovation happens for 10 percent of the people. We shall try to help the 90 percent downtrodden of the population. For example, the standard [rural Indian stove] that is being used: 60 percent of Asia uses it, and 90 percent of Africa uses it. So basically half the world works with it...we develop a four times more efficient stove. A woman who collects wood at the roadside, she will have to collect once a month instead of weekly. Human energy can be used monthly instead of weekly," freeing her to devote that energy to other economic activities if she so requires.[19]

The Multiplier Effect of Economic Opportunity

Beyond the direct economic benefit the entrepreneur receives from disseminating the devices, there are two major beneficiaries: the end users of the devices and the future generations of entrepreneur families.

The economic impacts of disseminating energy-efficient biomass technologies extend to the rural end users, as the increased efficiency of the devices saves both fuel cost and time. "Previously our men had to carry lots of firewood from farms. And apart from the farms, they had to go to the forest and cut the wood. And many households will tell you what a difference this new stove has made because now the wood in the farm itself is self-sufficient, if we ever need wood [the increased heat at which the energy-efficient devices burn enables waste such as nut husks to be used instead of wood]. And previously while cooking food we just had to sit there in front of the stove because we always had to push the firewood in for more heat. But now, I just, while I am preparing food, I also go outside and work and come back."[11] What this means for those who use their stove for commercial purposes, such as preparing and selling food, is that after the initial investment, they are taking home profits with larger margins due to the fuel savings, which spell both money and time for the end user. Traditional devices demonstrate energy efficiencies between 5 and 10 percent. Devices that Savir's company is manufacturing and marketing have energy efficiencies between 40 and 60 percent. Based on data that the company has collected and analyzed, users are recovering the cost of the devices in less than 1 year—and in most cases much less than 1 year. For example, a top boiler that is used in many rural restaurants would typically cost between 10,000 and 13,000 INR, which is a substantial investment for many rural entrepreneurs. However, modern top broilers are most commonly fueled with liquid petroleum gas (LPG) cylinders, which typically cost about 1,900 INR per day. By switching to one of Savir's top boilers, the cost of wood to create the same heat for the same amount of time is about 250 INR. Thus, a restaurateur can recover the cost of his top boiler in less than 1 month.[19]

Families of TIDE's entrepreneurs are also seeing economic benefits from the income generation activities. Because of the increased income that TIDE entrepreneurs are able to generate, they gain the capacity to afford to send their children to better schools, or in some cases send them to school at all. Their children will have more employment opportunities as a result of their parent's entrepreneurial work. One of TIDE's female stove-building entrepreneurs talked about how before working with TIDE, "in our house, we could not sustain the fuel supplies regularly and I could not even afford the fees for my kids. I have three daughters and one son. I could not even send them to school." And now she was building 180–200 stoves per year and earning sums for those, while continuing to perform the same agricultural work she had done before. All of her children will get an education.[11]

Another stove-building entrepreneur described wanting better opportunities for her children as the driving force behind her entrepreneurial success. LalitaBai related: "I know that my fate had been decided but I at least wanted my kids to earn...so at that time I decided that by building stoves, I will ensure my daughter becomes a teacher."[26] Since that decision, LalitaBai has built over 10,000 stoves and won monetary prizes for her work. "Since I have learned the skill of installing a stove, I sent my daughter to do a TCH...for a teacher training course, and now she has a job. And now my son is studying and I also received an award worth 100,000 INR and with that, I renovated my house and one of my sons got the operation he needed, so I spent 50,000 INR on that." LalitaBai, like many other entrepreneurs interviewed through TIDE's program, speaks of her work and tells her story with glowing esteem but also with gratitude. She finishes softly but with strength: "So...I can say I am making a decent living out of this."[26]

HAVING AN IMPACT ON SOCIAL DEVELOPMENT

Although TIDE's program began with a focus on solving rural environmental and economic problems, social impacts beyond poverty alleviation have emerged. As a member of TIDE's leadership team explained: "But, if you look at the larger picture, then you realize that the social gain is much more than the financial."[16] Subjective measures, such as confidence levels, ambitions for a better future, or feelings of control over one's life, prove difficult to measure but exist as prevalent themes throughout the stories of TIDE entrepreneurs. Social benefits became a very important motivator in TIDE's program, for both TIDE leadership and also for the entrepreneurs. Having recognized what a powerful motivator these social impacts could be, TIDE made social improvement beyond financial gains a shaping force in the evolution of their entrepreneurship program. Among the positive changes observed within target communities and entrepreneurs, the most significant were gender equity and increased self-confidence and belief in a better future.

Promoting Gender Equity and Empowerment

When TIDE's entrepreneurship project began, the cohort of entrepreneurs consisted entirely of males. TIDE came to realize that by failing to target women, they were failing to harness the full social potential of their program.

> We wanted to reach out to women, because we found that if you are looking at overall social development of a household, then money in a woman's hand is spent differently than money in a man's hand. We found that typically, women, if they have money, spend more on education, health, nutrition...even if a man is earning more money, it is not leading to a better life for his family...So we just said that if you are looking at an economic indicator, you would have gone with men. But, if you are looking at a social indicator, then you have to go with women. So we simply went with the women.[22]

This realization has led TIDE to create demand-led programs for rural women. Their model consists of a three-stage approach of initial diagnosis, identification and selection of interventions, and program design and convergence, to customize each program to the needs and wants of the community in which it is initiated. The customized model results in a sustainable and useful program for the community that will yield long term outcomes. TIDE chose to focus their gender equity promotion on rural women because "that's where the need for livelihood is highest."[29] One of the greatest difficulties that an outside organization trying to reach out to rural communities encounters is assimilation into or gaining the trust of the local community. To circumvent this problem, TIDE has partnered with grassroots-level NGOs and established self-help groups (SHGs) in rural India. The SHGs are groups of fewer than 20 people, usually women, that meet on a regular basis to support each other in a certain discipline. Membership in SHGs usually involves some sort of regular fee contribution to build a source of microcredit for members. The grassroots-level NGOs assist TIDE in identifying SHGs that focus on income generation, therefore targeting a subset of the demographic with a preexistent interest in livelihood generation. This strategy ensures local specificity and support, and enables a regular setting for data collection, analysis, training, and support, with an already established and locally trusted organizational body. This is why TIDE "ha[s] to choose these nonprofits very carefully, where they have a mandate for a sustainable livelihood program."[22] Through these networks, TIDE is able to leverage the credibility and trust of the SHG with which they connect, enabling them to provide the women with comprehensive training and support in establishing a sustainable livelihood designed to suit their community life, including familial obligations and geographic location.

TIDE's program designs the trainings with a holistic approach. The trainings teach the women about the technology that TIDE delivers to them and provides them with the skills and knowledge with which to make a living using the technology, but more important to TIDE, the trainings also address the many barriers that women must face to conduct this type of work, preparing and inspiring women with tools to help them overcome these obstacles. Social barriers that women entrepreneurs in TIDE's program encounter include lack of family support, mobility, cross-gender communication, cross-caste communication, and community norms. To address these barriers, TIDE's trainings are women only and focus on small group (10–15 members) engagement and include what they call "ice-breaker" activities. The trainings vary in length from 3 days to 7 days, but in general they follow a similar format with the first course focusing on a mix of life skills and microenterprise development and the latter part of the training on technical skills. The most important goal of the training is "To develop an attitude. The most important thing...to develop in a person, it will be attitude...positive, confident attitude."[30] This is done through various interactive small group activities, as well as through a video featuring the story of TIDE's most successful woman entrepreneur, Lalita Bai.

All these modalities are meant to convey the idea that with the right attitude, the women are capable of greatly improving their lives. Another major focus for empowering the women is developing their communication skills: "The skill to speak. It's a psychological approach. First...they are to...open up their minds, their ideas, their concepts. It's a kind of counseling also."[30]

One of the main barriers to women's participation in the entrepreneurship program can be lack of support from their family. TIDE participants spoke of some of these barriers specifically, including objections from "the household, the objection of the kids, the husband, the inlaws."[28] "I myself have seen many women having a problem. They will be very much interested as I am, but there are a lot of troubles at home and objections."[11] For the most part, this barrier is so large that TIDE has begun assessing family support as a prerequisite for enrollment in their program and has included how to negotiate personal wishes with family as a part of the training.

Even though empowering women to overcome social barriers could seem to be a conflict-laden process, TIDE is careful to be as sensitive as possible to the concerns of the villages and homes of its entrepreneurs. In fact, one of TIDE's founding principles is that whatever they do "must be socially and culturally acceptable...As society changes slowly, let us change, but let us not bring it into sharper conflict. In the sense that we would follow kind of a consensus-building rather than conflict-dissolving approach."[8]

TIDE's programs have already made substantial differences in the lives of the women involved. One female entrepreneur talked about how this program has given her the opportunity to explore her curiosity about different people and places:

> I always wanted to go out and know about the people—as to how they think and how they think in other villages and how our thinking changes once we set our foot out of the house.[11]

Many women spoke about learning how to cope with derision that they may encounter when they begin to behave differently as a result of pursuing their goals. One woman relayed:

> If I go to the villages...we do have to listen to a lot of harsh words...They ask us, "How does your husband let you go out?" And "How much you make for a stove?" And sometimes they really hurt us, but I take only the positive aspect and we choose to ignore the rest and we hardly talk and we mainly focus on the work aspect. But some people will never change however much you tell them.[11]

TIDE meets with experts in development and women's empowerment from around the country to exchange ideas, lessons, and best practices. As a means of expanding their program, TIDE has produced a consultative version designed to enable them to replicate their work with the women entrepreneurs in other fields. The program is summarized on a compact disc entitled "Reaching Rural Women," that addresses "designing demand-led programmes for rural women," as TIDE hopes to continue to expand their work in this area. Despite the difficulty in quantifying the outcomes of a program that targets gender equity and the empowerment of women, the stories of the women participating in TIDE's women's entrepreneurship program speak volumes about its importance.

Promoting Self-Confidence and Goals for a Better Future

One of the main social development issues that emerged during TIDE's entrepreneurship programs was self-confidence as a crucial factor in the success of an entrepreneur. For both TIDE's men's and women's projects, they "realized that the limitation there is their own personal limitation. And that they don't have higher aspiration levels."[22] With TIDE's women's programs, building confidence and setting goals in order to address the additional challenges they faced has been a central component for some time. TIDE recognized very early in the program that having a strong goal was a necessary motivating factor for women entrepreneurs. "Women [participants] who succeed are the ones…[who] have a particular goal. Like Lalita Bai, she wanted her daughter to become a teacher, so she found this is a good way to earn money to finance that."[31] Women's trainings use examples such as Shilpa, one of TIDE's most ambitious entrepreneur, to try to encourage women to set ambitious goals for their enterprises. At women-only trainings, Shilpa spoke openly and assertively, sharing her ambitions and dreams of marketing her products internationally, and teaching other women about how she is currently independently pursuing the certifications by which to do so. Women entrepreneurs spoke often of how participating in TIDE's programs had increased their overall confidence and changed the way they interacted with people. In the words of a female entrepreneur in the Sarala stove-building program: "Now actually I have just studied to fifth standard and even while studying I was not that bold and I did not know how to conduct myself. But now, I know how to communicate with people, how to deal with them, and how I will grow from inside once I talk to so many people."[11]

For male entrepreneurs, greater self-confidence was mostly gained through TIDE's regular training and support programs. Many male entrepreneurs told of how gaining technical expertise and soft skills through TIDE's trainings resulted in increased confidence in their own abilities. Madhav, an entrepreneur in Kerala, explained that he had initially had doubts about his capacity to carry out this work. After joining the program, he received training in soft skills such as how he should introduce himself to the client and how to give information about his products in addition to learning how to manufacture the stoves and driers. The skills gained during the training sessions followed by his experience as a successful entrepreneur have changed his view of his own potential: "So he is saying that when he went to the training program, he was not able to believe that he can be a professional like this. He was not dreaming that he would reach such a position. Now he is full-time professional, he is doing it very happily, he is very successful. But he was not able to even think that it will be a full-time job, even a full-time job. Now he has many things, he has reached a higher level than he expected."[32] Furthermore, TIDE's training program had given Madhav the confidence to communicate the importance of environmental sustainability to his village and surrounding communities.

TIDE has now set in place a program that specifically targets the need to build greater self-confidence in participants. In 2010, TIDE was approached by

BetterFuture (http://www.betterfutureindia.com), a Dutch management consultancy firm offering a GStar Corporate Social Responsibility–funded pilot project for personal development of entrepreneurs in Bangalore, India. The Better Future training of June 2010 was the first of its kind within TIDE's program. An introductory 1-day training session was focused entirely on personal and professional development, with aspiration building being the theme that ran through the day. The training took place in Bangalore, with entrepreneurs traveling as far as 14 hours from their villages to attend. The course, spread over a 1-year period, would focus on the areas of personal development, entrepreneurial skills, expectations and connections, microcredit, coaching, and evaluation and reflection.[33] During the introductory training session, participants took part in a series of exercises designed to have them reflect on and share their personal and business goals. At the end of the day, the group sat in a circle and participants openly shared their thoughts on the utility of the day's training with the group. One of the male entrepreneurs shared how he saw his situation as analogous to the roads in Bangalore, where the streets are winding, often unnamed, and where it is difficult to navigate. He considered BetterFuture as giving the entrepreneurs a navigation system, and now it was up to the entrepreneurs to use the navigation system to greatly improve their ability and efficiency in getting from point A to point B.[34]

LESSONS FOR SUCCESSFUL DISSEMINATION

Since beginning its green enterprise projects in 1998, TIDE has seen both successes and challenges, and it has adapted its approach to better incorporate these experiences. TIDE's work can provide valuable lessons for organizations implementing similar programs. TIDE's sustainability and impact have been largely determined by three main lessons TIDE has adopted: the importance of focusing on teaching entrepreneurial skills; the potential of the social benefits of the program as an important motivator for its participants; and the need to respect the local context.

Enterprise Trainings Should Include a Focus on Entrepreneurial Skills

TIDE's original project concept focused on recruiting and training individuals who already possessed the technical skills needed to construct TIDE's devices and to have them market and disseminate the products to create their own sustainable product and service enterprise. This focus on technical skills soon proved inadequate. "Initially we made the mistake that we thought we should go with engineers . . . or technically trained people. But very quickly we realized that technology is easier to accept, whereas entrepreneurial skills are very difficult to come by."[22] TIDE found that individuals with previous sales or business experience were able to pick up the technical aspects of the devices and were more adept at succeeding independently with their sale and distribution. Whereas technically trained individuals had a much harder time succeeding when it came time to set up their independent enterprises, despite receiving introductory trainings on how to start a small business. From this observation, TIDE realized that there was more to the equation than simply providing accounting, marketing, and finance education.

As a consequence, both TIDE's recruitment and training strategies were modified. They no longer recruited engineers and masons, but rather actively recruited individuals with sales and/or business experience. In addition, for those without previous sales or business experience, TIDE began to analyze what it was that made certain participants successful in sales and incorporate these lessons into the construction of trainings that emphasized the transmission of these entrepreneurial soft skills.

As an additional challenge, TIDE's trainees include people with a broad spectrum of literacy rates and educational backgrounds. Thus, TIDE's training programs focus on brief yet evocative lessons that use interactive modalities such as video presentations and group activities. In TIDE's current trainings, the entrepreneurial soft skills taught include developing confidence through disciplined action, improving communication skills, and harnessing aspirations and igniting motivation. Confidence in skills and abilities, and how diligence and persistence can build confidence, are woven into the trainings through group discussions and examples of other entrepreneurs. Goal setting and action steps are addressed at this time, and the training encourages participants to find what motivates them. Through group activities and role playing, TIDE's participants also practice communication skills in scenarios they are likely to encounter in a typical business day.

Social Benefits as a Powerful Motivator

The extent to which program participants embraced the social benefits of the program and were motivated by them was not something that TIDE initially anticipated. At the beginning of their program, TIDE saw financial benefits as the primary motivator for participants to become involved. Their recruitment efforts and trainings used financial gains to motivate trainees. They also educated them on the environmental benefits, which they saw as being a potential secondary motivation for some participants. What was unanticipated, however, was the powerful motivator that the social benefits of the program would become. While TIDE focuses on giving entrepreneurs opportunities to improve their own economic conditions, the feeling of working toward the greater good was repeatedly mentioned by entrepreneurs as an important motivation and source of satisfaction. TIDE suspected that of their two programs, the women would be more motivated by improving the well-being of their family, and this was what led to the creation of the women's project—money in a woman's hand would be spent on her family. However, through the interviews with male participants, it became apparent that the social benefit brought to their family and village was important for many. When hydroelectricity entrepreneur Ranveer talked about his motivation, he explained that he primarily aims to earn a living but that he also feels good when he can earn a living by making the lives of others better.[18] Ranveer related a story about how, as a boy, he was pushed by his village to get an education so that he could make a difference in the world. He describes this as the root of his social motivations: his village pushed him so he would be able to accomplish what he has, so in all he does he thinks about giving back to his village and ones like his own. He relayed how TIDE had given him the tools to help villages become electrified, and how in helping others, he can feel good about himself.[18] Women involved in running greenhouses and a midday meal scheme talked about how running village education programs was an enjoyment for them.[20] TIDE has since incorporated social benefits as an additional tool to motivate participants in the training and recruitment process. Future programs could benefit by continuing to harness the social benefits of the program during recruitment and training as well as during ongoing interactions that require motivating entrepreneurs.

Respecting the Local Context to Promote Sustainability

TIDE has recognized that in order for their projects to be sustainable over time, they must respect and adapt to the variable geographic, economic, and cultural milieus in which they operate.

Geographically, TIDE's projects take into account the resources available in each of their project locations when considering a technological intervention. For example, in Kerala, which is a coastal state, TIDE selected the biomass drier, which could process the abundant seafood resources available in Kerala. In Karnataka state, however, where the agricultural season is limited to the short monsoon months, Sarala stove building was chosen because it offered the stove builder year-round income generation, if necessary.

Economically, TIDE conducts a survey of local biomass-utilization process industries prior to selecting a technology in a given area. In this way, TIDE strategically identifies which industries it can profitably enter, and which should be avoided due to market saturation or other barriers.[9]

Culturally, TIDE has learned, especially through its women's project, that activities must be culturally acceptable. Specifically, this means that for women, activities required should generally not fall outside of existing gender norms. TIDE discovered that "even if women are temperamentally entrepreneurial, there are a lot of social obstacles they have to overcome."[22] TIDE respects the context in which their trainees exist and adapts their programs to meet the needs of their trainees while not overstepping boundaries that will cause them problems. For example, the women's program involves TIDE helping out with a lot of linkage building with suppliers and purchasers, as it is not always socially acceptable for women to be out on their own doing this type of networking. TIDE has also seen that women prefer to be near their families, have work that enables them flex time in which they can meet their domestic responsibilities, and also that the nature of the work should not require them to give up agricultural work, if that is their main source of income. As a response to this, TIDE focused on creating groups of women who could share responsibilities within an enterprise rather than having them run by individuals.

CONCLUSION

TIDE's green enterprise model brings together the creation of income-generating opportunities with environmental improvements. Giving rural individuals and groups the means to improve their income while improving their environment has led to a range of beneficial outcomes for participants and their families and communities, including health improvements through reduced air pollution, increased self-confidence, and gender equity. The sustainability demonstrated by TIDE's programs depends on their ability to adapt to local contexts and offer designs and technologies that are locally appropriate. In this way, green social enterprises can continue to promote greater health and well-being through environmentally sustainable economic growth.

NOTES

1. *The Millenium Development Goals Report, 2010*, United Nations, accessed April 30, 2013, http://www.un.org/millenniumgoals/pdf/MDG%20Report%202010%20En%20r15%20-low%20res%2020100615%20-.pdf#page=8
2. *Millenium Development Goals Indicators, 2012*, United Nations, accessed May 26, 2013, http://mdgs.un.org/unsd/mdg/Default.aspx
3. *Census Data, 2001: Rural-Urban Distribution*, Government of India, accessed May 29, 2012, http://censusindia.gov.in/Census_Data_2001/India_at_glance/rural.aspx
4. *Census Data, 2001: Number of Literates and Literacy Rate*, Government of India, accessed May 29, 2012, http://censusindia.gov.in/Census_Data_2001/India_at_glance/literates1.aspx

5. D. G. Bassani et al., "Child Mortality from Solid-Fuel Use in India: A Nationally-Representative Case-Control Study," *BMC Public Health* 10 (2010): 491. doi: 10.1186/1471-2458-10-491.

6. A. W. Johnson, "The Association of Household Pollutants and Socio-Economic Risk Factors with the Short-Term Outcome of Acute Lower Respiratory Infections in Hospitalized Pre-School Nigerian Children," *Annals of Tropical Paediatrics* 12, no. 4 (1992): 421–32.

7. V. Mishra, R. Retherford, "Cooking Smoke Increases the Risk of Acute Respiratory Infection in Children," *National Family Health Survey Bulletin* no. 8 (1997): 1–4.

8. Interview with Technology Informatics Design Endeavour Leadership, July 16, 2010, Bangalore, India.

9. Technology Informatics Design Endeavour, "Project Performance Report," in *Diffusion of Efficient Biomass Utilization Technologies in Non-formal Industries in Kerala and Karnataka*, ed. TIDE (Bangalore, India: ETC/TTP Netherlands, 2004).

10. Technology Informatics Design Endeavour, "Third Quarterly Report on the Program," in *Extension for the Technical Training in Household Stove Construction and Pilot Training in Charcoal Making from Waste Biomass*, (Bangalore, India: ETC/TTP/Netherlands, 2004-2005).

11. Translated interview with Female Stove Entrepreneur 2, June 7, 2010, Gubbi District, Karnataka, India.

12. Technology Informatics Design Endeavour, *Technology Report* (Bangalore, India: ETC/TTP Netherlands, 2003).

13. Interview with Sarala Stove Customer, June 19, 2010, Nagasumudra Village, India.

14. Translated interview with Female Stove Entrepreneur 1, June 7, 2010, Gubbi District, Karnataka, India.

15. Department of Science and Technology Grant Officer 2, *Memo of Personal Interview* (New Delhi, India: Department of Science and Technology, SEED Program, 2010).

16. Interview with Technology Informatics Design Endeavour Leadership, June 4, 2010, Bangalore, India.

17. Translated interview with Male Production Entrepreneur, June 20, 2010, Shimoga, India.

18. Interview with Hydroelectricity Entrepreneur, June 20, 2010, Shimoga, India.

19. Interview with Production Entrepreneur, June 30, 2010, Bangalore, India.

20. Interview with Female Polyhouse Entrepreneurs, June 7, 2010, Byapura Village, India.

21. Translated interview with Male Entrepreneur, June 30, 2010, Bangalore, India.

22. Interview with Technology Informatics Design Endeavour Leadership, May 24, 2010, Bangalore, India.

23. Technology Informatics Design Endeavour, "Final Report," in *Extension of the Technical Training in Household Stove Construction and Pilot Training in Charcoal Making From Waste Biomass* (Bangalore, India: ETC/TTP Netherlands, 2006).

24. Interview with Technology Informatics Design Endeavour Leadership, July 9, 2010, Bangalore, India.

25. *Woman Exemplar Award*, Confederation of Indian Industry, accessed January 23, 2011, http://www.cii.in/AwardsDetail.aspx?enc=Y724SUiQraY7VcDZjgBoGO+FafhuVoTI1PIzPlzbMbY=

26. Interview with Lalita Bai, June 7, 2010, Tiptur, Karnataka, India.

27. Translated interview with Entrepreneur, B. D. W., June 26, 2010, Bangalore, India.
28. Translated interview with Female Solar Product Entrepreneur, June 7, 2010, Tiptur Taluk, India.
29. Interview with Technology Informatics Design Endeavour Leadership, June 9, 2010, Bangalore, India.
30. Translated interview with Kudumbashree Trainer, May 27, 2010, Puruva, India.
31. Interview with Technology Informatics Design Endeavour Leadership, June 1, 2010, Bangalore, India.
32. Translated Interview with Male Entrepreneur 2, May 27, 2010, Peruva, India.
33. S. Lockhart, Field Journal 1 (June 26, 2010).
34. Memo: Better Future Entrepreneurial Training, June 26, 2010. Memo author: Shannon Lockhart, company name: Better Future, place of distribution: Bangalore, Karnataka, India.

SECTION 2

Addressing Specific Environmental Challenges in an Economically Sustainable Way

Moving Toward Sustainable Urban Transport

How Can We Integrate Environmental, Health, and Equity Objectives Globally?

DAVID BANISTER AND JAMES WOODCOCK

Transport and travel can bring enormous benefits, as economies have become globalized, and as many transactions are now facilitated through relatively cheap networks and communications infrastructures. In high-income countries and among the growing middle classes of middle-income countries, expectations of travel have accelerated, and aspirations have been raised through media coverage, education, and increasing income.[1] But we also live in a carbon-dependent society, and carbon emissions are affecting the global climate with irreversible long-term consequences. Transport is the one major sector that has not made any contribution to a reduction in energy use and emissions. Equity is also a major issue, as many of the new opportunities for greater mobility have occurred very unequally across the global population, with lower income groups typically suffering more of the adverse consequences without reaping the benefits. The environmental limits and social inequities of the current transport situation make it economically and socially unsustainable and lead to detrimental impacts on population health. Rather than improve, the situation has worsened since global awareness of the potential impact of climate change was recognized at the Rio Summit (1992).

This chapter has two main aims. The first aim is to describe some of the major changes that are taking place in global cities, which with their huge increases in population are the economic powerhouses of the 21st century. Although economic growth and increased wealth is important for development, particularly in lower income countries, it will be argued that cities need to give equal value to issues relating to the environment, quality of life, and the health and well-being of the population. Such a change in thinking can be encompassed within the sustainable mobility paradigm,[2] which links together reduced dependence on carbon-based energy sources with broader societal benefits.

The second aim is to move the debate on sustainable transport forward to cover healthy, equitable, and sustainable transport by arguing strongly for more active transport. High-income countries have long suffered from physical inactivity, which both directly increases the risk of chronic disease and indirectly throws energy metabolism out of balance, thereby increasing overweight and obesity.[3] In the lower income countries, urbanization and motorization are bringing about a rapid increase in diseases associated with inactivity, air pollution, and road traffic injuries. The more active forms of transport (walking, cycling, and bus and rail—where these include a walk or cycle stage) can be at the core of the accessible city, while at the same time contributing to better health, social equality, and reducing emissions of carbon and other more local pollutants. Although investment is required, these options are comparatively inexpensive and can be accommodated in the new megacities that will be a global feature by 2050. However, while the problems of urban growth, traffic congestion, environment, health, and equity objectives could theoretically be resolved at a low cost through initiatives targeting increased use of active transport and decreased dependence on personal vehicles, it seems that in practice there is an inexorable move away from such initiatives.

CITIES AND SUSTAINABLE TRANSPORT

Over 50 percent of the world's population are now classified as urban dwellers (2005), and it is expected that this will increase to 70 percent by 2050,[4] as globally, the rate of urbanisation is 3 million per week. These levels of urbanization are already apparent in Europe, North America, and Latin America.[5]

In lower and middle-income countries the largest cities, megacities (population over 10 million) are generally characterized by high population growth, both from natural increase and inward migration, and a huge expansion in the urban area with substantial new requirements for both housing and jobs, in addition to transport. These megacities have tremendous potential for economic growth, but simultaneously they are centers for potential unrest, as there is substantial inequality and poverty.[6,7] The challenges for governments are daunting—with little space for expansion in the original cities, there is extensive urban sprawl with increased distances between where the people live, their jobs, and other facilities. The concept of monocentric cities is becoming less relevant, as they are rapidly developing as polycentric urban agglomerations, often absorbing smaller cities in the process. Many local governments have taken on a leadership role in addressing the transport problems as they relate to carbon emissions, but there is considerable variation between cities. For example, more than half the total energy consumption in Mexico City, Hong Kong, and Cape Town is land transport based,[8] while it remains at approximately one-quarter in many European cities (for example, London and Paris). This reflects the different strategies adopted by city planners, such as promoting the use of the car through investment in roads and free parking, to demand management and constraints on the use of the car, and investment in local facilities and in public transport.

Given the rise in urbanization around the world and the increased access to motor vehicles, the rate of increase in the supply of motorized transport infrastructure will never match the growth in demand. Attempting this would have enormous environmental, social, and health implications and would not "solve" the problem, as can be seen in many cities in high-income countries.

Current investment in transport infrastructure and services does not benefit all groups equally. Typically greater benefits are realized by higher income groups who have the means to take advantage of the improved transportation. In the United Kingdom the Sustainable Development Commission estimated that the richest 10 percent of the population effectively receive four times greater public expenditure on transport than the poorest 10 percent.[9] This inequality is even more pronounced in many lower income cities where investment is spent on infrastructure for cars, access to which is limited to higher income groups. In many low- and middle-income cities, public transport largely consists of informal vehicles, often with little consideration given to safety. The poorest cannot afford public transport and so have no option but to walk.[10] While walking can be a natural, healthy, and pleasant way to travel, it is often experienced as a necessity traversing a polluted and dangerous environment in which the pedestrian is seen as a second-class citizen.[11]

The environmental and public health needs of higher income and lower income cities contain both similarities and differences. In higher income cities quality of life, air pollution, and noncommunicable diseases resulting from excessive energy intake and inactivity are the most pressing burdens. In many lower income cities there remain basic unmet needs for clean water, electricity, waste management, and sanitation. However, it must not be forgotten that in many rapidly motorizing middle and lower income cities, air pollution is worse and the burden from noncommunicable diseases greater than in higher income cities.

All cities contribute, if unequally, to global emissions, and they have a responsibility to reduce these, but the desire for economic growth often takes precedence over other priorities. High-income cities have the opportunity to substantially reduce emissions through investment in clean technology, energy efficiency, and a switch from energy-intensive to lower carbon modes. For low-income cities, the challenges are even greater, as they have other pressing social needs to address, but investment in sustainable transport is still possible. Some of these low-income cities until recently have had high levels of walking and cycling, but this is being rapidly lost through motorization and the increased distances needed to reach desired destinations (Table 7.1); in particular, cycling has suffered as cars and powered two wheelers dominate the roads.

Climate change and related natural hazards will have a major impact on cities, many of which are located on the coast or along the major rivers, as historically they have been centers of trade. These locations are increasingly prone to flooding, caused by storm surges and high winds, and accentuated by global warming (+2°C) and sea level rise.[12] About 40 percent of the world's cities (1–10 million) and 15 of the 20 megacities lie on the coast. Their vulnerability to flooding has been substantially increased, and some have taken action to reduce the potential impacts, but 40 million or 10 percent of the total population are exposed to a 1 in 100 year coastal flood event, and this is predicted to rise to 150 million in 2070.[13]

Though some cities are moving away from active transport options, there are good examples where development has been seen as investment, with the basic infrastructure such as transportation and improved housing for low-income residents being provided as part of the urbanization process, as in Guangzhou City (Pearl River). Conversely, higher densities can be achieved through compactness and integrated approaches that combine investment in high-capacity public transport and development, as in Hong Kong or Singapore (around their metro systems) or in Curitiba (around its bus rapid transit system). Strong city-level governance is essential, where there is a clear vision about the future of the city, and where there is both the power and resources for action. But above all, there is a need for leadership and for all stakeholders

Table 7.1. MODAL SPLIT IN SOME SOUTH ASIAN CITIES (2001)

	Total Trips (%)		
Cities	Private Transport	Public Transport	Nonmotorized Transport
Lahore	24	16	60
Karachi	27	23	50
Delhi	18	40	42
Mumbai	18	60	22
Kolkata	5	78	17

Source: A. K. Jain (2011), "Sustainable Urban Mobility in Southern Asia," Regional study prepared for Sustainable Urban mobility, Global Report on Human Settlements 2013, UN Habitat, Nairobi.

to engage with the process of city building, so that responsibilities and actions are both supported and implemented effectively. This is the only way to move toward the sustainable city. The alternative is one of weak governance, where there is no direction and the consequences are huge sprawling divided cities— this is the inefficient and unsustainable city.

To summarize, there are four major urban transport issues, which impact on its sustainability. First, urban transport is totally dependent on nonrenewable fuels, with about 62 percent of global oil now being used in the transport sector (over 70 percent in the OECD countries[14]). This brings up generic issues relating to the availability of oil, the notions of "peak oil," volatility in oil prices, the costs of subsidy to oil in some countries, and energy security.[15] Irrespective of the wider environmental imperative, transport needs to diversify its sources of energy and to decarbonize.

Secondly, there are the impacts of urban transport on climate change. Climate change poses a major threat to human health and development. The IPCC fourth report estimates that the resilience of many ecosystems may well be exceeded this century. By mid-century there will be a 10–30 percent decline in water availability in some already water-stressed areas. Even earlier, by 2020, in Africa an additional 75 million and 250 million people could face increased water shortages. As well as increasing water stress, millions of additional people could be affected by flooding every year due to sea-level rise by the 2080s. Low-lying areas with high population density and high levels of poverty are at greatest risk. Africa, the area with the lowest per capita greenhouse gas emissions, is particularly vulnerable to climate change due to the combination of multiple environmental stresses and poverty. There is also a considerable intergenerational inequity with future generations expected to bear the cost of current emissions. Overall the global impact on health is anticipated to be predominately harmful, particularly in developing countries, and is expected to become considerably larger from the middle of the 21st century. In this context there is a strong argument for reducing greenhouse gas emissions in all sectors, including transport.

As one important example, the United States produces over 21 percent (2006) of the carbon emissions from energy (including transport), yet it is not part of any international agreement to reduce its emissions.[16] Over the recent past it has increased its CO_2 emissions by 14 percent, while global levels of CO_2 increased by 24 percent (1995–2005). Although only 5 percent of the world's population lives in the United States, it has 30 percent of the cars and produces 45 percent of global car-based CO_2 emissions.[17] It is crucial that the United States is fully engaged in the international debates about reducing levels of carbon emissions. Only very recently has the US motor industry seemingly become aware of the need to produce a range of fuel-efficient vehicles. The American Recovery and Reinvestment Act (2009) has allocated more than US$80 billion to the generation of renewable energy, investment in clean technology, advancing vehicle and fuel technologies, and building a smarter electric grid. There are also new efficiency standards for cars and trucks.[18]

Third, urban transport is energy intensive, and one of the principal means by which energy use in transport can be made more efficient is through using the most efficient technologies available and ensuring that all transport is operating at capacity. Running empty cars and buses is not efficient, and full public transport is more efficient than full cars. Table 7.2 shows the typical transport energy characteristics in cities in developing countries where the fuel consumption characteristics of the vehicles are combined with occupancy levels to give the energy intensity figures.

Fourth, there has been a striking growth in car dependence of cities and urban sprawl. The central issue here is the role that increasing levels of motorization can have in promoting decentralization, and the second round effects that to live in suburban areas requires the ownership of a car. Motorization and congestion can form a vicious circle. In congested streets the car offers more control than public transit to those who can afford it as alternative routes can be used. As the distance between services and facilities (including homes and work) becomes longer, so it consequently becomes more difficult to walk or cycle, further increasing the pressure to use a car.

This chapter now addresses some of these issues from the perspective of health and equity. At one level the alternatives are clear, namely that there should be a much greater emphasis placed on the active forms of transport, for environmental, health, and equity reasons, as well as cost of investments. As the following sections will show, the current reality of transport policies is the opposite. The growth of motorized transport is still totally dependent on carbon energy sources, it is hugely expensive in terms of infrastructure costs, there are substantial negative health implications, and its availability is inequitable. The last sections of the chapter describe potential solutions and recommendations for moving forward toward sustainable transport.

Table 7.2. ENERGY EFFICIENCY CHARACTERISTICS FOR TRANSPORT MODES IN DEVELOPING COUNTRIES

	Fuel Consumption (l/100 km)	Energy Use (MJ/vkm)	Vehicle Occupancy (pkm/vkm)	Energy Intensity (MJ/pkm)
Urban bus	23–53	8.2–19	50	0.16–0.44
Motorcycle	2.2–2.3	0.71–0.74	1.5	0.47–0.49
Car	8.5–14	2.7–4.5	2.5	1.1–1.8

MJ, mega joules; pkm and vkm are passenger and vehicle kilometres traveled, respectively.

HEALTH AND EQUITY IMPACTS OF TRANSPORT

Local Air Pollution

Issue

Local air pollution is a key concern in many cities. Included here are particulate matter ($PM_{2.5}$, PM_{10}); nitrous oxides (NO_x, NO_2); volatile organic compounds (VOCs), which can react to produce ozone; and sulphur dioxide (SO_2). The oxides of nitrogen and sulphur contribute to acid rain, while other pollutants directly and indirectly affect health. A systematic review of the effects of transport pollution found good evidence for an increase in all-cause mortality, respiratory morbidity, allergic illness and symptoms, cardiopulmonary mortality, nonallergic respiratory disease, and myocardial infarction plus a possible link to lung cancer.[19] Long-term decreases in air pollution are associated with reduced bronchial hyperactivity and respiratory and cardiovascular disease, and consequent gains in life expectancy.

According to the World Health Organization (WHO) Global Burden of Disease study, lead exposure, primarily from transport sources, led to the loss of 12.9 million DALYs[20] in 2002.[21] After lead, the strongest evidence for a specific pollutant is for particulate matter (PM) in particular particles with an aerodynamic diameter 2.5 μm or less ($PM_{2.5}$).[22] In addition to tail pipe emissions, motor vehicles can produce particulate matter through resuspension of road dust, and break and tire wear.[23] Recent modeling evidence concludes that anthropogenic $PM_{2.5}$ is associated with approximately 3.5 million cardiopulmonary and 220,000 lung cancer mortalities annually, resulting in an estimated 30 million years of life lost.[24]

The same study estimated that global ozone pollution was responsible for approximately 700,000 respiratory mortalities.[25] Through emission of the precursors, transport indirectly is a source of ozone emissions. Time series studies have linked short-term variation in ozone to mortality, and there is also some evidence on longer term exposure.[26] Rising temperatures from climate change may exacerbate these problems of ozone pollution.

Road transport produces approximately 20 percent of black carbon emissions, a type of particulate matter,[27] which is of increasing concern to both climate scientists and epidemiologists. Its color and distribution make it a significant short-lived greenhouse gas pollutant,[28] while it might be more harmful to health than other types of particulate matter.[29]

The health impacts of local air pollution are linked to socioeconomic equity. Since traffic-related air pollution is unevenly distributed, exposure varies and lower income urban populations tend to live in the more polluted environments. For example, a recent study in London found that mean air pollution concentrations were generally higher in areas of low socioeconomic position.[30] There is also evidence that people of lower socioeconomic status living in the most deprived areas suffer more from the same exposure.[31]

In the transport sector in Europe, the main policy mechanism to tackle air pollution at the local level has been through regulations on emission standards, set by the European Union (EU) through a gradual increase in the quality of fuel used and through the increased effectiveness of add-on technologies.[32] In large part due to these standards, the EU-27 managed to achieve considerable reductions in transport-related emissions of NOx, CO, and VOC, with a small reduction in $PM_{2.5}$, between 1990 and 2005.[33]

However, since 2000 there has been no overall fall in the population-weighted exposure to the two pollutants most strongly associated with adverse health impacts, PM_{10} or ozone.[34] The steps from emissions to exposure are complex, but much of the explanation lies with urbanization combined with increasing vehicle distance traveled and dieselization of the vehicle fleet. It is predicted that compared with 2008 levels, EU-27 emissions of primary $PM_{2.5}$ are currently similar or even slightly higher, although substantial reductions could be achieved. To achieve the hoped-for reductions, some cities have designated areas as low emissions zones where only "clean" vehicles are permitted to enter, and these areas are now being used to meet air quality obligations as nonconforming vehicles are either excluded or charged for entry.

Although low-emission zones are likely to benefit all city populations, there is conflicting evidence as to whether they disproportionately benefit lower income or higher income groups. A health impact modeling study of the socioeconomic distribution of mortality benefits from reduced air pollution due to the London Congestion Charge estimated the largest health benefits in the most deprived areas of London.[35] On the other hand, a study of the effect of the low emission zone in Rome found that it benefited people in the highest socioeconomic group (1,387 years of life gained per 100,000 people) more than those in the lowest group (340 years of life gained per 100,000 people).[36] Low emission zones have been found to be cost effective in terms of health benefits. For Germany it was estimated the health benefits of low emission zones (based on statistical value of a human life) were around double the cost (of replacing vehicles).[37]

Trends in emissions are largely determined by the competing trends of cleaner vehicles and longer distances. In the case of particulate matter even when tail pipe emissions have been reduced, tire and brake wear contribute to emissions. If strategies can actually halt the rise in vehicle distances in lower income countries and reduce distances in higher income countries, then it becomes far easier to see substantial improvements in air quality.

Although regulations and standards have costs associated with them, the benefits to the local affected population are seen to outweigh those costs. The main benefit is from the direct improvement in population health, but there could also be fewer working days lost due to sickness, and benefits from a more general increase in the attractiveness of city living. Attention needs to be paid to ensure that those benefits reach the entire population, particularly lower income groups that are disproportionately affected by local air pollution.

Road Traffic Injuries

Issue

The WHO World Report on Road Traffic Injury Prevention estimated that 1.2 million people were killed and 50 million people injured in road traffic crashes in 2002.[38] Although road traffic injuries have been falling across many higher income countries (10.3 fatalities per 100,000 population), within the more populous lower to middle-income countries rates have generally been on the rise (21.5 in lower income and 19.5 in middle-income countries), and road traffic injuries feature among the leading causes of disease burden in many developing countries. The global status report suggests that these impacts equate to US$518 billion or about 1–2 percent of global gross domestic product.[39] In the United Kingdom, the total impact of road crashes (2009) has been put at equivalent to £15 billion per year, with 78 percent of this figure being attributed to urban areas (with speed limits under 40 mph). Much of this cost is quantifying the loss of human life in monetary terms; the rest relates to the casualty in terms of loss of output, medical and ambulance treatment, and the costs of dealing with the crash, including policing, administration, and damage to property (33 percent of total).

The highest road death rate is in the African continent (28 deaths per 100,000 population per year), and the highest national rates are in El Salvador (42 per 100,000 per year) and the Dominican Republic (41 per 100,000 per year).[40] In India the rate of road traffic fatalities increased by an average of 5 percent per year between 1980 and 2000. Since then the rate of increase has accelerated to around 8 percent per year, with, in 2006, 105,725 people killed.[41]

In lower and middle-income countries, the majority of those killed are pedestrians, cyclists, and users of two-wheeled motor vehicles, in other words, those less likely to have the means to have access to a car. A recent systematic review found that 45 percent of road traffic fatalities in low-income countries were among pedestrians, compared with an estimated 29 percent in middle-income countries and 18 percent in high-income countries. In absolute terms an estimated annual total of 228,000 pedestrians die from traffic-related injuries in low-income countries, 162,000 in middle-income countries, and 23,000 in high-income countries.[35] Current policy is inadequate to protect these road users, with only 29 percent of countries meeting basic criteria for reducing speed in urban areas, and less than 10 percent rating their enforcement of traffic laws as effective.[42,43] High-income countries also present inequalities in traffic-related injuries and deaths. In the United Kingdom among children these are over 20 times higher in the lowest socioeconomic group for pedestrians and cyclists.

The differing trend in the direction of road traffic injuries between the high- and lower income countries is part of a global picture in which road traffic injuries rise and then fall with increasing motorization and economic growth. Cross sectional and time series studies have found that at low levels of motor vehicle ownership road traffic fatalities increase, while at higher levels of motor vehicle ownership road traffic deaths decline in absolute terms, giving an inverse U-shaped relationship (see Fig. 7.1).[44] Recent models have tended to focus on the relationship between per capita income and road traffic injuries and deaths, and have found a similar inverse U-shaped relationship.[45]

One recent cross sectional study, including data from 44 countries, found that mortality peaked among low-income countries at about 100 motor vehicles per 1,000 people and a per capita income of US$2,200.[46] It found that most of the increase in deaths below 100 motor vehicles per population was due to increasing occupant, pedestrian, and motor cyclist deaths, with the decline at higher rates coming mainly from decreasing number of pedestrians.

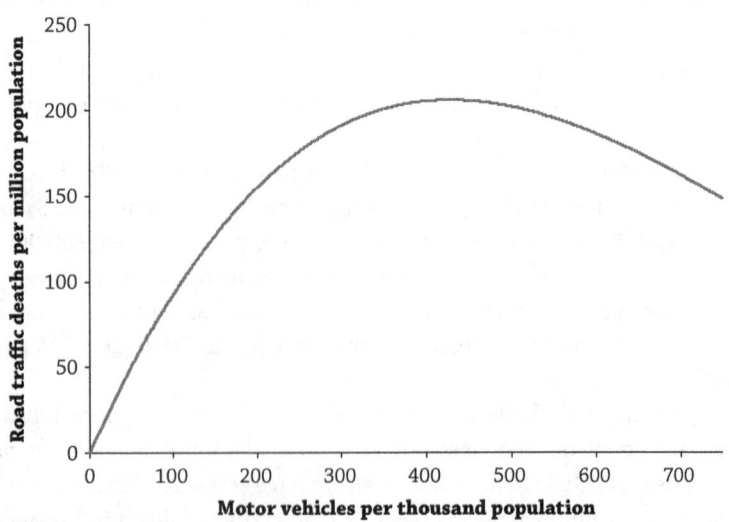

Figure 7.1:
Inverse U-shaped relationship between motor vehicle ownership and road traffic deaths. (From C. Koren and A. Borsos, "Is Smeed's Law Still Valid? A World-Wide Analysis of the Trends in Fatality Rate," *Journal of Society for Transportation and Traffic Studies* 1, no. 1 (2010): 64–76.)

Many countries are still in the upward phase of this trend, and it is likely that road traffic injuries will continue to increase with the rise in motor vehicle use. However, if injury rates start to fall because modal shift from walking to motor vehicle has passed the threshold described earlier, then the environmental effects are likely to be devastating, as this implies a vast increase in motor vehicle use. The resulting effects on physical activity levels would also be extremely detrimental for population health.

However, not all the fall in injuries in higher income countries can be attributed to less walking and cycling. In the EU, 57,691 people died in road traffic collisions in 1999, but by 2008 the number of fatalities had fallen to 38,875.[47] This huge reduction in road deaths can be attributed to a range of factors, including improved health care and the taking of concerted action at the European level.

Responses

Policies can play a vital role in decreasing road traffic accidents and deaths, as seen in the case of European standards and regulations. To begin with, cars are now safer for their occupants due to their heavier construction, crumple zones and airbags, and driving tests, and standards are considerably higher. The introduction and enforcement of severe penalties for drinking and driving, the use of penalty points for driving, enforcement of speed limits, the compulsory use of seat belts, and more general education programs have all helped. The explanation for the fall in fatalities among pedestrians and cyclists is less clear than that for motorists. Although danger reduction (e.g., lower speeds and less drunk driving) has played a role, there is also likely to have been a contribution from behavior modification on the part of the pedestrians and cyclists. In some countries this has meant less total walking and cycling and in many countries activity restriction, such as reduced independent mobility of children has continued (see section on "Physical Activity, Overweight, and Obesity"). In some countries, such as the United Kingdom, fewer young drivers may also have reduced the injury burden. It should also be noted that even in countries where overall injuries are falling the number of injuries is still sensitive to changes in traffic volume.[48]

Within the EU, fatality rates vary greatly by country. The lowest death rates from road collisions are in the Netherlands, Sweden, and the United Kingdom, with rates in Italy and France twice as high, and rates in Greece, Poland, and Latvia more than three times as high. It is interesting to note that there may be different ways to achieve a low rate. The two countries with the lowest overall road traffic fatality per million population in Europe are the Netherlands (39 deaths per million people) and the United Kingdom (38 deaths per million people) in 2009, despite the much higher rates of cycling in the Netherlands.[49] Although the United Kingdom has taken steps to reduce road danger (e.g., speed cameras and 20 mph zones[50]), it appears to be much safer to cycle and to walk in the Netherlands. The low injury risk in the Netherlands for cyclists is a result of a number of factors, including provision of a high-quality infrastructure for cyclists, priority for cyclists at junctions, and strict liability legislation in favor of cyclists and pedestrians.[51] The large number of cyclists has acted both as a spur for better provision for cyclists and itself increases the awareness of drivers of cyclists. Safety in numbers may play a part in making walking and cycling safer, but the relative contribution of direct measures to reduce risk compared with a pure safety in numbers effect is not yet clear.[52]

The aim of policy should be road danger reduction rather than an approach to safety that restricts the mobility of pedestrians and cyclists. Speed reduction is a vital policy tool for reducing road danger. At 20 mph the risk of a pedestrian fatality in a collision with a car is 5 percent, while at 40 mph it is over 80 percent. The WHO advocates a combined approach to speed reduction and lays out practical measures for measuring and tackling the problems in its manuals. Tackling speed involves appropriate speed limits starting from a safe system approach; considering the safety of the most vulnerable road users, roads with large numbers of vulnerable road users should not exceed 20 mph. Limits need to be enforced both through legislation but also through design. Low- to medium-cost engineering options have demonstrated benefits. A UK study found that 20 mph speed zones with physical enforcement reduced overall road traffic injuries with the greatest benefit in younger children.

Other measures include provision of high-quality infrastructure for pedestrians and cyclists and legislation and enforcement to stop drunk driving.[53] Speed cameras can also play an important role. A systematic review of speed cameras demonstrated effectiveness in reducing crashes (from 8 percent to 49 percent for all crashes) and fatal and serious injuries (11 percent to 44 percent).[54] Educational campaigns can have a positive effect in some circumstances. Public education campaigns to win community support by highlighting the dangers of speeding and drunk driving and promoting support for enforcement can be effective. However, providing more training for drivers is unlikely to work.[55] School-based driver education has been found to lead to an increase in injuries by leading to people driving at a younger age, while in existing drivers increases in skill can lead to taking of greater risks.

Physical Activity, Overweight, and Obesity

Issue

Physical activity arises from two sources, bodily movement and resistance activity. Walking is perhaps the most obvious form of bodily movement, while cycling combines both bodily movement and resistance activity. Over the past century, in many settings, oil has displaced food as the main energy source for human movement with the subsequent danger from motor vehicles acting as an additional disincentive to active transport.[56] Lack of physical activity is a risk factor for many chronic diseases and obesity and comes with wider social and economic costs.

The Global Burden of Disease (GBD) study estimated that 17 percent of the global population was inactive[57] and that this ranged from 10 percent in Africa D region[58] to 25 percent in the European C region,[59] while 41 percent of the world's population was insufficiently active, varying between regions from 32 percent to 52 percent.[60]

This study was not able to estimate inequalities based on socioeconomic group. It is likely that in lower income countries high-income people are less likely to be active, because lower income groups have to walk for transport and are more likely to be working in manual jobs, while in higher income countries the picture is different as higher income populations have better access to sports and leisure facilities and are more attuned to health promotion messages. However, the picture in many lower income urban environments is changing with the rapidly growing obesity epidemic and burden of noncommunicable diseases.

The example of the United Kingdom gives a clear indication of what has happened in terms of the move from active to motorized transport, and this picture is reflected in most other rich countries, and increasingly in the poorer countries as well. In the United Kingdom in 1949 the total distance traveled by bicycle was greater than the vehicle distance traveled by car but, while the distance traveled by car has subsequently increased 20 fold, the distance cycled fell by a factor of 6 between the early 1950s until the early 1970s,[61] and the distance cycled has not risen substantially since (Fig. 7.2).

For walking, national statistics for the United Kingdom are only available since the 1970s. These figures indicate that since the mid-1970s there has been a decline of around a third in minutes per day walking for transport (Fig 7.3). Given longer term trends in availability of motorized transport, it is likely that time spent walking has fallen over a much longer period. There are few good-quality direct data on long-term trends in physical activity, but many other trends in physical activity are likely to have exacerbated declining physical activity from active transport. Walking provides an important contribution to children's physical activity, with walking to school expending more energy than from organized sports and physical education.[62] Children are more likely to be taken by car to structured activities, while they are more likely to walk to unstructured activities. With rising motorization children's independent mobility has been radically curtailed.[63] Even in the short period between 2002 and 2008, the percentage of children aged 7 to 10 years in the United Kingdom not allowed to cross the road alone increased from 41 percent to 50 percent.[64] In 2008, 58 percent of adults gave traffic danger as the reason for accompanying their children to school.

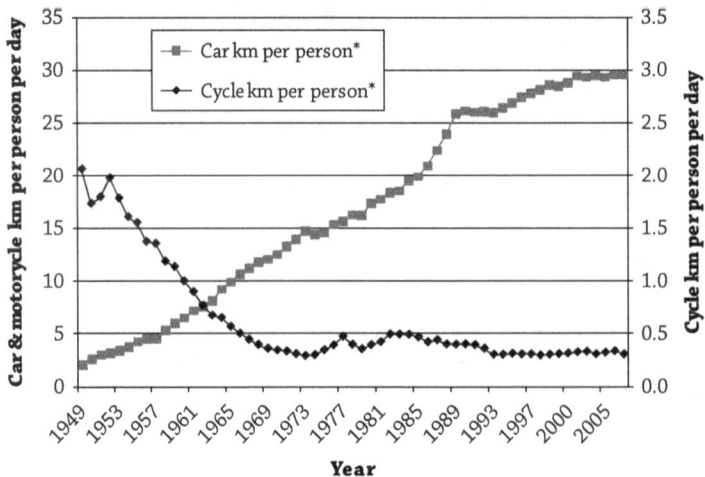

Figure 7.2:
Comparison of trends in distance cycled and driven in the United Kingdom. (Department for Transport, "National Travel Survey: 2007," [London: National Statistics; 2008].)
These figures show the total distance traveled by each type of vehicle in the United Kingdom in 1 year divided by the population in that year. On the right-hand axis we see the distance traveled per person by bike and on the left-hand axis (using a 10 times greater scale) we see the distance traveled by car and motorcycle.

Though there are fewer data available on walking and cycling in low- and middle-income countries, similar trends away from active transport are becoming evident. In many cities in developing countries, cycling rates have fallen substantially. Urban India has seen a substantial drop in cycling,[65] while

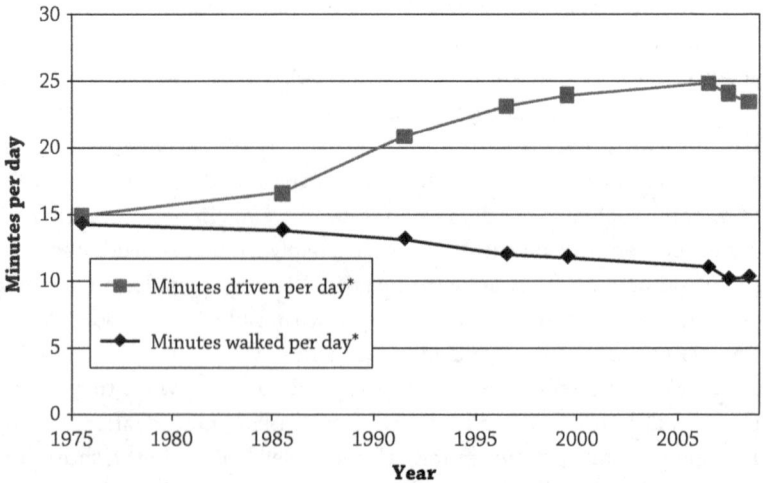

Figure 7.3:
Comparison of trends in time spent walking and driving in the United Kingdom. (Department for Transport, "National Travel Survey: 2007," [London: National Statistics; 2008].)
Estimate of total time spent walking or driving for transport in the United Kingdom per day divided by the population size (does not include time spent as a car passenger).

in Nairobi bicycle share fell from 20 percent in the 1970s to 0.5 percent in 2004.[66] Even where cycling has fallen many lower income cities retain a large, captive, walking population who do not have the option of using motorized transport, particularly if public transport systems are unavailable or expensive.[67] As discussed in a previous section, though more physically active, this population is often at greater risk of injury.

The GBD study estimated that compared with a scenario in which everyone was active, current levels of inactivity and insufficient activity were responsible for 3.3 percent of deaths and 19 million (DALYs) worldwide. The condition-specific burden was estimated at 21.5 percent of the burden from ischemic heart disease, 11 percent of ischemic stroke, 14 percent of diabetes, 16 percent colon cancer, and 10 percent of breast cancer. A more recent systematic review found strong evidence of links between physical inactivity and the risk of diabetes, heart disease, colon cancer, strokes and breast cancer, depression, dementia, hypertension, and osteoporosis.[68]

Health burdens associated with inactivity are not just problems in high- but also in lower income countries. In low-income and middle-income countries, urbanization is associated with an increased health burden from noncommunicable diseases.[69] The prevalence of Type 2 diabetes in urban adults in India is reported to have increased from less than 3 percent in 1970 to around 12 percent by 2000.[70] Cardiovascular disease accounts for 27 percent of deaths in low-income countries. By contrast, HIV/AIDS, tuberculosis, and malaria combined account for 11 percent of deaths.[71] In China, a recent study found that the age-standardized prevalence of diabetes was 9.7 percent, equivalent to 92.4 million adults.

Physical activity is not only directly beneficial to human health but also forms one side of the energy equation. According to the GBD study, obesity accounts for 30 million DALYs lost,[72] and it accounts for an additional health burden beyond that of physical inactivity. If energy consumption exceeds energy expenditure, then an increase in body mass index (BMI) is the result. Conversely, increasing physical activity increases energy expenditure; and if energy intake remains constant, then mass will fall until energy balance is restored at a new lower mass. Because for many people food-energy intake has not fallen in line with declining physical activity, many countries are experiencing an epidemic of obesity.[73,74] A cross sectional study in Atlanta (Georgia, USA) found that each additional hour spent in a car per day was associated with a 6 percent increase in the chances of obesity.[75]

Studies have linked the rise in obesity to the level of inequality within a country[76] and to the market-liberal welfare regimens.[77] These studies have focused on the energy side of the equation, but the rise in obesity is always a result of the imbalance between the inputs and outputs. In addition to these between-country differences, within a country obesity tends to follow a socio-economic gradient.

The problem is not just those who exceed the threshold for obesity but a population BMI distribution that has shifted to the right due to the changing nature of the environment. A focus on the obese can lead to questions on why they are obese and not others. This means that factors such as genes are likely to play a role, while a focus on the shifting distribution leads to an understanding of the social and environmental causes.

Responses

Recommendations for a healthy life focus on achieving four or five sessions per week of at least 30 minutes of moderate or vigorous physical activity, with greater amounts of physical activity likely to be required to avoid the build-up of obesity. Brisk walking and cycling both count as such activity. However, all walking appears to be beneficial. The relationship between physical activity and all-cause mortality appears to be nonlinear, with the greatest gain coming from moving from a sedentary lifestyle to a small amount of activity, although there is no obvious threshold.

Policy responses need to address inactivity by making walking and cycling a viable option, and ensuring that the benefits of active transport are not outweighed by the risk of injury or death. Research has found that increased levels of walking or cycling are associated with safer walking or cycling.[78,79] However, uncertainties remain about the causal direction of this relationship, the scale at which it occurs, and whether a threshold in cycling levels is needed to realize it.[80] Increasing the attractiveness of cycling requires making cycling both objectively and subjectively safer. Well-designed segregated infrastructure with attention to junction design is likely to play an important role in making cycling feel safer, particularly for more marginal cyclists, and may make cycling objectively safer.[81] The low injury risk in the Netherlands and in Copenhagen, where there are high rates of walking and cycling support this view.[82,83] The high expenditure and focus on a continuous and integrated network for cyclists, particularly in the Netherlands, is likely to have played a major part both in the safety of cyclists and in increasing cycling.

It has been suggested that across Europe replacement of short trips in cars by walking or cycling would enable most motorists to achieve the recommended levels of physical activity described earlier. In London (2001), 16 percent of car trips were shorter than 1 km, 67 percent shorter than 5 km and 80 percent shorter than 8 km. There may also be a benefit from replacing car trips with public transport as public transport trips usually include a walking component.

The differences in walking and cycling between countries can make an important contribution to the physical activity of the population. Comparison of travel surveys from Germany and the United States found that in 2008/2009 in Germany 21.2 percent and 7.8 percent achieved more than 30 minutes walking or cycling compared to 7.7 percent and 1.0 percent in the United States. In both countries differences in walking and cycling by household income were not substantial, with some tendency for more walking and cycling among lower income groups in both countries. This indicates the potential for walking and cycling as an inclusive form of physical activity, more so in Germany than the United States. Perhaps of particular benefit for health, activity among older adults was notably higher in Germany than in the United States (29 percent vs. 6 percent walked for more than 30 minutes per day).[84]

Other Health and Equity Effects

Health could be affected by changes to traffic noise. There is an extensive scientific literature on the health effects of noise. Although the health evidence is not as strong as for air pollution, the evidence supports an impact on cardiovascular disease, in addition to other harms, including sleep disturbance, reduced cognition, and annoyance.

Achieving high levels of access to retail, employment, education, health services, and social and community networks is vital for health, quality of life, and social inclusion. However, transport policy often promotes mobility rather than accessibility. High motor traffic volume can act as a barrier to access to services, employment, and social support networks. Urban sprawl can negatively impact community cohesion, reducing social capital and further impinging on the access of those without private motorized transport.

Economic and resource use effects of climate change mitigation in the transport sector may also have implications for health. Private motorized transport is highly resource intensive. This resource use can be conceived as having a health-related opportunity cost, as the resources could in theory be spent in other ways that would benefit health. On a macro scale, indirect effects are possible through resource-use-related conflict and effects on socio-economic development.[85] Climate change is occurring in the context of wider ecological stresses,[86,87] which are also affected by transport-related resource use, in particularly oil production.

THE ROLE OF RESEARCH IN PLANNING FOR SUSTAINABLE TRANSPORT

Health Impact Modeling of Increasing Active Transport and Reducing Greenhouse Gas Emissions from Transport

Modeling has indicated the potential for substantial health benefits from greenhouse gas mitigation in the transport sector. Studies initially focused on the link between greenhouse gas emissions and air pollutants harmful to human health.[88,89,90,91] However, more recently a number of studies have considered the impact on health from increases in physical activity and changes in road traffic injury risk from increases in walking and cycling and less use of cars.[92,93,94,95,96] These studies have consistently found that the health benefit from increasing physically active travel and reducing car use are likely to be greater than the effects from changes to air pollution or injury risk. Studies have modeled for Delhi (India), London (England), the Netherlands, New Zealand, Midwestern United States, Barcelona (Spain),[97] and Paris (France).[98] For physical activity, all the health gain is experienced directly by those who change their behavior, whereas for air pollution and road traffic injuries, although the total level of air pollution and road danger may be reduced, those changing their behavior may face a higher risk. Taking the differential impacts into account, studies have modeled the impact on whole population health,[99] the impact on the population of people who change their behavior,[100,101] and both.[102]

A range of studies, from modest to ambitious, have assessed the impact of increased physical activity on health outcomes.[103,104] For physical activity studies most studies have used a version of or values from the WHO HEAT tool[105] calculating changes in premature deaths, in some cases using the values from HEAT in a more sophisticated life table analysis to estimate changes in life expectancy. Another approach by Woodcock et al.,[106] using a comparative risk assessment method, compared changes in age- and sex-specific population distributions of walking and cycling times and estimating changes in disease burden (premature mortality and morbidity).

For road traffic injuries most studies assumed that the risk per distance faced by cyclists and pedestrians remained constant and estimated the change in injuries based only on the change in internal risk for those that changed their mode.[107] This approach is suitable if only small changes in driving are envisaged, but if large changes in driving are modeled, then an approach should be used that also allows for the external risk, that is, the change in risk faced by other road users due to reductions in distance traveled by motor vehicles.

Studies comparing the health impact of active transport to the impact of changes to air pollution have consistently found that the health benefit from increasing physically active travel and reducing car use are likely to be greater than the effects from changes to air pollution or injury risk. Studies have modeled for Delhi (India), London (England), the Netherlands, New Zealand, Midwestern United States, Barcelona (Spain),[108] England and Wales,[109] and Paris (France).[110]

One study that compared some of the most ambitious scenarios directly compared the health impact of lower emission motor vehicles with that from substituting car travel with active travel.[111] It found that in both Delhi and

London an increase in active travel and less use of motor vehicles had considerably larger health benefits per million population than from the increased use of lower emission motor vehicles. However, achieving the substantial reductions in emissions climate scientists argue are necessary would require implementation of both strategies. The largest health gain would be from substantial reductions in ischemic heart disease (10–19 percent in London, 11–25 percent in Delhi). In London the vast majority of the benefit came from the increases in physical activity. In Delhi although again the largest benefit was from increased physical activity, there were also large benefits from reductions in air pollution, and from reduced road traffic injuries. This study was also the only to specifically include the health impacts of change to freight.

In all cases the studies have found the health benefits from increased physical activity were larger than those from changes to air pollution or injury risk both at the whole population level and for the population of those changing behavior. However, the contribution of these three pathways to health impacts appears to vary by setting.

The potential for reduction in greenhouse gas emissions depends on the reduction in vehicle distance and the use of cleaner fuels, but reducing shorter trips may have a larger than anticipated impact due to the higher emissions from cold starts.[112] Achieving large reductions is likely to also require changes in land use that reduce travel distances. As of yet studies have not considered the potential for second-order effects as money saved on petrol is spent in other activities with emission factors.

Including a Cost–Benefit Analysis

Estimating the economic and social effects of a move toward a physically active, low-carbon transport system is difficult and to some extent notional, for a number of reasons. First, the attempt to place a real economic cost on the changes in lifestyle and physical activity remains controversial. This is both because of the controversies on valuing human health and life but also because the positive health effects of greenhouse gas reduction strategies have appreciable macroeconomic impacts, which vary by sector, rapidity of implementation, and other factors. Second, investment studies have found that fiscal instrument and regulation with stringent climate targets can induce investment and lead to more rapid technological change toward a low-carbon society.[113] In this context a narrowly considered cost–benefit analysis will not provide the right evidence for social decision making. Third, cycling is a low-cost transport mode for the user and for society more broadly. Investment in infrastructure in cycling is likely to be considerably cheaper than investment in infrastructure for motor vehicles, and it often gives benefit–cost ratios over 10 to 1.[114]

Fourth, further controversy also exists over how to value changes in travel times. Travel time savings traditionally provide a large proportion of the benefit from schemes for motorized road transport, but these benefits may be transient as changes to speed can lead to increased geographical separation of activities with no limited appreciable benefit. A shift to walking and cycling could mean slower transport, but it could also mean reduced congestion. This introduces the dampening loop on mode shift that reduced congestion could make driving more attractive and increase injury risk from higher speeds. Fifth, in the context of economic crises and high unemployment facing many countries, the potential for job creation in the move to a more active travel can be seen as a benefit, not a cost. However, active travel jobs are frequently marginalized, the UNEP (2008)[115] stating that walking and cycling are overlooked by most traffic planners and economists. In particular, it is important to note that investment in active travel is more likely to be more labor intensive than investment for private motorized travel (hence creating more jobs) and is more likely to create local jobs.

The WHO HEAT tool is specifically designed to monetize the reductions in premature mortality using the statistical life and to feed into cost–benefit analyses. Three of the modeling studies[116,117] mentioned earlier have included some form of economic evaluation. Rabl suggested that the Paris bike hire scheme (Vélib) would be cost effective based on assumptions that 14,500 out of 160,000 daily trips by Vélib represented a shift from cars to bikes. It suggested that in economic terms the largest benefits would come from reductions in noise pollution and congestion, and increases in physical activity. However, in no case was a full cost–benefit analysis attempted.

The greater issue is not the affordability of the change but how to achieve it. Beyond changes to the built environment an equal or greater focus on culture is imperative.[118] The cultural changes required may not be costly and are certainly very difficult to cost, but they may still be difficult to achieve.

Turning Research into Policy

Health impact models have the potential to effect change by strengthening the case in the mind of the public and policy makers. Future studies will be expected to improve the modeling methods and parameterization. Important questions include further considering the impact of changes in behavior of different population groups, the choice of dose–response function, and inclusion of the impact of additional pathways.

Improving the methods for estimating potential gains from physical activity is important because the impact may well be considerably larger than for air pollution or for injuries.[119] In quantifying the potential health impacts of climate change mitigation, the size of the effect is sensitive to the potential for active travel to replace motorized travel, including whether travel distances remain constant. If it is to be assumed that people transfer from faster to slower modes, then a reduction in travel distances is required to compensate for an increase in travel times.[120] Another important variable is on the takeup of active travel at different ages. It might be anticipated that increasing activity among older adults is more difficult, but these groups have higher health risks so have the greatest potential absolute benefits from increasing their activity. Estimating the size of the health benefits and the beneficiaries is important, primarily in its own right but also for the wider economic and social impact.

For injuries the most important issue may be how to reduce the road traffic danger that currently acts as a disincentive to walking and cycling. It is possible for the risk faced by pedestrians and cyclists to go down, while injuries to go up if there are many more pedestrians and cyclists on the roads. However, in some settings it may be the case that the reduction in danger, if accompanied by strong policies to improve the active travel environment and limit speeds, is sufficient to lead to an actual absolute reduction in the number of injuries.[121] The effect may well depend on baseline walking and cycling levels; the higher these are, the more people will benefit from danger reduction. The inclusion of additional health impact pathways is also important. The study by Rabl,[122] although not doing a full noise analysis, suggested the value of the social benefits may be particularly large from reductions in noise.

One area of future research will be around the effects on health inequalities. In lower income cities it might be anticipated that the main physical activity benefits would be to higher income groups who currently are less active, while the lower income groups might benefit more from reduced road injury risk as they are still walking for transport and leading more physically active lives. In higher income cities the potential for reductions in air pollution to reduce inequalities has already been noted.[123]

Modeling of the health impact of scenarios is important because it shows what potentially could be achieved if the political and social will were there. The potential size of the benefits (and on the downside the size of the harms) makes a strong case for looking for ways to move toward these scenarios. Furthermore, as the modeling methods improve, it allows policy makers, researchers, and the public to answer more detailed, "What if?" questions.

A review of evidence to support integrated health impact assessment of transport policies recommended that future modeling and evaluation should consider in more detail the kind of policy packages required to achieve the scenarios, both to increase realism and to allow the assessment of a wider range of potential harms and benefits.[124]

However, the impact modeling studies cannot, on their own, answer the question as to how we make the changes. There is good evidence from international and interurban comparisons of large differences in levels of walking, cycling, and car use between areas at similar levels of economic development.[125] In locations with high walking and cycling populations, such as the Netherlands, inequalities in transport-related physical activity are low (inclusive). The differences between the best European cities and many North American cities are large and have been associated with differences in the built environment. Although causality is difficult to establish, issues of culture and habit clearly also play an important role. For example, deeply rooted negative perceptions of cyclists in many low-cycling countries act as a barrier to normalization of cycling.[126] The evidence from well-conducted studies on what interventions can achieve is modest.[127] Well-conducted prospective evaluation of changes in the built environment (e.g., construction of new infrastructure) is vital for improving the evidence base.[128] However, it is only possible to evaluate interventions once they have been implemented. It is imperative, therefore, that strong interventions on a sufficient scale are implemented and evaluated over a period of time, linking together the goals of reducing car use and increasing physically active travel. An analogy can be made with the bans on smoking in public places. In this case strong measures were adopted, following campaigns to raise public and political support, and when these measures were evaluated over a period of time large benefits were found.[129]

THE SUSTAINABLE MOBILITY PARADIGM AS THE WAY FORWARD

The sustainable mobility paradigm provides a framework within which to investigate the complexity of cities, and to strengthen the links between land use and transport.[130] Such urban forms would keep average trip lengths to below the thresholds required for maximum use of cycle and walk modes. It would also permit high levels of innovative services and public transport priority, so that the need to use the car would be minimized. Cities would be designed at the personal scale to allow both high-quality accessibility and a high-quality environment. The intention is to design cities of such quality and at a suitable scale that people would not need to have a car.

This approach (Fig. 7.4) requires clear and innovative thinking about city futures in terms of the reality (what is already there) and the desirability (what we would like to see), and the role that transport can (and should) play in achieving these objectives. The sustainable city must balance the requirements along the physical dimensions (urban form and traffic) against those concerning the social dimensions (people and proximity). The sustainable mobility approach requires actions to reduce the need to travel (fewer trips), to encourage modal shift, to reduce trip lengths, and to encourage greater efficiency in the transport system. A sustainable transport system means that overall we need to travel less and inequalities in travel patterns are reduced.

The key to such a shift in thinking is the creation of spaces and localities in the city that are attractive and affordable, as neighborhood quality is central

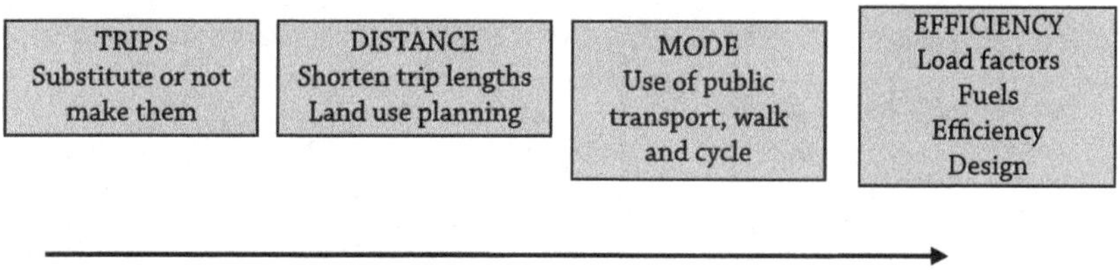

TRIPS	DISTANCE	MODE	EFFICIENCY
Substitute or not make them	Shorten trip lengths Land use planning	Use of public transport, walk and cycle	Load factors Fuels Efficiency Design

Figure 7.4:
The Sustainable Mobility Paradigm.

to sustainable mobility. Transport planning must involve the people, so that there is an understanding of the rationale behind the policy changes and an increased likelihood that behavioral change follows. Public acceptability is central to successful implementation of radical change, and it must involve community and stakeholder commitment to the process of discussion, decision making, and implementation.

The sustainable mobility paradigm has been designed to provide a platform against which the conventional transport planning model that has been in use for the last 50 years can be reassessed, and to use the same arguments to question the need for such high levels of motorized mobility, as this has substantial environmental, safety, and health outcomes.[131] It challenges the importance of speed and travel time savings, through emphasizing the need for sustainability, which means slower travel, reasonable travel times, and travel time reliability.

Within this paradigm, health is affected in three main ways, as less motorized traffic and "cleaner" vehicles improve local air quality, as slower travel leads to road danger reduction, and as more active transport results in increased physical activity. In addition, these improvements are likely to have a positive effect on climate change through reductions in the use of carbon-based fuels and fewer CO_2 emissions. Priorities for sustainable transport in cities need to be reconsidered within the framework of the sustainable mobility paradigm, and its extension through the health and equity agendas.

At the same time, the transition to an active, low-carbon transport system has the potential to improve social and health equity through linking affordable and inclusive transport to affordable and inclusive opportunities for physical activity, while at the same time reducing the inequality in direct and indirect harms from transport. Such an approach has strong benefits for improving health and in reducing levels of inequality in cities.

The CO_2 and other emissions reductions will be contingent upon the reduction in car use and the uptake of lower emission motor vehicles. The health benefits will primarily come through increases in active travel, even though this is unlikely to be achieved without measures to reduce road traffic danger. How each part of the sustainable mobility paradigm might be anticipated to play out in terms of health effects is shown in Table 7.3.

Table 7.3. LINKAGE DIAGRAM BETWEEN COMPONENTS
OF SUSTAINABILITY AND HEALTH OUTCOMES

	Fewer Trips	Shorter Distances	Modal Shift	Efficiency
Physical activity	—	—	⇧	—
Air pollution	⇩	⇩	⇩	⇩
Road traffic injuries	⇩	⇩	?*	—
Greenhouse gas emissions	⇩	⇩	⇩	⇩

*The effect of modal shift on road traffic injuries is unclear because there are different potentially conflicting factors at play. Increased walking and cycling means greater exposure to road vehicle danger, although there could be a safety in numbers effect, while reduced motor vehicle use reduces the source of danger. Policies to induce modal shift may also have the effect of making walking and cycling safer.

Concerted actions are needed across all policy dimensions that are both consistent and mutually supporting, so that a change in culture is developed that places equal importance on the accessibility for all within the urban area to services and facilities. Although the evidence on how to achieve large-scale changes is limited, the most effective approaches are likely to combine strong implementation of a wide range of measures. In the Netherlands, the country with the highest levels of cycling, the focus has been on providing integrated and continuous networks for cyclists.[132] However, there is clearly also a cultural component that may be harder for policy makers to act upon. Transport mode choice is strongly affected by both habit[133] and cultural norms. Provision of high-quality infrastructure without also changing these social norms is likely to have modest effects. However, encouragement can be drawn from the number of major cities that have recently seen substantial increases in cycling, including London, Paris, Barcelona, Berlin, and Copenhagen. Only in the last two (and particularly last one) can this increase be attributed to an already strong cycling culture. Unfortunately, even in the Netherlands with high cycling rates greenhouse gas emissions from transport are far above sustainable levels. To achieve the largest gains, strong measures should be implemented and simultaneously rigorously evaluated, thereby improving the evidence base and allowing for further implementation of the most effective measures.

Central to the success of any scheme must be the reallocation of space in the city to pedestrians and cyclists—this is the key to sustainable mobility. Cities provide us with the best opportunity for moving toward sustainable transport. The starting point needs to be a view as to the sustainable city of the future, in terms of its economic functions (e.g., employment, government, housing, education, and health), as well as its attractiveness (e.g., cultural, social, and community). The city should be inclusive and cater to all sections of the population. The quality of life should be high, with city living based around good-quality affordable housing, strong neighborhoods, and good facilities that are easily accessible. The city must be seen as a place for people, providing opportunities for all, in a safe and secure neighborhood, with green space and other recreational facilities accessible to all. It is then that we consider what sort of sustainable transport system might be most appropriate to fit this vision of the city, following the idea that transport serves the city.

Effective leadership must look at new visions of the city and implement effective strategies that are both politically and publicly acceptable. It is unlikely that there is going to be any substantial increase in the supply of city infrastructure for transport, and so the biggest challenge for urban planners is to decide how that infrastructure can be managed in the most sustainable way. This includes the allocation of space to different types of use (perhaps by time of day and day of week), substantial increases in the costs of access by car to that space, and decisions about who actually owns that space.

In many lower income countries urbanization and motorization are leading to a rapid increase in both the burden of diseases associated with inactivity and in road traffic injuries. While here a large majority cannot afford access to private motorized transport, road traffic danger and social stigma are leading to use of private motorized transport when it can be afforded. Walking and cycling could provide the opportunity for equity in access to high levels of physical activity. Achieving this in practice will require provision of urban environments that are conducive and inclusive to these activities. To encourage real change requires a well-connected and safe network of routes for cyclists and pedestrians that are of a sufficient quality, and this physical infrastructure needs to be supported by skills and awareness programs to teach drivers that the responsibility for safety lies with the user of the most dangerous vehicle, not with the most vulnerable. The links between health and active transport need to be emphasized through education programs and the involvement of doctors. Copenhagen is often cited as a good example of a cycling city; 68 percent of Copenhagen residents cycle at least once a week. While cycling has increased, the number of cyclists seriously injured has fallen by more than 60 percent since 1996, and over 90 percent of the population think of the city as good place for cyclists.[134] Both subjective and objective safety of cyclists is measured and acted on. New cyclists cited speed, convenience, health, and cost as their main reasons for starting cycling.

The basic dilemma facing society in terms of climate change and sustainable transport is that many people like traveling, particularly to distant locations (by air), and much more travel is being undertaken. Yet there is also an awareness of the environmental and social costs of traveling, and individual responsibilities, and this is present in many actions that are now being taken in cities to reduce travel distances and even the need to travel, as well as investing in the low-carbon infrastructure (for walking, cycling, and public transport). This chapter has clearly outlined the range of solutions that are available to creating sustainable transport within world cities, and there are many examples cited of good practice that make sense in economic terms, as well as improving the health of people and in reducing inequities caused by limited access to transport. The best practice needs to be rolled out in all cities, and cities need to learn from each other so that society can benefit from sustainable urban transport.

NOTES

1. D. Banister, "The Trilogy of Distance, Speed and Time," *Journal of Transport Geography* 19, no. 4 (2011): 1538–1546.
2. D. Banister, "The Sustainable Mobility Paradigm," *Transport Policy* 15, no. 2 (2008): 73–80.
3. I. Roberts and P. Edwards, *The Energy Glut The Politics of Fatness in an Overheating World* (London and New York: Zed Books, 2010).
4. UN Habitat, *State of the World's Cities 2008/2009: Harmonious Cities* (Nairobi, Kenya: UN Habitat, 2008).
5. Ibid.
6. UN Habitat, *State of the World's Cities 2010/2011—Cities for All: Bridging the Urban Divide* (Nairobi, Kenya: UN Habitat, 2010).
7. UN Habitat, *State of the World's Cities 2008...*
8. Ibid.
9. Sustainable Development Commission, *Fairness in a Car Dependent Society* (London, England: Sustainable Development Commission, 2011).
10. G. Tiwari, "Transport and Land-Use Policies in Delhi," *Bulletin of the World Health Organ* 81, no. 6 (2003): 444–450.
11. M. Khayesi, H. Monheim, and J. M. Nebe, "Negotiating 'Streets for All' in Urban Transport Planning: The Case for Pedestrians, Cyclists and Street Vendors in Nairobi, Kenya," *Antipode* 42, no. 1 (2010): 103–126.
12. CO_2 concentrations are currently about 385 ppmv and with other greenhouse gases being included, this value increases to 430 ppmv CO_2e (2009). A level of 450 ppmv CO_2e means that there is a 26–78 percent chance of exceeding 2°C. A level of 550 ppmv CO_2e means that there is a 63–99 percent chance of exceeding 2°C. If global concentrations of greenhouse gases stabilize at 560 ppmv CO_2e, it is "likely" that global mean surface temperatures will rise by 3°C above preindustrial levels.
    Meinhausen, M. (2006) 'What does a 2C target mean for greenhouse gas concentrations? A brief analysis based on multi-gas emission pathways and several climate sensitivity uncertainty estimates', In H.J. Schellnhuber, W. Cramer, N. Nakicenovic, T. Wigley and G. Gohe (eds) *Avoiding Dangerous Climate Change*, Cambridge University Press, Cambridge, pp. 253–279.
13. N. Adger et al., "IPCC, 2007: Summary for Policymakers," in *Climate Change 2007: Impacts, Adaptation and Vulnerability. Contribution of Working Group Ii to the Fourth Assessment Report of the Intergovernmental Panel on Climate Change*, eds. M. L. Parry et al. (Cambridge, England: Cambridge University Press, 2007), 1–22.

14. International Energy Agency, *World Energy Outlook* (Paris, France: OECD/IEA, 2009).
15. R. Gilbert and A. Perl, *The Transformation of Travel and Freight Movement in a Post-Peak-Oil World* (Vancouver, Canada: Vancouver New Society Publishers, 2010).
16. European Commission (EC) DG for Energy and Transport, *EU Energy and Transport in Figures 2007/2008* (Luxembourg, Belgium: European Commission, 2008).
17. J. DeCicco and F. Fung, F. *Global Warming on the Road: The Climate Impact of America's Automobiles* (Washington, DC: Environmental Defense, 2006).
18. The National Fuel Efficiency Policy (2012–2016) requires an average fuel economy standard of 35.5 mpg in 2016, and it will save 1.8 billion barrels of oil over the life of the program. The fuel economy gain averages more than 5 percent per year and will result in a reduction of approximately 900 million metric tons in greenhouse gas emissions.
19. M. Krzyzanowski, B. Kuna-Dibbert, and J. Schneider, eds., *Health Effects of Transport-Related Air Pollution* (Geneva, Switzerland: World Health Organization, 2005).
20. The DALY (disability adjusted life year) is a measure of disease burden that combines years of life lost through premature mortality with years of healthy life lost through living with a disease, injury, or disability.
21. A. Prüss-Üstün et al., "Lead Exposure," in *Comparative Quantification of Health Risks*, eds. M. Ezzati et al. (Geneva, Switzerland: World Health Organization, 2004), 1295–1352.
22. A. Cohen et al., "Urban Air Pollution," in *Comparative Quantification of Health Risks*, eds. M Ezzati et al. (Geneva, Switzerland: World Health Organization, 2004), 1353–1434.
23. Krzyzanowski et al., *Health Effects of Transport-Related*
24. S. C. Anenberg et al., "An Estimate of the Global Burden of Anthropogenic Ozone and Fine Particulate Matter on Premature Human Mortality Using Atmospheric Modeling," *Environmental Health Perspectives* 118, no. 9 (2010): 1189–1195.
25. Ibid.
26. M. Jerrett et al., "Long-Term Ozone Exposure and Mortality," *New England Journal of Medicine* 360, no. 11 (2009): 1085–1095.
27. K. R. Smith et al., "Public Health Benefits of Strategies to Reduce Greenhouse-Gas Emissions: Health Implications of Short-Lived Greenhouse Pollutants," *The Lancet*, 374, no. 9707 (2009): 2091–2103.
28. V. Ramanathan and G. Carmichael, "Global and Regional Climate Changes Due to Black Carbon," *Nature Geoscience* 1, no. 4 (2008): 221–227.
29. Smith et al., "Public Health Benefits of Strategies. . ."
30. A. Goodman et al., "Characterising Socio-Economic Inequalities in Exposure to Air Pollution: A Comparison of Socio-Economic Markers and Scales of Measurement," *Health and Place*, 17, no. 3 (2011): 767–774.
31. S. Deguen and D. Zmirou-Navier, "Social Inequalities Resulting from Health Risks Related to Ambient Air Quality—A European Review," *European Journal of Public Health* 20, no. 1 (2010): 27–35.
32. European Commission, *European Climate Change Change Programme—EU Action against Climate Change*, (Brussels, Belgium: European Commission, 2006).
33. European Environment Agency, *Impact of Selected Policy Measures on Europe's Air quality* (Copenhagen, Denmark: European Environment Agency, 2011).

34. European Environment Agency, *The European Environment State And Outlook 2010 Air Pollution* (Copenhagen, Denmark: EEA, 2010).

35. C. Tonne et al., "Air Pollution and Mortality Benefits of the London Congestion Charge: Spatial and Socioeconomic Inequalities," *Occupational and Environmental Medicine* 65, no. 9 (2008): 620–627.

36. G. Cesaroni et al., "Health Benefits of Traffic-Related Air Pollution Reduction in Different Socioeconomic Groups: The Effect of Low-Emission Zoning in Rome," *Occupational and Environmental Medicine* 69, no. 2 (2011): 133–9.

37. H. Wolff and L. Perry, *Keep Your Clunker in the Suburb: Low Emission Zones and Adoption of Green Vehicles* (Seattle, WA: University of Washington, 2011).

38. M. Peden et al., *World Report on Road Traffic Injury Prevention* (Geneva, Switzerland: World Health Organization, 2004).

39. WHO Regional Office for Europe, *European Status Report on Road Safety: Towards Safer Roads and Healthier Transport Choices* (Copenhagen, Denmark: World Health Organization, 2009).

40. Peden et al., *World Report on Road Traffic...*

41. D. Mohan et al., *Road Safety in India: Challenges and Opportunities* (report no. UMTRI-2009-1, University of Michigan Transportation Research Institute, Ann Arbor, MI, 2009), 1–57.

42. WHO, *Global Status Report on Road Safety* (Washington, DC: World Health Organization, 2009).

43. A. Rabl and A. de Nazelle, "Benefits of Shift from Car to Active Transport," *Transport Policy* 19, no. 1 (2012): 121–131.

44. C. Koren and A. Borsos, "Is Smeed's Law Still Valid? A World-Wide Analysis of the Trends in Fatality Rate," *Journal of Society for Transportation and Traffic Studies* 1, no. 1 (2010): 64–76.

45. E. Kopits and M. Cropper, "Traffic Fatalities and Economic Growth," *Accident Analysis and Prevention* 37, no. 1 (2005): 169–178.

46. L. J. Paulozzi et al., "Economic Development's Effect on Road Transport-Related Mortality Among Different Types of Road Users: A Cross-Sectional International Study," *Accident Analysis and Prevention* 39, no. 3 (2007): 606–617.

47. *Fatalities by Transport Mode in EU Countries Included in CARE*, European Commission Road Safety, accessed May 2, 2013, http://ec.europa.eu/transport/road_safety/pdf/statistics/2008_transport_mode_graph.pdf

48. I. Roberts and I. Crombie, "Child Pedestrian Deaths: Sensitivity to Traffic Volume—Evidence from the USA," *Journal of Epidemiology and Community Health* 49, no. 2 (1995): 186–188.

49. *Fatalities by Transport Mode...*

50. C. Grundy et al., "Effect of 20 Mph Traffic Speed Zones on Road Injuries in London, 1986-2006: Controlled Interrupted Time Series Analysis," *British Medical Journal* 339, no. 3 (2009): b4469.

51. Public Works and Water Management Ministry of Transport, Directorate-General for Passenger Transport, and Fietsberaad (Expertise Centre for Cycling Policy), *Cycling in the Netherlands* (Den Haag and Utrecht, The Netherlands: Ministry of Transport, 2009).

52. R. Bhatia and M. Wier, "'Safety in Numbers'" Re-Examined: Can We Make Valid or Practical Inferences from Available Evidence?," *Accident Analysis and Prevention* 43, no. 1 (2011): 235–240.

53. Peden et al., *World Report on Road Traffic Injury...*

54. C. Wilson et al., "Speed Cameras for the Prevention of Road Traffic Injuries and Deaths," *Cochrane Database of Systematic Reviews* 11 (2010). Cochrane Database Syst Rev. 2010 Oct 6;(10):CD004607. doi: 10.1002/14651858.CD004607.pub3.

55. I. Kwan, I. Roberts, and the Cochrane Injuries Group Driver Education Reviewers, "School-Based Driver Education for the Prevention of Traffic Crashes," *Cochrane Database of Systematic Reviews*, accessed http://www. cochrane.org/reviews/en/ab003201.html

56. J. Woodcock et al., "Energy and Transport," *Lancet* 370, no. 9592 (2007): 1078–1088.

57. It defined inactivity as "doing no or very little physical activity at work, at home, for transport, or in discretionary time" and insufficiently active as "doing some physical activity but less than 150 minutes of moderate-intensity activity or 60 minutes of vigorous activity accumulated across work, home, transport, or discretionary domains" over 1 week.

58. Countries of the Africa D region include Algeria, Angola, Benin, Burkina Faso, Cameroon, Cape Verde, Chad, Equatorial Guinea, Gabon, Gambia, Ghana, Guinea, Guinea-Bissau, Liberia, Madagascar, Mali, Mauritania, Mauritius, Niger, Nigeria, Sao Tome and Principe, Senegal, Seychelles, Sierra Leone, and Togo.

59. Countries of the European C region include Belarus, Estonia, Hungary, Kazakhstan, Latvia, Lithuania, Republic of Moldova, Russian Federation, and Ukraine.

60. F. Bull et al., "Physical Inactivity," chap. 10 in *Comparative Quantification of Health Risks*, eds. M. Ezzati et al. (Geneva, Switzerland: World Health Organization, 2003).

61. Department for Transport, *National Travel Survey: 2007* (London, England: National Statistics, 2008).

62. R. L. Mackett et al., "The Therapeutic Value of Children's Everyday Travel," *Transportation Research Part A: Policy and Practice* 39, no. 2-3 (2005): 205–219.

63. M. Hillman, J. Adams, and J. Whitelegg, *One False Move: A Study of Children's Independent Mobility* (London, England: PSI, 1990).

64. Department for Transport, *National Travel Survey: 2008* (London, England: National Statistics, 2009).

65. G. Tiwari and H. Jain, "Bicycles in Urban India," *Urban Transport Journal* 7, no. 2 (2008): 59–68.

66. J. Heyen-Perschon, *Non-Motorised Transport and Its Socio-Economic Impact on Poor Households in Africa: Cost-Benefit Analysis of Bicycle Ownership in Uganda* (Wohltorf, Germany: ITDP Europe, 2005).

67. Tiwari, *Transport and Land-Use Policies...*

68. D. Warburton et al., "A Systematic Review of the Evidence for Canada's Physical Activity Guidelines for Adults," *International Journal of Behavioral Nutrition and Physical Activity* 7, no. 1 (2010). doi:10.1186/1479-5868-7-39.

69. R. Kumar et al., "Urbanization and Coronary Heart Disease: A Study of Urban-Rural Differences in Northern India," *Indian Heart Journal* 58, no. 2 (2006): 126–130.

70. K. Srinath Reddy et al., "Responding to the Threat of Chronic Diseases in India," *Lancet* 366, no. 9498 (2005): 1744–1749.

71. K. Anderson and A. Bows, "Reframing the Climate Change Challenge in Light of Post-2000 Emission Trends," *Philosophical Transactions of the Royal Society B* 366, no. 1882 (2008): 3863–3882.

72. W. James et al., "Overweight and Obesity (High Body Mass Index)," in *Comparative Quantification of Health Risks*, eds. M. Ezzati et al. (Geneva, Switzerland: World Health Organization, 2004), 2191–2230.

73. A. M. Prentice and S. A. Jebb, "Obesity in Britain: Gluttony or Sloth?", *British Medical Journal* 311, no. 7002 (1995): doi: http://dx.doi.org/10.1136/bmj.311.7002.437.

74. A. Colin Bell, K. Ge, and B. Popkin, "The Road to Obesity or the Path to Prevention: Motorized Transportation and Obesity in China," *Obesity Research* 10 (2002): 277–283.

75. L. D. Frank, M. A. Andresen, and T. L. Schmid, "Obesity Relationships with Community Design, Physical Activity, and Time Spent in Cars," *American Journal of Preventive Medicine* 27, no. 2 (2004): 87–96.

76. K. E. Pickett et al., "Wider Income Gaps, Wider Waistbands? An Ecological Study of Obesity and Income Inequality," *J Epidemiol Community Health* 59, no. 8 (2005): 670–674.

77. A. Offer, R. Pechey, and S. Ulijaszek, "Obesity Under Affluence Varies by Welfare Regimes: The Effect of Fast Food, Insecurity, and Inequality," *Economics and Human Biology* 8, no. 3 (2010): 297–308.

78. P. L. Jacobsen, "Safety in Numbers: More Walkers and Bicyclists, Safer Walking and Bicycling," *Injury Prevention* 9, no. 3 (2003): 205–209.

79. R. Elvik, "The Non-Linearity of Risk and the Promotion of Environmentally Sustainable Transport," *Accident Analysis and Prevention* 41, no. 4 (2009): 849–855.

80. Bhatia and Wier, "'Safety in Numbers' Re-Examined . . ."

81. K. Teschke et al., "Route Infrastructure and the Risk of Injuries to Bicyclists: A Case-Crossover Study," *American Journal of Public Health* 102, no. 12 (2012): 2336–43.

82. Netherlands Ministry of Transport, *Cycling in the Netherlands* (Rotterdam, The Netherlands: Ministry of Transport, Public Works, and Water Management, 2006).

83. Danish Public Works and Water Management Directorate-General for Passenger Transport, *Copenhagen City of Cyclists- Bicycle Account 2008* (Copenhagen, Denmark: DPW and WMD-G, The Technical and Environmental Administration,Traffic Department, 2009).

84. R. Buehler et al., "Active Travel in Germany and the U.S.: Contributions of Daily Walking and Cycling to Physical Activity," *American Journal of Preventive Medicine* 41, no. 3 (2011): 241–250.

85. J. Sachs and A. Warner, "Natural Resources and Economic Development: The Curse of Natural Resources," *European Economic Review* 45 (2001): 827–38.

86. A. McMichael, "Population, Environment, Disease, and Survival: Past Patterns, Uncertain Futures," *The Lancet* 359 (2002): 1145–1148.

87. Adger et al, "*IPCC, 2007: Summary for Policymakers.*"

88. L. Cifuentes et al., "Assessing the Health Benefits of Urban Air Pollution Reductions Associated with Climate Change Mitigation (2000-2020): Santiago, Sao Paulo, Mexico City, and New York City," *Environ Health Perspect* 109, supp. 3 (2001): 419–425.

89. S. Syri et al., "Low-CO2 Energy Pathways and Regional Air Pollution in Europe," *Energy Policy* 29, no. 11 (2001): 871–884.

90. G. McKinley et al., "Quantification of Local and Global Benefits from Air Pollution Control in Mexico City. *Environmental Science and Technology* 39 (2005): 1954–61.

91. P. Wilkinson et al., "Energy, Energy Efficiency, and the Built Environment," *Lancet* 370, no. 9593 (2007): 1175–1187.
92. J. Woodcock et al., "Public Health Benefits of Strategies to Reduce Greenhouse-Gas Emissions: Urban Land Transport," *Lancet* 374, no. 9705 (2009): 1930–1943.
93. D. Rojas-Rueda et al., "The Health Risks and Benefits of Cycling in Urban Environments Compared with Car Use: Health Impact Assessment Study," *British Medical Journal* 343 (2011): d4521.
94. G. Lindsay, A. Macmillan, and A. Woodward, "Moving Urban Trips from Cars to Bicycles: Impact on Health and Emissions," *Australian and New Zealand Journal of Public Health*, 35, no. 1 (2010): 54–60.
95. Rabl and de Nazelle, "Benefits of Shift from Car..."
96. J. J. de Hartog et al., "Do the Health Benefits of Cycling Outweigh the Risks?" *Environmental Health Perspectives* 118, no. 8. (2010): 1109–1116.
97. Rojas-Rueda, D., de Nazelle, A., Teixido, O., Nieuwenhuijsen, M. J., "Replacing car trips by increasing bike and public transport in the greater Barcelona metropolitan area: A health impact assessment study," *Environ. Int.* 2012; 49C: 100–109.
98. Rabl and de Nazelle, "Benefits of Shift from Car..."
99. Woodcock et al., "Public Health Benefits of Strategies..."
100. Rojas-Rueda et al., "The Health Risks and Benefits of Cycling..."
101. de Hartog et al., "Do the Health Benefits of Cycling..."
102. Rabl and de Nazelle, "Benefits of Shift from Car..."
103. Rojas-Rueda et al., "The Health Risks and Benefits of Cycling..."
104. M. L. Grabow et al., "Air Quality and Exercise-Related Health Benefits from Reduced Car Travel in the Midwestern United States," *Environmental Health Perspectives* 120, no. 1 (2012): 68–76.
105. WHO Europe, *Health Economic Assessment Tools (HEAT) for Walking and Cycling: Economic Assessment of Transport Infrastructure and Policies* (Geneva, Switzerland: WHO, 2011).
106. Woodcock et al., "Public Health Benefits of Strategies..."
107. Ibid.
108. Rojas-Rueda et al., "The Health Risks and Benefits of Cycling..."
109. J. Woodcock, M. Givoni, and A. Morgan, "Health Impact Modelling of Active Travel Visions for England and Wales Using an Integrated Transport and Health Impact Modelling Tool (ITHIM)," *PLoS One* 8, no. 1 (2013): e51462.
110. Rabl and de Nazelle, "Benefits of Shift from Car..."
111. Woodcock et al., "Public Health Benefits of Strategies..."
112. Grabow et al. "Air Quality and Exercise-Related..."
113. T. Barker and S. S. Scrieciu, "Modeling Low Climate Stabilization with E3MG: Towards a 'New Economics' Approach to Simulating Energy-Environment-Economy System Dynamics," *The Energy Journal* 31, (2010): 137–164.
114. J. Macmillen, M. Givoni, and D. Banister, "Evaluating Active Travel: Decision-Making for the Sustainable City," *Built Environment* 36, no. 4 (2010): 519–536.
115. *Green Jobs: Towards Decent Work in a Sustainable, Low-Carbon World*, UN Environment Programme, Accessed 16th May 2013 http://www.ilo.org/wcmsp5/groups/public/@ed_emp/@emp_ent/documents/publication/wcms_158727.pdf
116. Lindsay et al., "Moving Urban Trips..."

117. Rabl and de Nazelle, "Benefits of Shift from Car..."
118. R. Aldred and K. Jungnickel, *Cycling Cultures Final Report* (project report, University of East London, London, England, 2004).
119. Woodcock et al., "Public Health Benefits of Strategies..."
120. Banister, "The Trilogy of Distance..."
121. Woodcock et al., "Health Impact Modelling of Active Travel..."
122. Rabl and de Nazelle, "Benefits of Shift from Car..."
123. Tonne et al., "Air Pollution and Mortality..."
124. de Nazelle et al., "Improving Health Through Policies that Promote Active Travel: A Review of Evidence to Support Integrated Health Impact Assessment," *Environment International* 37, no. 4 (2011): 767–777.
125. J. Pucher, J. Dill, and S. Handy, "Infrastructure, Programs, and Policies to Increase Bicycling: An International Review," *Preventive Medicine* 50, supp. 1 (2010): S106–S125.
126. R. Aldred, "Incompetent or Too Competent? Negotiating Everyday Cycling Identities in a Motor Dominated Society," *Mobilities* 8, no. 2 (2013): 252–271.
127. D. Ogilvie et al., "Promoting Walking and Cycling as an Alternative to Using Cars: Systematic Review," *British Medical Journal* 329, no. 7469 (2004): 763.
128. D. Ogilvie et al., "Evaluating the Travel, Physical Activity and Carbon Impacts of a 'Natural Experiment' in the Provision of New Walking and Cycling Infrastructure: Methods for the Core Module of the iConnect Study," *British Medical Journal Open* 2 (2012): e000694.
129. P. Goodman et al., "Are There Health Benefits Associated with Comprehensive Smoke-Free Laws," *International Journal of Public Health* 54, no. 6 (2009): 367–78.
130. Banister, "The Sustainable Mobility Paradigm..."
131. Ibid.
132. Ministry of Transport (2009) Cycling in the Netherlands, Published by the Ministry of Transport, Public Works and Water Management, Den Haag. Accessed 16th May 2013 from http://www.fietsberaad.nl/library/repository/bestanden/CyclingintheNetherlands2009.pdf
133. C. Domarchi, A. Tudela, and A. González, "Effect of Attitudes, Habit and Affective Appraisal on Mode Choice: An Application to University Workers," *Transportation* 35, no. 5 (2008): 585–599.
134. City of Copenhagen, The Technical and Environmental Administration, *Copenhagen City of Cyclists: Bicycle Account 2010* (Copenhagen, Denmark: The Technical and Environmental Administration, Traffic Department, 2011). Published in May 2011. Accessed 16th May 2013 from http://www.cycling-embassy.dk/wp-content/uploads/2011/05/Bicycle-account-2010-Copenhagen.pdf

CHAPTER 8

The New Challenges of Rapid Urban Growth

Imperatives and Strategies for Transport in India

MADHAV BADAMI

As examined in Chapter 7, transportation has a critical impact on the environment and health globally. Addressing its impact is made all the more important by the continuing rapid rise in motor vehicle activity. The number of motor vehicles in use globally grew from roughly 250 million in 1970 to around 800 million in 2000, not counting motorized two-wheeled vehicles, of which there were an estimated 200 million in 2000. This more than three-fold growth in just three decades, which demonstrates rapid global motorization, far exceeds the growth during the same period in the human population, both globally as well as in urban areas.[1,2]

The countries comprising the Organization for Economic Development (OECD) even now account for the bulk of motor vehicle numbers and use globally, but motor vehicle growth has been occurring most rapidly in the low-income countries; so much so that, while these countries now account for around 35 percent of the global motor vehicle fleet, their share will likely grow to around 50 percent by 2040. The growth in motor vehicle numbers has been particularly high in South and East Asia, owing to rapid urbanization and growing urban incomes.[3,4] The overall relationship between transportation and health and equity having been examined earlier, this chapter will focus on one country, India, which has had a particularly rapid increase in motorization. India is now the seventh largest producer globally of passenger cars and commercial vehicles. If motorized two-wheeled and three-wheeled vehicles, which account for nearly 80 percent of India's motor vehicle production, are included, the country's global ranking as a motor vehicle manufacturer would very likely be much higher.[5] Moreover, the growth in motor vehicle production in India has been dramatic—it has doubled three times since 1990, and it currently stands at around 18 million annually.[6] Correspondingly, the number of motor vehicles on India's roads has doubled every 6 or so years, from merely 5.4 million in 1981, to as many as 98 million in 2008.[7]

Rapid growth in motor vehicle production and activity provides significant societal benefits by offering mobility to millions, contributing to the development of technological know-how and skills, providing employment, and benefiting the economy at large. At the same time, the rapid growth in motor vehicle ownership and activity has serious implications for a wide range of issues at the local, regional, and global scales, ranging from resource use, environmental degradation, compromised health and welfare, and negative socioeconomic impacts, especially for the poor. It is for these reasons that it is important to focus policy attention on urban transport in India as well as on urban transport globally.

ROAD TRAFFIC ACCIDENTS

Perhaps the most serious impacts of rapidly growing motor vehicle activity are the deaths and injuries that result from road traffic accidents. Road traffic deaths in India, which stood at 14,500 in 1970, have increased rapidly to 54,100 in 1990, 78,911 in 2001, and 119,860 in 2008.[8] India, with around 10 percent of the total global road fatalities, has the dubious distinction of being the country with arguably the world's worst road safety record.[9] India's traffic fatalities are considerably more than twice those in the United States, yet Indian motor vehicle activity represents only a fraction of that of the United States. Per capita traffic fatalities in urban areas are similar in the two countries; however, the rates of per capita traffic fatalities in urban areas and per capita traffic fatalities nationally continue to increase in India (and other Asian countries), while declining in the United States and other high-income countries.[10,11,12]

The sad irony is that the road users and modes that are the least responsible for traffic fatalities (and other urban transport issues) are the most adversely affected. Pedestrians and cyclists, the most vulnerable road users, and two-wheeled motor vehicle users account, respectively, for 50–67 percent and 25 percent of road fatalities, while car users comprise only around 5 percent of road fatalities.[13,14,15] Traffic fatalities, already the ninth leading cause of death globally, are likely to become the fifth, ahead of all cancers, by 2030.[16] As tragic as traffic deaths are, traffic injuries are no less so, since they can economically devastate families. Yet attention to the serious problem of traffic accidents focuses on fatalities. In India, it is estimated that for every traffic death, there are around 20 serious injuries and 70 minor injuries.[17] Injuries pose a significant threat to socioeconomic well-being for a number of reasons. First of all, traffic injuries typically occur during the most economically productive phase of life; secondly, they can force family members to give up their jobs in order to care for traffic injury victims; and lastly, because many people who are injured lack medical insurance coverage, medical bills can become financially crippling.[18] Because of the large and growing number of traffic fatalities, and the considerably larger number of traffic injuries, road accidents are a major—but largely neglected—public health issue. So also is traffic noise, which is given virtually no attention.

CONGESTION AND VEHICLE EMISSIONS

The urban transport issues that have perhaps attracted the most serious policy attention are congestion and vehicle emissions. Congestion levels are high, especially in the large metropolitan centers, with average peak hour speeds reported to be around 17 km/hr.[19] As for vehicle emissions, they contribute significantly to the poor air quality in Indian cities.[20,21] In Delhi, for example, suspended particulate matter levels have exceeded World Health Organization (WHO) guideline limits[21a] almost daily since the 1990s. Particulates below 10 microns diameter (PM_{10}) levels, which are strongly linked with respiratory and cardiovascular illnesses and deaths, also exceed the WHO limits, particularly in high traffic areas.[22] The poor often suffer the highest exposures to urban air pollution, since many of them live and work roadside, where air pollution levels are typically higher than in areas farther away. It is also worth noting that, for many, exposure to high outdoor air pollution levels is in addition to the high levels of indoor air pollution caused by the use of low-quality cooking fuels that are used by a significant number of low-income urban households.[23] Furthermore, the poor are also the most affected by, and least capable of, coping with the impacts of air pollution because of synergies between pollution, poverty, nutritional deficiency, and poor access to health care.[24,25]

A wide range of policies, including increasingly stringent vehicle emission and fuel quality standards, vehicle inspection and maintenance (I&M) to control in-use emissions, the phasing out of commercial vehicles older than 15 years, and the conversion of public and for-hire vehicles to compressed natural gas (CNG) in some cities, have been implemented since the early 1990s.[26,27,28,29] Notwithstanding these measures, PM_{10} levels at the busy ITO intersection in Delhi, where the air pollution is predominantly if not exclusively transport generated, have still exceeded the WHO guideline daily limit almost every day since 2000. It has been argued that this situation is likely due to the increase in motor vehicle activity, which has compensated for emission reductions on a vehicle-kilometer basis due to the policies. But even if this is so, the ITO data demonstrate that technological solutions can be neutralized by increased activity.

ENERGY CONSUMPTION

The local impacts of rapid motorization in India are of course serious, but there are also important regional and global implications resulting from increased motorization in terms of energy security and climate change. The growth in energy consumption in road transport, which accounts for 90 percent of energy consumption for all transport modes, has been the most rapid of all sectors except for agriculture; energy consumption in road transport has tripled since 1981 in India. Globally as well, energy consumption has been increasing the most rapidly in road transport. Furthermore, while the residential and industrial sectors consume the most in terms of total energy use, road transport consumes the most in terms of petroleum products. While the shares of the other major sectors in petroleum consumption have declined since 1971, the share of road and other transport modes has grown significantly. In India, road transport accounts for 9 percent of all energy consumption, but it accounts for as much as 30 percent of the consumption of petroleum products. The transport sector is by far the most dependent on petroleum products, which supply nearly all of its energy needs. Globally the bulk of the growth in petroleum consumption is also due to transport; while road transport now accounts for a fifth of all energy consumption, and the transport sector as a whole for about 28 percent, these two sectors account for as much as 45 percent and 60 percent of global petroleum consumption.[30,31]

The high dependence on petroleum in the transport sector raises concerns from an energy security standpoint. Transport systems are vulnerable to potential oil supply disruptions, especially given that petroleum resources are unevenly distributed globally and are increasingly supplied from hard-to-access and politically volatile sources. This is particularly important in India and similar countries; although the OECD accounts for 65 percent of energy consumption in road transport, growth in this sector is by far the most rapid in Asia. In India, petroleum consumption, which supplies about 30 percent of all energy needs, has been doubling every 12 or so years since 1971. The future is daunting, given increasing trends in motor vehicle use and other energy-intensive activities: over two-thirds of India's oil requirement is imported, leaving India especially vulnerable to world oil prices.[32,33,34]

PEDESTRIAN AND CYCLIST ACCESSIBILITY

But of all the urban transport issues in India, the loss of accessibility, in particular for pedestrians, is perhaps the most critical. First of all, this is because the loss of accessibility adversely affects the most vulnerable road users. The pedestrian environment in Indian cities is so vitiated that walking, the most natural of human activities, has become an extremely unpleasant, indeed hazardous activity, as evidenced by the traffic fatality data. Indeed, the pedestrian has been rendered a third-class citizen in a nation of pedestrians.

The loss of pedestrian and cyclist accessibility not only severely affects the most vulnerable road users, it contributes to and exacerbates other serious urban transport impacts. It is because it is so time consuming, if not unsafe, for people to walk even short distances, that many trips over these distances are needlessly—and by force of circumstance—conducted by motor vehicles. This is especially true of the elderly, who often need to resort to hiring an auto-rickshaw or be driven just to cross the road; and if neither option is available, they suffer greatly by way of restricted activity, lost opportunities for social interactions, and so on. Also, because school children can no longer walk safely to school (or because parents are too wary of letting them do so), and because of the lack of school buses, children are driven to school. The increased congestion that results from these needless motor vehicle trips sets up a vicious circle, whereby accessibility and public transit viability are even more compromised than before, necessitating even greater use of motor vehicles. The largely avoidable use of motor vehicles for short-distance trips, which account for a significant proportion of all urban trips, exacerbates congestion, which in turn increases air pollution and energy consumption, because stop-go traffic typical of congested conditions increases vehicle emissions and worsens fuel economy.

Though levels of vehicle ownership in India are significantly lower than those in the OECD, as these levels rise the already serious urban transport issues discussed, including the loss of accessibility, intensified pollution and oil consumption, and increasing road traffic accidents, among others, will likely become even more serious. Tragically, the growing impacts affect all, including motor vehicle users.

WHY BUSINESS AS USUAL IS FUTILE

It is important to note that the loss of pedestrian accessibility is the result both of rapidly growing motor vehicle activity and transportation policy that privileges motor vehicle activity, while not only ignoring pedestrians and cyclists but actively discriminating against them. The loss of safe and convenient pedestrian and cyclist accessibility constitutes a user-on-nonuser externality, because, while pedestrians and cyclists benefit little from the provision of transport infrastructure, they bear the bulk of the burdens of motor vehicle activity; it is precisely because of the lack of pedestrian and cyclist infrastructure and facilities, and therefore the inability to walk and cycle safely, that such an overwhelming proportion of traffic fatalities are accounted for by these two modes of transport. This user-on-nonuser externality is rendered all the more serious by being caused as a result of discriminatory transport policy.

Policy making related to urban transport pays scant attention to the provision of infrastructure and facilities for pedestrians and cyclists, notwithstanding the National Urban Transport Policy,[35] which stresses the importance of these modes. Instead, it has focused predominantly on measures such as road widening, flyovers, limited access expressways, synchronized signals, and area traffic control systems to accommodate and improve the traffic characteristics of motor vehicles, and on technological measures to mitigate the impacts of motor vehicle activity per vehicle-kilometer, with a particular focus on congestion and air pollution. Urban road infrastructure projects are being implemented at great public expense. For example, Mumbai's 50-odd flyovers, completed about a decade ago, cost around US$440,000 each, and in Delhi, 30 new flyovers had been approved at the same time, at about US$70,000 to US$660,000 each. In Pune, a 5.5 kilometer four-lane elevated highway, projected to cost US$43 million per kilometer, was recently proposed.[36,37]

The US Example

While policy makers focus on road infrastructure development as the principal response to traffic congestion, building our way out of the problem is not only very expensive, it is, even worse, an exercise in futility, even in resource-rich contexts such as the United States. Capital and maintenance expenditures on US highways have increased 15 and 19 percent per annum since the 1970s, while annual growth in motor vehicles was only 3–4 percent. In 2000, US highway expenditures amounted to an astounding US$350 million every day.[38] Notwithstanding this massive investment, congestion has worsened, and is expected to continue to do so, particularly on urban highways.[39]

This trend in congestion despite continuous road building is not surprising—as international experience has shown, road building may improve speeds for motor vehicles and ease congestion in the short term, but these benefits tend to be neutralized over the longer term by attracting traffic from other routes, times, and destinations; shifting trips from public transit and other modes to personal motor vehicles; and by causing longer and new vehicle trips.[40] This process becomes an irreversible vicious spiral over time, as public transit and the nonmotorized modes become less viable due to increased congestion, and pedestrian and cyclist accessibility becomes even more compromised due to highway capacity additions, leading to automobile use becoming even more inevitable, and the need to build more roads. The net result is that road building as a means of addressing congestion is not only futile, it is counterproductive, since it worsens congestion as well as the other negative urban transport impacts discussed earlier. The conclusion reached by the Texas Transportation Institute, based on monitoring traffic congestion for decades in the United States, is instructive in this regard: "Additional roadways reduce the rate of increase in congestion. It appears that the growth in facilities has to be at a rate slightly greater than travel growth in order to maintain constant travel times, if additional roads are the only solution used to address mobility concerns."[41]

The Indian Context

If road building is futile in the United States, despite massive investments, one can only imagine the likely success of this approach in combating traffic congestion in India, given resource constraints, and ever-growing multiple demands on those resources. Furthermore, in the Indian context, addressing congestion through large-scale road building on an ongoing basis—including limited-access highways and flyovers—would not only be infeasible, it would also be highly undesirable, given the high population densities and poverty levels of Indian cities. Construction would displace large numbers of poor people, cause considerable social disruption, and further compromise access for nonmotorized mode users, who are already the most affected in this regard. Beyond the futility of construction to combat congestion, there is the peril of becoming locked into an inflexible and therefore highly vulnerable system. For example, in the event of oil supply disruptions or exorbitant pricing, personal vehicle use would be compromised, effectively crippling a transport system that caters to motorized vehicles.

Massive investments have also been devoted to rail-based metro systems since the late 1990s as a means of addressing rapidly growing traffic congestion. Delhi's metro system, and the one currently being built in Bangalore, cost roughly $40-45 million per kilometer to build.[42,43] Several Indian cities, following Delhi's example, are building, or are proposing to build, metro rail systems.[44]

In the Indian context, this approach presents several challenges. First of all, because of the high cost per kilometer and constrained resources, metro systems are likely to be highly circumscribed in terms of the extent of the network, relative to the size of rapidly growing metropolitan regions in low-income countries like India. Even these circumscribed systems take a long time to construct and become fully operational, and they are highly disruptive while being constructed, particularly in densely populated cities in low-income countries. Delhi's system, when fully operational in the "horizon year" of 2021, is planned to be 200–400 km long; in that year, the National Capital region is projected to cover an area of roughly 34,000 square kilometers and house as many as 64 million people. The network length of the first phase of Bangalore's system is 42 kilometers, in a metropolitan region that is one of the most rapidly growing in Asia, and currently extends to around 8,000 square kilometers.[45,46,47,48]

Secondly, metro systems need to be both widespread and fine-grained in order to attract a high ridership. Studies the world over have shown that, if motor vehicle users have to travel farther than about 500 meters to access metro, or indeed, any mass transit system, they will likely prefer to commute in their personal motor vehicles rather than use public transit. Given this fact, the number of motor vehicle–owning commuters who would use circumscribed metro networks is likely to be quite limited, relative to the total number of motor vehicle users in rapidly growing and motorizing metropolitan regions. This situation is only likely to be further exacerbated because access to public transit is compromised in the Indian context.

Furthermore, the potential for high ridership is even more constrained because metro systems are not competitive with personal motor vehicles in terms of door-to-door journey times over the short- and medium-distance trips that form the bulk of urban trips (see later), and because many commuters need to combine different trip purposes.[49] Also, while fares have to be high in order to recoup their costs, a very small proportion of urban commuters can afford even subsidized fares. Scooters and motorcycles, the bulk of the motor vehicle fleet, offer their highly price-sensitive users door-to-door capability, unmatched navigability in congested road conditions, ease of parking, and the ability to carry passengers and luggage at very low cost. Given all of these factors, it is not clear to what extent metro rail systems can cost-effectively mitigate congestion and other urban transport impacts over the long term in Indian cities.

URBAN TRANSPORT IN INDIA—CHARACTERISTICS AND CONSIDERATIONS

Vehicle Ownership

Rapid urbanization and growth in urban incomes, and the fact that vehicle manufacturing is increasingly shifting to Asia, are of course important contributors to the rapid growth in motor vehicle ownership and activity in India. Sociocultural forces, by way of the aspiration of middle-class Indians to first own a motorcycle or scooter, and then replace it as quickly as possible with a car, also play a crucial role. These forces are only strengthened by marketing that projects cars as status symbols, by easily available credit, buy-back schemes, and the like. Changing demographics also contribute to rapidly growing personal motor vehicle ownership and activity, including the increasingly atomistic family structure, and growing female workforce participation.

Equally important in the Indian context is the fact that motorcycles and scooters form the bulk of the motor vehicle fleet, since, in addition to their high maneuverability in congested traffic, these vehicles cost a fraction of what cars do to own and operate, especially as they have become more fuel efficient.[50] The marginal cost of operating a scooter or motorcycle, even at current gasoline prices, is a little more than a rupee per kilometer. These factors explain the preponderance of these vehicles and demonstrate why, although India has a much lower motor vehicle ownership than the industrialized West, it has a considerably higher per capita motor vehicle ownership than countries such as Mexico did when at the same levels of per capita income.[51]

The rapid growth in motor vehicle ownership and use is also due to force of circumstance. Many people have been forced to live in areas poorly served by transit in the urban periphery because they have been priced out of the land market in the inner cities. But even in areas covered by public transit, service is unreliable, inconvenient, and increasingly expensive. Consequently, because of increased traffic congestion and compromised access and safety, many people have been forced to purchase and use personal motor vehicles, if they can afford them.

Poverty

While incomes are growing for many, Indian cities are also characterized by poverty. Even in Delhi, one of the most affluent cities in India, the average annual income per capita in 2008 was roughly US$1540, or about US$4.20 per day.[53] Nearly half of Delhi's population lives in unauthorized settlements, rural villages, and slums.[54] This means that, even as motor vehicle ownership and activity continue to grow, significant sections of the population cannot afford even the least expensive motor vehicles, and indeed, even public transit fares, which for a round trip average around 50 cents.[55,56,57] Delhi's motor vehicle ownership—including motorized two-wheeled vehicles—was under 300 per 1,000 people in 2008,[58,59] despite it being by far the most motorized Indian city; in the same year, by comparison, Canada's motor vehicle ownership—excluding motorized two-wheeled vehicles—was over 600 per 1,000 people.[60]

The confluence of growing incomes and motorization on the one hand, and low affordability and poverty (and consequently, low motor vehicle ownership) among a significant proportion of the urban population on the other, has important implications for urban transport. While the high levels of impacts imposed on the large populations in Indian cities give rise to significant and serious health and welfare effects, there are important synergies between urban transport impacts and poverty. The significant proportion of the population that is poor hardly benefits from motor vehicle activity while bearing the lion's share of its adverse impacts. Furthermore, these impacts exacerbate their poverty. That the urban poor are likely the most exposed to, affected by, and least capable of coping with the impacts of air pollution has been already discussed, as has the fact that road traffic deaths and injuries and the serious associated economic impacts are suffered disproportionately by pedestrians and cyclists, many of whom are poor. Additionally, it should be noted that because of inadequate accessibility in the periphery, the poor face higher travel-related time and monetary costs. Poor accessibility in the periphery also has implications for gender equity. Low-income women in the periphery are particularly affected by the lower accessibility, poorer employment opportunities, and inadequate public transit provision relative to the central areas, as these barriers limit their transportation choices and income-generation possibilities. Lastly, it should be noted that road building and other urban transport projects cause social disruption, further compromise access for non-motorized mode users, and displace large numbers of poor people; indeed, thousands of poor families have been displaced to the periphery, as a result of such projects, and in the name of "urban beautification."[61,62,63,64]

Urban Geography

The low per capita incomes—indeed the high levels of poverty—in Indian cities, coupled with their geographical layout, also have important implications for the characteristics of urban travel in India. Because of low average per capita incomes, and an urban geography characterized by high densities and intensive mixed use, there is proportionally little discretionary trip making in Indian cities. Importantly, a significant proportion of trips are conducted over short and medium distances. Consequently, even though the trip shares of the non-motorized modes and public transit have declined over time, the majority of trips continue to be made by these modes. In Delhi, by far the most motorized Indian city, as many as 40 percent of all trips are conducted within a distance of 2.5 km. As many as 33 percent of all trips are made on foot or bicycle, and 42 percent by public transit, with only 19 percent of trips being made in personal motor vehicles.[65,66] In Mumbai, an even larger, and on average, wealthier city than Delhi,[67] more than half of all household trips are made on foot, and 30 percent by public transit; personal motor vehicles account for a mere 10 percent of all trips.[68] This is in spite of the increase in motorization, the poor quality of the pedestrian environment and public transit service, and the degradation of the natural advantages of a high-density, mixed-use urban geography that is the result of planning that discriminates against walking and cycling.

Resource Allocation

In addition to the implications of low affordability and poverty on the part of the majority in its cities, urban transport policy in India must consider the serious resource constraints. The provision and maintenance of physical infrastructure is not the only cost; administrative and financial resources are also required for effective regulation, monitoring, and enforcement to control the impacts of rapidly growing motor vehicle activity. In this regard, note that traffic congestion is growing, even in Delhi, despite the city enjoying the largest supply of roads of any Indian city and the massive investments that continue to be made in its transport infrastructure. Lastly, important as urban transport is, Indian cities face a multitude of serious challenges, including provision of drinking water, adequate sanitation, and housing, among others, and therefore multiple growing demands on limited resources.

The urban transport challenge in Indian cities is how to cater to rapidly growing mass mobility needs while minimizing adverse resource use, environmental, health and welfare, and socio-economic impacts at the local, regional, and global scales, and being mindful of the urban travel needs and priorities, and capabilities and constraints, in the context.

Because resources are constrained, and there are multiple growing demands on them, we must aim to achieve synergies by developing urban transport solutions that mitigate the wide range of impacts in a cost-effective manner. For the same reason, we need to develop urban transport systems that promote resilience—or in other words, that reduce vulnerability to disruptions of various kinds. And because health, broadly defined, is not merely the absence of disease, and because the purpose of public space is not merely to enable the conveyance of vehicles and people from one point to another, urban transport policy ought to strive not only to minimize the various adverse impacts discussed but also to promote well-being (in terms of liveability and livelihoods). Given socioeconomic realities, it is important for urban transport policy and planning in India to pay particular attention to the needs of low-income groups and the poor, and the modes on which they depend. This is important because these groups represent a significant share of the urban population, and the modes that they rely on—in many cases, as a matter of necessity—account for the bulk of urban trips, despite adverse circumstances. More generally, since different groups in society are differentially affected by motorization, and the costs and benefits of motorization and policies to accommodate it are unevenly distributed across society, urban transport policy and planning in India must cater to a wide range of road user groups with conflicting needs and objectives, and multiple modes of transport with differing characteristics. Finally, while the bulk of policy attention tends to be focused on the urban transport situation in the metropolitan centers, it should be noted that both population and motor vehicle growth are at least as rapid in the medium-sized towns and cities, in which the urban transport situation is far more stressed, and the resources to deal with transport far more constrained, than in the metropolitan centers.

With all this in mind, how can we develop an urban transport policy that is sensitive to these considerations in the Indian context? Personal motor vehicles play a vitally important role in urban transport, since they fulfill mobility needs for millions; so do various technological measures to accommodate and mitigate the impacts of motor vehicle activity. What is problematic is the excessive use of cars and other personal motor vehicles for easily avoidable trips; even more problematic is privileging motor vehicles in urban transport policy, at the expense of the nonmotorized modes, which in fact leads to excessive vehicle use and all of the negative impacts that it entails. Because of this, and also since continuous infrastructure building to accommodate motor vehicles is in the end infeasible and futile, and technological measures to mitigate negative impacts on a per-kilometer basis can be neutralized with increased activity, the primary objective of urban transport policy ought to be to minimize the need for motor vehicle ownership and activity, and restrict the use of motor vehicles to their most highly valued purposes. Urban transport policy should not privilege mobility for the few but ensure accessibility for the benefit of all. To the extent that motor vehicles are used, urban transport policy must aim to have as much of it as possible occur in high-occupancy modes; it is only for the residual motor vehicle activity that technological measures to mitigate its impacts ought to be applied.

What we need, therefore, in order to effectively address the urban transport challenge over the long term, is an integrated approach that encompasses a range of interlocking actions. As shown in Figure 8.1, land use-transport integration must be the very foundation of transport policy. But it should be noted that in the Indian context, while sprawl and haphazard development on the urban periphery due to poor land use regulation is of concern and needs to be controlled especially because of its urban transport implications, and transport corridors need to be optimally routed and integrated with land use to maximize transit ridership, the high densities and intensely mixed land use in Indian cities generally facilitate a minimized need for personal motor vehicle use. Indeed, it is the increasingly motor vehicle-centered planning that is destroying this natural advantage. Nonmotorized transport (NMT) should be the next greatest priority in preventing excessive motor vehicle use. At the other end of the spectrum, technological measures to mitigate per-vehicle impacts and solutions such as traffic engineering and management are curative rather than preventive. All policy action must take place with effective coordination across these different initiatives and be sensitive to the relevant geographic limitations, time scales, and agencies involved. For these reasons, the subsequent discussion focuses on public transit that is reliable, convenient, affordable, and widespread; pricing of road use to internalize the social costs of urban transport and provide incentives for minimizing motor vehicle

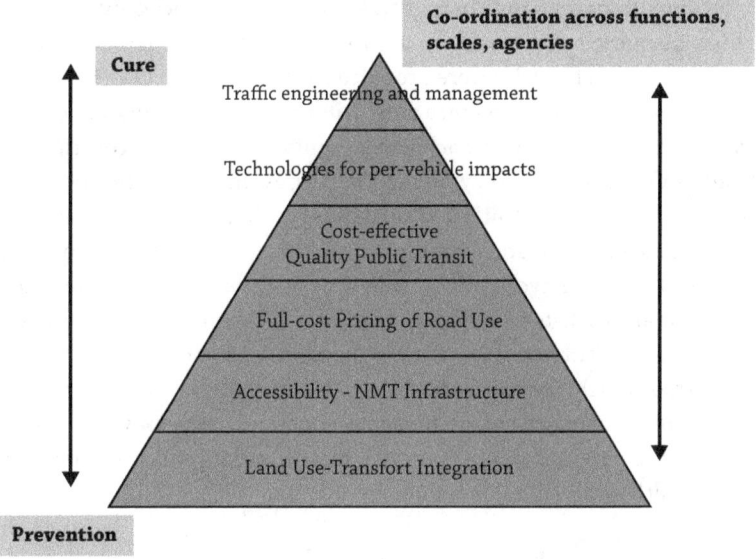

Figure 8.1:
Policy and Planning Pyramid for An Integrated Approach to Urban Transport

activity; and last but not least, accessibility for all, in particular pedestrians. Indeed, these measures should be seen as comprising a three-legged stool, with each measure depending on the other two.

Accessibility and Infrastructure for Nonmotorized Modes

Accessibility for all, and in particular pedestrian accessibility, should be the very foundation of urban transport policy and planning, if we are to achieve the objectives discussed at the end of the last section. Providing adequate infrastructure and facilities for pedestrians (and cyclists) is only logical and fair, given that the majority do not own personal motor vehicles, and the fact that a large proportion of trips are conducted by these modes. Furthermore, given that the majority of road fatalities, perhaps the most serious urban transport issue in India, are pedestrians and cyclists, it is imperative that safe accessibility for these modes be ensured. Just as importantly, making walking and cycling safer and easier by providing adequate infrastructure and facilities for these modes would reduce short-distance motor vehicle trips, which are both the most avoidable and the most energy-consuming and polluting on a per-kilometer basis, thereby contributing to reductions in congestion, emissions, and energy consumption with high cost-effectiveness, and obviating the need for expensive (and futile) end-of-pipeline technological cures. Lastly, as the European experience described in Chapter 7 demonstrates, walking and cycling are potentially competitive with motor vehicles over short and medium distances, and would be used even more than they already are, if infrastructure and facilities were provided for them.

The provision of infrastructure and facilities for pedestrians and cyclists in Indian cities is important for achieving equity objectives by contributing to easy and safe access to employment and other essential services for the poor. It will also help address multiple urban transport impacts and be of great benefit for all, including personal motor vehicle users, for while the poor have no choice but to walk or cycle, not all who walk are poor. Furthermore, whereas pedestrians and cyclists fare extremely poorly and are in fact highly vulnerable to various urban transport impacts in a system designed to cater for motor vehicles, motor vehicles can in fact operate efficiently in a system that takes the needs of pedestrians and cyclists into account. Lastly, providing adequate infrastructure and facilities for safe walking and cycling will promote liveability, and health and well-being for all.

Cost-Effective, Quality Public Transit Provision

Maintaining and enhancing the delivery of public transit service that is reliable, convenient, affordable, and widespread is vitally important for meeting rapidly growing mass mobility needs in Indian cities. First and foremost, this is because low-income commuters, the vast majority, have no choice but to use public transit if they can afford it, however inconvenient and time consuming it may be, and will likely continue to depend on it for their economic survival. Affordable mobility is particularly important for this group, because low-income households already spend large shares of their income on transport, thus affecting their expenditure on health, shelter, and food. In Mumbai, for example, the lowest income groups spent 15 percent of their income on transport against an average of about 10 percent for all income groups.[69,70] At the same time, quality public transit is essential in order to have a chance of attracting personal motor vehicle users and curbing motor vehicle activity. Finally, public transit accounts for significantly lower emissions, fatalities, and road space use on a passenger-kilometer basis than personal motorized modes. These characteristics are extremely important in a context in which transport impacts already overwhelm scarce resources, and expanding road infrastructure is difficult on account of high population densities.

While urban rail projects are either being built or considered for various Indian cities, it remains to be seen how effective and financially viable they will be in the long run, as discussed earlier. Even if they are effective, it will be several years before they become fully operational, and motor vehicle activity will likely grow in the meantime. Finally, it is unlikely that urban rail would be economically viable in medium-sized cities, in which per capita incomes are low and population growth and mobility needs are increasing rapidly. Bus-based systems have the potential to be a low-cost transit solution appropriate to the realities of the Indian context.[71] Besides, even if urban rail systems are implemented, efficient feeder buses will be needed in order for these systems to be truly effective. Lastly, Indian cities rely predominantly on buses for their public transport needs, with the exception of Mumbai, where rail plays a major role, and are likely to continue to do so over the coming years. For all of these reasons, bus transit systems will be vitally important for meeting mass mobility needs at low cost.

However, the state of India's urban bus transport systems leaves much to be desired in terms of user satisfaction. Urban bus transit corporations have suffered heavy losses owing to increasing input costs and declining productivity; the losses have persisted despite rapidly increasing fares, and ridership has declined even as capacity has increased.[72] Despite subsidized fares, bus travel has been simply unaffordable for a significant proportion of urban residents.[73,74] If bus transit use is high despite the poor service, it is because of the lack of viable alternatives for the bulk of users. Apart from jeopardizing the ability to meet rapidly growing mass mobility needs, the poor urban bus transit situation will likely cause accelerated growth in private motor vehicle ownership and activity, particularly in the case of scooters and motorcycles, given their advantages relative to public transit. The situation is rendered more acute by the large accumulated losses and reduced government contributions to urban transit, leading to a vicious spiral in which poor service levels contribute to declining ridership and accelerated personal motor vehicle use, which in turn further compromise bus service levels. Small and medium-sized cities face a particularly serious challenge in sustaining public transit ridership. This challenge is demonstrated by the fact that, while public transit mode shares have declined over the last couple of decades in all Indian cities, these shares are both much lower, and have declined even more sharply, in small and medium-sized cities than in the metropolitan centers.[75,76]

It is of course important to improve the management of bus operations in order to meet the aforementioned challenges. It is worth noting that some urban bus operations in India have performed significantly better than their counterparts under similar circumstances, which demonstrates the possibility for improvement. But it is also important to recognize that buses, important as they are for affordably meeting mass mobility needs, perform inefficiently in congested, mixed traffic. One response to this challenge is to implement, wherever appropriate and possible, bus rapid transit (BRT) systems operating on dedicated busways, with passengers boarding and alighting rapidly. BRT systems are a promising means of improving service to maintain and enhance ridership, since such systems can potentially carry significantly more people per hour than conventional bus systems, and indeed, as many per hour as some rail systems. Furthermore, because BRT systems involve buses and other modes using road space in their own lanes with minimal conflicts with one another, all modes are able to operate more efficiently, therefore potentially allowing the movement of a significantly higher number of people per hour overall, while also significantly reducing vehicular energy consumption, air pollution, and accident rates. And because they are significantly less expensive than equivalent rail-based mass transit, a far more widespread network may be provided with BRT than with metro systems for the same investment. A survey of BRT systems worldwide showed that, for the same ridership levels, BRT systems cost one-sixth to one-eighteenth per kilometer.[77] Also, BRT can be constructed and expanded more readily and flexibly using existing road infrastructure. BRT systems are therefore ideally suited, when properly designed and implemented, to be low-cost mass transit solutions that are appropriate for cities in India and other rapidly motorizing, low-income countries. Of course, rail-based mass transit can play an important role in certain circumstances, as in Mumbai. And where rail-based mass transit is being built, as in Delhi, such systems and BRT can, and should, be designed to complement each other. Lastly, the provision of public transit in the rapidly growing urban periphery will need particular attention.

Rational Pricing of Road Use

The effectiveness of efforts to minimize motor vehicle activity and its adverse impacts depends importantly on the rational pricing of road use. When the monetary costs associated with the provision of transport infrastructure and the environmental and social costs due to motor vehicle activity are not fully borne by road users, the perceived cost of motor vehicle activity to them is low. Without government intervention to ensure cost internalization, there will likely be ever-increasing motor vehicle activity, leading to an excess of associated negative externalities. Rational pricing of road use in order to internalize the costs of motor vehicle activity as far as possible is therefore important for limiting this activity to its most valued uses. At the same time, while measures like BRT would help improve the time-competitiveness of bus transit, internalizing the costs of motor vehicle use would render public transit more attractive, and therefore effective, by increasing the marginal cost of motor vehicle use relative to transit (this is especially true of scooters and motorcycles, given their low operating costs). Also, by curbing motor vehicle use, this measure would allow transit to operate more efficiently in mixed traffic.

Pricing policies that target variable rather than fixed costs (by, for example, taxing motor vehicle use instead of only ownership) are likely to be far more effective in influencing commuter choices that favor reduced personal motor vehicle use and increased public transit use. In this regard, one aspect of motor vehicle use that needs serious attention in Indian cities is parking. It is well recognized that parking availability and pricing are major determinants of automobile use. As long as parking is abundant and free or inexpensive, personal motor vehicle users will have little incentive to consider mass transit, high quality though it may be.[78,79,80,81] Parking control and pricing will undoubtedly be difficult to implement in Indian cities, especially for scooters and motorcycles since they can be parked easily anywhere, but it would help curb motor vehicle use, free up road and sidewalk space to render traffic flow more efficient for all modes, and make mass transit more attractive. In addition, appropriate pricing policies can serve as a means of funding public transport.

Maintaining and enhancing quality public transit service, rational pricing of road use, and accessibility for all, particularly pedestrians, are vitally important measures that depend on each other for their individual and overall effectiveness. Improving the attractiveness and effectiveness of public transit depends importantly on measures to curb personal motor vehicle use through pricing to increase its marginal cost relative to transit. Additionally, promoting safe and convenient walking and cycling would contribute significantly to enhancing the effectiveness of public transit, both by improving access to it and by helping improve its operational efficiency by segregating and minimizing conflicts between modes in mixed traffic. At the same time, however, measures to curb personal motor vehicle use would be politically unacceptable without the provision of convenient and affordable transit options, and safe and easy pedestrian accessibility. Though the pricing of transport infrastructure will be politically if not technically challenging, implementation difficulties may be eased by strategically phasing in pricing, along with the other measures. Finally, increasing the attractiveness of walking and cycling depends not only on the provision of adequate infrastructure and facilities for these modes but also on reducing motor vehicle congestion. Because this, in turn, depends on more effective public transit, and rational pricing of road use, one can see how these measures not only depend on, but also reinforce, each other.

SUMMARY AND CONCLUSIONS

Rapid motorization in India delivers significant societal benefits, in terms of providing mobility to millions, but it also contributes to a range of serious resource use, environmental, health and welfare, and socioeconomic impacts at the local, regional, and global scales. This situation, which is already serious despite motor vehicle ownership and activity levels that are significantly lower than those in the OECD, will likely become even more so as these levels rise. These impacts particularly affect the urban poor, who benefit little from motor vehicle activity. The situation in medium-sized cities, in which population and motorization rates are growing very rapidly, is particularly concerning.

The loss of accessibility, in particular for pedestrians, is perhaps the most important urban transport issue because it not only severely affects the most vulnerable road users but also contributes to and exacerbates other serious urban transport impacts. This is the result of rapidly growing motor vehicle activity as well as transportation policy that privileges motor vehicles, and not only ignores pedestrians (and cyclists) but actively discriminates against them. Motor vehicle–centered planning, which assumes we can build our way out of congestion and other impacts, is futile, as well as counterproductive, even in resource-rich contexts like the United States, since this approach only makes motor vehicle activity ever more inevitable, leading to a vicious circle of ever-increasing motorization and impacts, which affect all, including motor vehicle users and pedestrians. In the Indian context, not only would this approach be infeasible, it would be highly undesirable, because of the access loss and social disruption it would cause.

The urban transport challenge in Indian cities is how to cater for rapidly growing mass mobility needs while minimizing adverse resource use, environmental, health and welfare, and socioeconomic impacts at the local, regional and global scales, and being mindful of the characteristics of the context that have important implications for urban transport—low motor vehicle ownership, high poverty levels, an urban geography characterized by high densities and intensive mixed use, and multiple demands on constrained resources.

Personal motor vehicles play a vitally important role in urban transport, since they fulfill mobility needs for millions, as do technological measures to accommodate and mitigate the impacts of motor vehicle activity. But given the foregoing contextual characteristics, and the fact that continuous infrastructure building to accommodate motor vehicles is futile and technological measures can be neutralized with increased activity, the primary objective of urban transport policy ought to be to minimize the need for motor vehicle ownership and activity, and restrict the use of motor vehicles to their most highly valued purposes. Furthermore, urban transport policy ought not to privilege mobility for the few but ensure accessibility for the benefit of all; in particular, it ought to pay attention to the needs of low-income groups and the poor, and the modes on which they depend.

Achieving these objectives will call for an integrated approach that encompasses a range of interlocking actions, including in particular reliable, convenient, affordable, and widespread public transit; pricing of road use that internalizes the social costs of urban transport, and provides incentives for minimizing motor vehicle activity; and last but not least, accessibility for all, in particular pedestrians, as the very foundation of urban transport policy. Such an approach will help lead to an urban transport system that is cost effective, health promoting, resource conserving, environmentally benign, and of great benefit for all, including personal motor vehicle users as well as the urban poor.

NOTES

1. A. Faiz et al., *Air Pollution from Motor Vehicles: Issues and Options for Developing Countries* (Washington, DC: The World Bank, 1990).
2. M. Walsh, *Global Trends in Motor Vehicle Pollution Control* (Falconer Lecture, May 2005), accessed May 20, 2011, http://www.walshcarlines.com/pdf/Falconer%20 Lecture2.pdf.
3. *EIU Data Services*, Economist Intelligence Unit, accessed March 10, 2011, http:// www.eiu.com/Default.aspx.
4. G. Plouchart, *Energy Consumption in the Transport Sector* (Paris, France: IFP, 2005).
5. Organisation Internationale des Constructeurs d'Automobiles. *World Motor Vehicle Production by Country and Type 2009-2010, OICA Correspondents Survey* (Paris, France: Organisation Internationale des Constructeurs d'Automobiles, 2011).
6. *Automobile Production Trends*, Society of Indian Automobile Manufacturers, Delhi, accessed January 2012, http://www.siamindia.com/scripts/ production-trend.aspx
7. *Statistical Year Book 2012*, Ministry of Statistics and Programme Implementation, Government of India, accessed May 19, 2013, http://mospi. nic.in/mospi_new/upload/statistical_year_book_2012/htm/index1.html
8. Ministry of Road Transport and Highways, *Road Accidents in India, 2009* (New Delhi, India: Ministry of Road Transport and Highways, Government of India, 2011).
9. World Health Organization, *Global Status Report on Road Safety: Time for Action* (Geneva, Switzerland: World Health Organization, 2009).
10. E. Kopits and M. Cropper, "Traffic Fatalities and Economic Growth," *Accident Analysis and Prevention*, 37 (2005): 169–78.
11. National Crime Records Bureau, *Crime in India* (New Delhi, India: Ministry of Home Affairs, Government of India, 2001).
12. V. M. Nantulya and M. R. Reich, "The Neglected Epidemic: Road Traffic Injuries in Developing Countries," *British Medical Journal* 324 (2002): 1139–41.
13. Central Institute of Road Transport, *State Transport Undertakings— Profile and Performance 2005-2006* (Pune, India: Central Institute of Road Transport, 2007).
14. D. Mohan, *The Road Ahead: Traffic Injuries and Fatalities in India* (Delhi, India: Indian Institute of Technology, 2004).
15. The Sundar Committee, *Report of the Committee on Road Safety and Traffic Management* (New Delhi, India: Ministry of Road Transport and Highways, Government of India, 2007).
16. World Health Organization, *Global Status Report* . . .
17. M. Varghese, "Long-Term Health and Welfare Effects of Traffic Accident Injuries," (presentation, Workshop on Transport, Health, Environment, and Equity in Indian Cities, TRIPP, Delhi, India, December 17–19, 2007).
18. Ibid.
19. Wilbur Smith Associates, *Study on Traffic and Transportation Policies and Strategies in Urban Areas in India—Final Report* (Bangalore, India: Wilbur Smith Associates, 2008).
20. *Ambient Air Quality Data*, Central Pollution Control Board, New Delhi, accessed May 2013, http://cpcb.nic.in/

21. A. Gertler et al., *Hyderabad Source Apportionment Study* (Washington, DC: US Environmental Protection Agency, 2007).

21a. The World Health Organisation guidelines on particulate matter are as follows: $PM_{2.5:}$ 10 μg/m³ annual mean, 25 μg/m³ 24-hour mean. $PM_{10:}$ 20 μg/m³ annual mean, 50 μg/m³ 24-hour mean. World Health Organization, *Air Quality and Health Factsheet (2011),* accessed August 2012, http://www.who.int/mediacentre/factsheets/fs313/en/index.html.

22. Central Pollution Control Board, *Ambient Air...*

23. The Energy Research Institute, *TERI Energy Data Directory and Yearbook 2001/2002* (New Delhi, India: Energy Research Institute, 2002).

24. Centre for Science and Environment, *Slow Murder—The Deadly Story of Vehicular Pollution in India* (New Delhi, India: Centre for Science and Environment, 1996).

25. Faiz et al., *Air Pollution...*

26. Centre for Science and Environment, *State of India's Environment—The Citizens' Fifth Report, Part I: National Overview* (New Delhi, India: Centre for Science and Environment, 2002).

27. Bureau of Indian Standards, *Motor Gasolines—Specification, IS 2796: 2000*, 3rd rev. with amendments (New Dehli, India: Bureau of Indian Standards, 2002).

28. M. Kojima, C. Brandon, and J. Shah, *Improving Urban Air Quality in South Asia by Reducing Emissions from Two-stroke Engine Vehicles* (Washington, DC: The World Bank, 2000).

29. The Energy Research Institute, *TERI Energy Data...*

30. International Energy Agency, *Energy Balances of OECD Countries*, (Paris, France: International Energy Agency, 2009).

31. International Energy Agency, *Energy Balances of Non-OECD Countries*, (Paris, France: International Energy Agency, 2009).

32. International Energy Agency, *Energy Balances of OECD...*

33. International Energy Agency, *Energy Balances of Non-...*

34. *Full Country Analysis Brief on India*, US Energy Information Agency, accessed October 1, 2010, http://www.eia.gov/countries/cab.cfm?fips=IN.

35. *National Urban Transport Policy*, Ministry of Urban Development, Government of India, accessed May 1, 2009, http://urbanindia.nic.in/policies/TransportPolicy.pdf

36. G. Tiwari, "Urban Transport Priorities—Meeting the Challenge of Socio-economic Diversity in Cities: A Case Study of Delhi, India," *Cities* 19 (2002): 95–103.

37. N. Patil and A. Khape, "Now, the Debate is on How 5.5 km Elevated Road Will be Funded," *Indian Express*, May 7, 2008.

38. *Highway Funding and Expenditures*, Federal Highway Administration, US Department of Transportation, accessed May 1, 2009, http://www.fhwa.dot.gov/ohim/onh00/onh2p10.htm

39. Texas Transportation Institute. *2007 Annual Urban Mobility Report*, (College Station, TX: Texas Transportation Institute, 2007).

40. T. Litman, *Generated Traffic and Induced Travel: Implications for Transport Planning* (Victoria, BC: Victoria Transport Planning Institute, 2007).

41. Texas Transportation Institute, *2007 Annual Urban...*

42. Delhi Metro Rail Corporation official website, accessed May 1, 2013, www.delhimetrorail.com

43. Bangalore Metro Rail Corporation official website, accessed May 1, 2009, http://www.bmrc.co.in/

44. D. Mohan, "Mythologies, Metro Rail Systems, and Future Urban Transport," *Economic and Political Weekly,* January 26, 2008, 41–53.
45. Delhi Metro Rail Corporation official website.
46. Bangalore Metro Rail Corporation official website.
47. *Draft Master Plan for Delhi-2021,* Ministry of Urban Development, Government of India, accessed May 1, 2009, http://www.urbanindia.nic.in/moud/what'snew/mps-eng.pdf
48. K. C. Sivaramakrishnan and A. Maiti, "Metropolitan Governance in India—An Overview of Selected Cities," (presentation, Workshop on Governance and Infrastructure Development Challenges in the Kathmandu Valley, Kathmandu, India, February 11–13, 2009).
49. Mohan, "Mythologies . . ."
50. N. V. Iyer and M. G. Badami, "Two-Wheeled Motor Vehicle Technology in India: Evolution, Prospects and Issues," *Energy Policy* 35 (2007): 4319–31.
51. R. Gakenheimer, "Urban Mobility in the Developing World," *Transportation Research Part A (Policy and Practice)* 33 (1999): 671–90.
52. RITES and ORG, *Household Travel Surveys in Delhi* (Rail India Technical and Economic Services Limited, New Delhi, and Operations Research Group, Baroda, India, 1994).
53. *Economic Survey of Delhi 2007-2008,* Government of the National Capital Territory of Delhi, accessed May 1, 2009, http://delhiplanning.nic.in/Economic%20Survey/ES2007-08/ES2007-08.htm
54. *Delhi—The Hot Spot,* National River Conservation Directorate, Ministry of Environment and Forests, Government of India, accessed May 1, 2009, http://yap.nic.in/delhi-slums.asp
55. M. G. Badami, G. Tiwari, and D. Mohan, "Access and Mobility for the Urban Poor in India," in *The Inclusive City: Infrastructure and Public Services for the Urban Poor in Asia,* eds. A. A. Laquian, V. Tewari, and L. Hanley (Washington, DC and Baltimore, MD: Woodrow Wilson Center Press, Johns Hopkins University Press, 2007), 100–121.
56. Tiwari, "Urban Transport Priorities . . ."
57. *Fare Stages and Fare Charts,* Delhi Transport Corporation, accessed February 1, 2012, http://www.delhi.gov.in/wps/wcm/connect/doit_dtc/DTC/All+Services/Fare+Stages+and+Fare+Charts
58. Government of the National Capital Territory of Delhi, *Economic Survey of Delhi 2007-2008.*
59. *Motor Vehicle Statistics,* Government of the National Capital Territory of Delhi, accessed May 1, 2009, http://transport.delhigovt.nic.in/info/info8.html.
60. *Motor Vehicles (per 1,000 People),* World Bank, accessed February 1, 2012, http://data.worldbank.org/indicator/IS.VEH.NVEH.P3
61. A. Arora, "Impact of Transport Projects on Accessibility and Mobility of the Urban Poor: Case of the Delhi Metro," (presentation, Workshop on Transport, Health, Environment, and Equity in Indian Cities, at IIT Delhi, New Delhi, India, December 17-19, 2007).
62. Tiwari, "Urban Transport Priorities . . ."
63. S. Srinivasan and P. Rogers, "Travel Behavior of Low-Income Residents: Studying Two Contrasting Locations in the City of Chennai, India, *Journal of Transportation Geography* 13 (2005): 265–74.
64. D. Mahadevia, "NURM and the Poor in Globalising Mega Cities," *Economic and Political Weekly*, August 5, 2006, 3399–403.

65. RITES and ORG, *Household Travel...*
66. Wilbur Smith Associates, *Study on Traffic and Transportation...*
67. Government of Maharashtra. *Economic Survey of Maharashtra 2003-04* (Mumbai, India: Government of Maharashtra, 2004).
68. J. Baker et al., *Urban Poverty and Transport: The Case of Mumbai* (World Bank Report 3693, Washington, DC: The World Bank, 2005).
69. Tiwari, "Urban Transport Priorities..."
70. Baker et al., *Urban Poverty and Transport...*
71. D. Mohan et al., *Delhi on the Move 2005: Future Traffic Management Scenarios,* (report prepared for the Central Pollution Control Board, Indian Institute of Technology, New Delhi, 1997).
72. M. G. Badami and M. Haider, "An Analysis of Public Bus Transit Performance in Indian Cities," *Transportation Research Part A (Policy and Practice)* 41 (2007): 961–81.
73. Tiwari, "Urban Transport Priorities..."
74. R. Carruthers, M. Dick, and A. Saurkar, *Affordability of Public Transport in Developing Countries* (transport paper TP-3, Washington, DC: World Bank Group, 2005).
75. RITES and ORG, *Household Travel...*
76. Wilbur Smith Associates, *Study on Traffic and Transportation...*
77. A. Ables, C. Huizenga, and B. Fabian, "Potential of Bus Rapid Transit in Improving Public Transportation in Metro Manila," (presentation, Capacity Building Program on Mainstreaming Environmentally Sustainable Transportation (EST) in Local and Metropolitan Development, at Makati City Hall, Manila, Philipines, March 3, 2006).
78. R. W. Willson and D. C. Shoup, "Parking Subsidies and Travel Choices: Assessing the Evidence," *Transportation* 17 (1990): 141–57.
79. D. C. Shoup, "The High Cost of Free Parking," *Journal of Planning Education and Research* 17 (1997): 3–20.
80. H. Knoflacher, "A New Way to Organize Parking: The Key to a Successful Sustainable Transport System for the Future," *Environment and Urbanization* 18, no. 2 (2006): 387–400.
81. P. Barter, "Parking Policy in Asian Cities," (consultant's report, Asian Development Bank, Lee Kuan Yew School of Public Policy, National University of Singapore, Singapore, 2010).

CHAPTER 9

Healthy and Sustainable Agriculture

Working with Farmers to Transform Food Production in

Latin America

DONALD COLE, GORDON PRAIN, AND WILLY PRADEL

Food production systems have a crucial impact on the supply of food as well as the health and well-being of those who produce food. Environmental processes and economic structures strongly influence how agricultural systems are organized.[1] In turn, systems of agricultural production, distribution, and consumption can be responsible for hugely variable impacts on economic equity and environmental processes that determine sustainability. Given that food is basic to life, it is no wonder that human food security and health are intimately bound up with the context, conditions, and forms in which we produce food.[2,3]

Globally, increasing concern has been expressed by diverse stakeholders on the multiple impacts of current agricultural technology and practices[4] and the effects of environmental and economic changes on global food security and agricultural sustainability, especially related to climate change and volatility in global food prices.[5,6] This chapter seeks to reflect the current landscape of challenges or issues on the one hand and responses on the other, drawing on multiple disciplines. Behind our exposition is a systems understanding of complex interactions among system parts, across different subsystems and levels. Farming and livelihood systems research linked with economic analyses have been essential for advancing understanding of the potential benefits of agricultural technologies in improving the well-being of poor people in low- and middle-income countries (LMICs).[7] A comprehensive literature has developed on food systems "which include not only [food] production but processing, distribution, use, recycling and waste disposal."[8] Food system links with environmental sustainability have been made in order to examine impacts on food security and social welfare[9] and in understanding how current models of globalization contribute to inequities in food availability, accessibility, and affordability.[10]

Each section of this chapter aims to use these systems understandings to summarize key points at the global level, followed by our experience in the Andes of Latin America. Andean countries exemplify not only the huge disparities in wealth that exist globally (the mean UN Gini coefficient for the Andean countries is 55, compared to a mean of around 43 for key East, West, and Central African countries) but also concerted country efforts to address these inequalities with economic and social development initiatives.[11] In the second section, we elaborate more on the Andean region and our program of agriculture, economics, and health research there. We then touch on two key underlying determinants for agricultural production—access to land and water. Crop management approaches follow, highlighting both the negative impacts of some current technologies and the positive environmental and economic outcomes that can be achieved with innovative practices. We explore the household food security and human health implications of these practices more explicitly in the next section. Then, we examine the relevance of markets, both local and further afield, conventional and alternative. Affecting each of these issues are the complex, often overlapping elements of governance, which can in myriad ways either impede or foster more environmentally sustainable, equitable, and ultimately healthy agricultural and food systems through a range of programs and policies.

FOCUS ON THE CENTRAL ANDEAN REGION IN LATIN AMERICA

Latin American countries have been the historical source of major world staple crops, for example, maize from Central America (http://maize.org/why-maize) and potatoes from the Andes (http://www.cipotato.org/potato/). They have also been important food and feed producers for world markets, for example, wheat and soybeans from Argentina, associated with volatility in food commodity prices.[12] Our own work has focused primarily on systems involving smallholder agricultural producers, who comprise the vast majority of farmers in Andean countries. An estimated 85 percent of them are farming on less than two hectares of land, and they are severely affected by environmental degradation and inequitable access to resources. Whilst these smallholders are not the poorest of the poor, adaptation of the Sustainable Livelihoods framework[13] has nevertheless helped us clarify how their limited assets can leave these households vulnerable to the economic, environmental, health, and political stresses and shocks that constitute the vulnerability context (see Fig. 9.1).

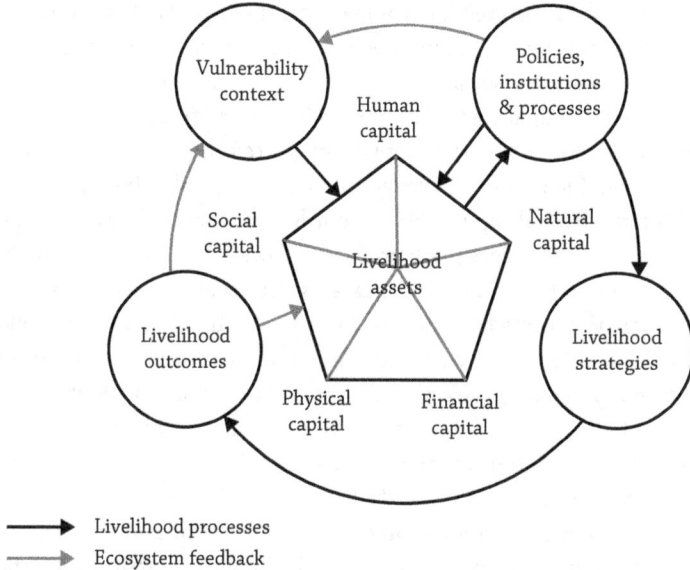

Figure 9.1:
Sustainable peri-urban agricultural smallholders' livelihoods framework. (From G. Prain and D. Lee-Smith. Urban Agriculture in Africa: What Has Been Learned? in G. Prain et al. (eds). African Urban Harvest. Agriculture in the Cities of Cameroon, Kenya and Uganda. Ottawa: Springer, International Potato Center (CIP), IDRC. 2010.)

In this framework, five types of capital assets are identified. Natural capital involves biodiversity and quantity and quality of accessible land and water. Physical capital includes buildings, equipment, seeds, transport, and animals. Human capital is composed of labor power, formally and nonformally acquired knowledge and skills, and health status. Available income and savings comprise financial capital. Social capital includes the access to networks, groups, trust, and support. The deployment of assets in household strategies is mediated through influences and impediments experienced in dealing with the institutional, policy, and cultural milieu of the society (structures and processes). These include the way markets function, the rules and regulations surrounding food handling, and the culturally accepted ways of making a living. The outcomes achieved through pursuit of livelihood strategies are part of livelihood processes, which in turn exert positive and/or negative ecosystem feedback on livelihood assets and the vulnerability context.[14]

In our gradually evolving agriculture, health, and economics research program in the Andes, we started by linking environmental and health impacts of pesticide and fertilizer inputs in potato production among small holders.[15] Using econometric models, we showed that greater use of highly hazardous pesticides (physical capital) had sufficient neurotoxic impacts (human capital) to reduce economic returns (financial capital), with variation across different agro-ecosystem niches (natural capital).[16] Scenario models of reduced pesticide use and greater farmer protection from exposure predicted both better economic returns and farmer health. We implemented such models through farmer field schools (FFSs) (building social capital) in which farmers conducted controlled agronomic trials, comparing potato plots using conventional crop management techniques with plots where they applied integrated crop and pest management (ICM and IPM) (gains in knowledge or human capital). Experimental plots required fewer external inputs (50 percent less fungicide, 75 percent less carbofuran, and 40 percent less methamidophos) and achieved similar production outputs (19 tonnes of potatoes per hectare), so they were more profitable (reductions in production costs from $80 to $104/ton).[17] In a longitudinal follow-up study, we were able to show that multipronged, intensive community-based interventions (processes) were plausibly associated with modest reductions in highly hazardous pesticide use, large improvements in pesticide use knowledge and practices, and significant positive changes in neurobehavioral function (human capital), adjusted for age and education.[18] However, when scaled up, the intensity of community-based strategies varied by local political leadership,[19] and their diffusion came up against entrenched policies, institutions, and processes that still favored substantial use of pesticides and other external inputs without adequate safeguards,[20] echoing other's findings.[21]

Partly as a result of these challenges, our most recent interdisciplinary action research project more explicitly included metropolitan region policy makers interested in shifting horticultural systems (including potatoes) toward greater human, environmental, and economic sustainability. Metropolitan regions (MRs) are an increasingly dominant form of physical, economic, and social integration through which agriculture and food systems are organized. They are defined as comprising rural and peri-urban areas and large urban centers, which are closely and interdependently connected through a multitude of economic, social, and ecological interactions[22] and are analyzable in terms of rural-urban linkages.[23] In the HortiSana project, our work took place in three MRs: "Cochabamba," Bolivia; "Huancayo," Peru; and "Pillaro," Ecuador (see Table 9.1 for MR administrative composition). Our aims were to describe current relationships among environmental, horticultural production and commercialization and health indicators; to experiment with production of safer inputs and implementation of alternative crop management approaches among collaborating small-scale farmers; to explore market opportunities for vegetables produced through safer and more sustainable production methods and develop alternatives; and to develop alliances with local organizations, including municipalities and regional authorities, to make positive changes in agro-ecosystems, food security, and health.[24]

We started with participatory appraisals in each MR, followed by baseline surveys of peri-urban vegetable farmers. As can be seen in Table 9.1, participants in the latter were small-scale producers with a median of half a hectare (5,001 square metres) and diversified livelihood strategies—41 percent of households reported off-farm income. Participants had low levels of income,

Table 9.1. RELEVANT DESCRIPTORS OF PERI-URBAN VEGETABLE FARM HOUSEHOLDS IN THREE METROPOLITAN REGIONS IN THE CENTRAL ANDES [MEDIAN, MEAN (STANDARD DEVIATION), OR PROPORTION] (N = 574)

Domain Variables	Metropolitan Region			
	Cochabamba	Huancayo	Pillaro	Total
Administrative composition of municipal region	Cochabamba city and province	Huancayo city and province, adjoining province of Chupaca, both Junin region	Pillaro town, Ambato city, and the province of Tungurahua	
Socioeconomic				
No. of economically active members	2, 2.8 (1.7)	2, 2.8 (1.5)	3, 2.8 (1.3)	3, 2.8 (1.5)
Access to off-farm income (proportion)	0.40	0.40	0.45	0.42
Amount of money available/month ($US)	71, 102 (59)	98, 99 (44)	125, 162 (109)	116, 123 (83)
Accessed loan for general household expenditures (proportion)	0.28	0.29	0.62	0.41
Agricultural production				
Access to sprinkler/drip irrigation (proportion)	0.00	0.01	0.16	0.05
Irrigated area (square meters)	5,000, 6,642 (6,798)	6,166, 11,565 (15,100)	5,001, 7,284 (10,133)	5,001, 8,742 (11,845)
Accessed loan for agricultural activities (proportion)	0.16	0.22	0.39	0.27
Received training on agricultural production (proportion)	0.19	0.42	0.91	0.43
Food security				
Not enough food eaten at home at least some of the year (proportion)	0.06	0.10	0.14	0.10

Source: HortiSana baseline survey, 2008.

estimated as a proportion of the monthly food basket costs. Our comparison of participants' monthly available funds (an indirect measure of income) to the monthly basic food basket costs estimated for each country showed that participants' income was 21 percent of an estimated food cost of US$470 in Peru, and 31 percent of US$520 in Ecuador (numbers were not available for Bolivia). Access to credit and training was greater among Pillaro MR farmers.

Throughout this chapter we provide examples from work with these farmers, their markets, and broader MR stakeholders to provide a window on the structural challenges for smallholder horticulture and innovative responses in programs and policies.

ACCESS TO FERTILE LAND AND CLEAN (ENOUGH) WATER

Land Issue

Despite centuries of struggle among social groups and decades of land reforms in low- and middle-income countries (LMICs), secure access to productive land remains a critical issue for millions of small-scale farmers *globally*.[25] In the pre-Columbian *Andes,* vertically integrated communal cultivation of different crops taking advantage of ecological niches at different altitudes provided indigenous peoples with a varied food supply for consumption and trade.[26] With Spanish colonization and allocation of people and lands to colonists in encomiendas, peasants were often forced off land in the fertile valleys and obliged to cultivate higher up the slopes, with consequent erosion and environmental degradation (see chapter 3 in Sherwood, 2009, regarding northern Ecuador).[27] Land reform in the 1960s and 1970s in Peru and Ecuador partially redistributed land, but formalization of tenure often remained incomplete in Peru. Adverse economic conditions, partially created by agricultural "modernization" policies, often drove smallholder farmers into debt and eventual sale of their land. With the continued urban sprawl in fertile Andean valleys, smallholder agriculture is losing prime agricultural land.

In our survey of smallholder households in peri-urban Huancayo, Peru, we found that 35 percent of 817 plots of land were held based on "inheritance," most often without any title deed. Across MRs, farmers cultivated a median of 5,000 m^2 of irrigated land (range 0–90,000 m^2) with 2,937 m^2 of nonirrigated land, very much depending on location (median total land, median irrigated land: around Huancayo, Peru = 8,417 m^2, 6,166 m^2; around Pillaro, Ecuador = 8,820 m^2, 5,292 m^2; and around Cochabamba, Bolivia = 7,100 m^2, 5,000 m^2). Such sizes of land are relatively small for sustaining households of a median of 4 persons (range 1–12), meaning family labor must be divided between farm work and nearby urban employment to make ends meet. Dividing time between farm and urban employment makes it difficult for peri-urban farm households to find the time to invest in soil management or find the investment worthwhile.[28]

Land Responses

Globally, land reform remains an unfinished agenda for many LMICs. International agencies have set out a wide range of policy changes and programs that could make a difference both in rural and peri-urban settings (see annex III in IFAD, 2008).[29] Of particular importance in Andean valleys is strengthening policy recognition of the mutually enriching relationship possible between urban centers and surrounding rural areas.[30] Including agriculture in urban development planning and protecting lands for agricultural purposes (crops and livestock) is one strategy that has been at least partially successful in areas surrounding Lima.[31]

The Hortisana team worked with regional-provincial and municipal stakeholders to make sure agriculture was part of economic and environmental planning. Policy statements were developed, emphasizing the mutual benefits for both urban consumers and peri-urban producers. For example, in Chupuro, Peru, a statement read: "Organic agricultural production is an alternative for taking care of our health and the environment, at the same time as providing an income for people with limited resources." In FFS, we promoted intensive, mixed production of higher value crops such as vegetables and herbs on small irrigated plots, to take maximum advantage of limited land availability. Considerable attention was paid to "growing a healthy crop" by focusing on crop rotation and soil management to boost or maintain the land's fertility. This included a special session on soils,[32] as well as the proactive development of soil amendments in Tungurahua and the hands-on preparation of liquid fertilizers in Junin (see later discussion). These initiatives have the potential to boost family incomes by increasing productivity and higher value agriculture, thereby promoting greater well-being for smallholder farms.

Water Issue

Globally, water use for agriculture in low-income countries (LICs) accounts for an estimated 87 percent of total extracted water, and 74 percent in middle-income countries (MICs).[33,34] Demand is expected to rise with increasing population and shifting dietary patterns.[35] With global climate change, greater variability in rainfall is causing wider variation in planting times from year to year and overall greater water scarcity.[36] An extensive assessment of water availability and use in the Andes highlighted the role of "land degradation with soil erosion and loss of [agricultural] productivity [in rural use and] for urban and industrial use, the main issues are of water quality and distribution (sanitation) and use conflicts (between for example, irrigation, domestic, and mining uses)."[37]

The HortiSana MRs experienced many of these challenges. The Andean Basin report[38] selected the Ambato subbasin as a case study highlighting problems of water scarcity—water demand in the basin exceeds supply by 40 percent. Around Huancayo deforestation continues apace according to the National Institute of Natural Resources in the Central Selva. Droughts in the highlands have resulted in declining crop yields, particularly for small-holders.[39] Few HortiSana farmers had permanent irrigation (see Table 9.1). Irrigation sources were primarily rivers around Huancayo (63 percent) and Cochabamba (55 percent) and canals from wetlands or lakes at higher elevations around Pillaro (70 percent). Around Huancayo, 55 percent of smallholder households complained of scarcity or unpredictability of irrigation water supply and 42 percent were concerned about irrigation water quality due to population increase and urban expansion (37 percent contamination by domestic clothes washing, 28 percent from sewage and garbage) or dumping of farm wastes (18 percent, including dung and dead animals).

Water Responses

Globally, greater emphasis will need to be placed on diversification of water sources (water harvesting, use of wastewater), plant breeding for drought resistance, and greater water use efficiency (drip irrigation methods).[40] Although no comprehensive global inventory of use of untreated wastewater exists, estimates range from around 6 million hectares to as much as 20 million hectares, nearly 7 percent of all irrigated land globally.[41] Safe use of wastewater, enabling farmers to "close the nutrient cycle," through recycling of accumulated nutrients in plant fertilization, will be an essential component of sustainable irrigation in the future.

Across multiple settings in the semi-arid Andes, "Katalysis" projects involving community-based colearning about water management have demonstrated the potential for both harvesting existing water, for example, through the construction of reservoirs lined with geomembranes (plastic) to store episodic rainwater, and retaining existing water in the ground, for example, through incorporation of organic matter into the soil.[42] For peri-urban farmers around Lima, low-cost water treatment with reservoirs, coupled with drip irrigation, has proven technically feasible, with economies of scale achieved via sharing of treatment reservoirs among several families.[43] During HortiSana FFS and field days, we emphasized the importance of adding organic matter to the soil, both to promote water retention in soil and increase nitrogen. These initiatives helped prolong growing seasons, increase yields, and integrate environmental benefits, resulting in higher incomes. These measures have the ability to create sustainable environmental and economic processes for vulnerable populations. As one northern Ecuadorian farmer explained:

> Once I learnt where the water was, I could grow that small plot of alfalfa. With
> the alfalfa, I could have cuy [guinea pig]. . . . with just the cuyes, we have already
> paid back our $200 investment in materials. Today we have 300 cuyes that are
> worth about $5.00 each or $1,500 in all. That is much more than I used to earn in

the city.... The cuy produced manure for my soil. With the manure, I've planted 75 mango and avocado trees. My farm has become an oasis.

APPROPRIATE CROP MANAGEMENT

Issue

From 1960 to 2005, substantial increases in yields per area were attained *globally*, partly due to increases in the use of external inputs and more intensive cropping and livestock systems.[44] Along with high-yielding varieties, fertilizer and pesticide use were promoted by agricultural development programs. Use of phosphorus-based fertilizers more than tripled, and use of nitrogen-based fertilizers increased over seven times. Exports of pesticides went from minimal to an over $US 15 million market. Yet declining productivity per unit area has been noted for crops such as cereal staples, while a host of other "externalities" have appeared with high external input agriculture.[45]

In the Andes,[46] researchers have collected evidence of decreasing yields per unit area in recent decades, despite substantial use of external inputs as part of "modernization." He attributed these to a combination of erosion and declining soil fertility in highland Ecuador. Work by International Potato Center and affiliated researchers showed that use of fertilizers and pesticides was often above recommendations, with potential for adverse environmental and human health impacts.[47] Paredes[48] showed wide variability in returns on external inputs among different kinds of farmers in potato cropping systems. Across communities in highland Ecuador, those more inclined to intensive market-oriented production with high external inputs had reduced net benefits from sale of their produce compared to those with lower external inputs.[49]

In HortiSana, we found that most farmers surveyed relied heavily on salespeople in local agricultural supply stores for crop management information—64 percent around Huancayo, 54 percent around Pillaro, and 48 percent around Cochabamba. Primarily they receive information on pesticide products and application rates, not on alternatives to pesticides. Such limited exposure to options was echoed by Ecuadorian smallholders, who critiqued the lack of adequate government extension services providing alternative information and the lack of alternative inputs, for example, insect traps instead of pesticides, in stores operating commercially in farming areas.[50]

We also assessed the impacts of insecticide use and structural complexity of the landscape on biodiversity and natural enemies using traps, nets, and direct observations primarily during the planting season.[51] Around Huancayo, parasitoid natural enemies were the insects most reduced by insecticide applications. Around Pillaro, very small populations of parasitoids, pollinators, and pest predators were found in potato fields receiving insecticides, while diverse ecological structures (hedges, trees, weed growth, etc.) around the fields increased these populations. The intensity of Andean potato weevil infestation was unaffected by insecticide applications, demonstrating resistance to currently applied insecticides, a common problem frustrating farmers. In other vegetable crops, foliage-eating beetles were less common in fields with multiple horticultural crops.

Responses

Globally, a host of options have been explored to transform high-external-in put-oriented-agriculture, including more sustainable use of local resources, greater use of indigenous and exotic agro-ecological knowledge, more environmentally sustaining practices, and lower impact biotechnologies.[52,53,54] In keeping with the principle, first do less harm, a recent UNCTAD working paper argued: "it is important to remove or modify the existing tax and pricing policies that generate perverse incentives...such as overuse of pesticides, fertilizers, water, and fuel or encouraging land degradation."[55] The working paper calls for a shift in policy toward replacing agrochemicals with production methods using biofertilizers and biopesticides. In addition to the environmental benefits, reduction in consumption of agrochemicals would also lead to reduction in imports of agricultural production inputs for developing countries.

Around pesticide use in particular, FAO's Global Integrated Pest Management (IPM) facility fostered a set of international, regional, and national efforts to reduce hazardous pesticide use.[56] FAO promotes IPM or "the careful consideration of all available pest control techniques and subsequent integration of appropriate measures that discourage the development of pest populations and keep pesticides and other interventions to levels that are economically justified and reduce or minimize risks to human health and the environment."[57]

In the Andes, we have been engaged in an extended research action process to shift potato-based agricultural production systems from a heavy dependence upon highly hazardous pesticides to less hazardous approaches.[58] In HortiSana, we aimed to reduce dependence on chemical fertilizers and pesticides, while promoting production and use of more locally produced inputs along with biological and cultural control methods. The rising costs of imported chemical fertilizers worked strongly in our favor—farmers were more willing to try alternative methods as the prices of many external outputs increased three- to four-fold from August 2007 to August 2008, though with some decline thereafter (see Fig. 9.2).

In the initiative around Huancayo, agronomy students conducted an inventory of diseases in different vegetable crops, distinguishing those aggravated by humidity and those most common during the dry season, and assisted farmers in understanding these problems and their control.[59] Following our

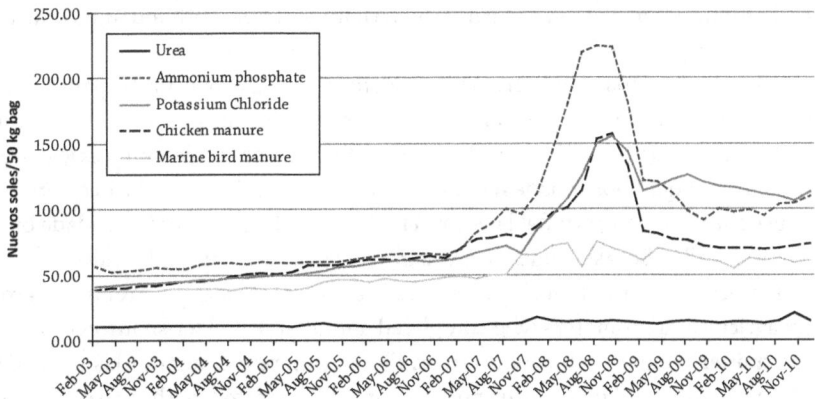

Figure 9.2:
Prices (in Nuevo soles, approx. US$0.37) of the main chemical and organic fertilizers used in Peru (produced by industries, not farm-level data) from 2003 to 2010. (From Huanuco Agrarian Agency of the Peruvian Government.)

assessments of impact of pesticide use, biodiverse landscapes, and mixed cropping on the presence of natural enemies of vegetable and potato pests, HortiSana recommended maintenance of variability in planted crops as well as the diversity of biological structures around fields as options for pest control without insecticides.

For control of damage to potatoes by late blight, project researchers around Pillaro evaluated several novel fungicide mixes and resistant potato seed clones. We used the Environmental Impact Quotient (EIQ), a relatively rapid assessment tool that integrates adverse effects on animal and plant species as well as farm worker and consumer health.[60] The use of phosphites (K,Ca y Cu), instead of the usual mutagenic dithiocarbamate fungicides, reduced EIQs by over 95 percent.[61] Application of integrated pest and disease management methods (rainfall-based threshold prediction methods) with shorter maturation clones could similarly reduce EIQs by over 10 times compared to current practices in Ecuador[62] with significant benefits for environment and health.

Responding to the demand for training in healthy, ecological production methods (both on the survey and in semistructured interviews with farmers), we drew on CIP and other stakeholders' experience with farmer field schools (FFS), an adult education approach to codiscovery of agroecological processes and alternative production methods. Prior work had shown positive results in enhancing knowledge, implementing IPM and applying less harmful, more efficient production methods.[63] Godtland and colleagues[64] formally compared farm productivity between participants and nonparticipants in Peru. Using sophisticated econometric models, which incorporated propensity scores to control for prior farmer characteristics, they estimated that participation in

FFS produced an increase in farm productivity of 32 percent and in income of US$236/ha per year.

FFS around Huancayo involved 26 women and 21 men participants who showed increased knowledge after the program, with mean pre- and posttest scores increasing from 67 percent correct to 86 percent correct. All participants tried using liquid homemade fertilizer-biocides called "Biols" and 21 continued to use them in their own fields. Another 14 were using another farm-made bio-fertilizer called Bocashi and 22 were using yellow insect traps or biocides to control insect pests, thus reducing their fertilizer and pesticide use. Around Pillaro, six agricultural promoters who completed a multistakeholder sponsored "train the trainer" course each conducted an FFS in different communities (total 65 FFS participants). An FFS focusing on potatoes field tested methods of reducing insecticide use, particularly highly hazardous products WHO Ia and Ib[65], using cultural control methods, biocides elaborated from local plants, and low toxicity insecticides (WHO category III). Another FFS validated methods of late blight control and a third planted multiple vegetable crops and used locally derived insect repellents to protect them. Around Cochabamba, 52 producers in three FFS in tomatoes, onions, and multiple crops assessed effectiveness of different "Biols" made with different kinds of animal manure, biofungicides, insect traps, parasitoids, and vegetable-based biopesticides. Both the latter provided adequate insect pest control. Following the FFS, meetings were held among FFS graduates to share ongoing experiences, learn additional techniques, and strengthen farmer organizations. Field days were also held for neighboring farmers in local communities to observe the different experiments conducted and thus extend the learning about low external input, safer vegetable farming.

Around Pillaro, we worked with the Santa Catalina women farmers' association in the preparation of proposals to municipal and national funders for contributions to the costs of construction of a biofertilizer facility. Having successfully acquired funding, women and agronomy students tested different methods of co-composting and humus production and used demonstration plots around the facility to test prototypes. Commercial production of biofertilizers began in 2010.[66] The 16 members of the Santa Catalina association received a total of US$4053.34 as income in 2010: 75 percent of this amount from the sale of 655 bags (40 kg) of organic fertilizer, mainly compost, 14 percent from membership fees, 8 percent from potato sales, and 3 percent from other income. Their costs were US$ 3745.45: 35 percent investments, 52 percent operations costs, and 13 percent administration. US$760 was used to pay part-time salaries between May and December 2010. Although their profit was not large (US$307.89), the female producers felt proud of having their own business and working together to strengthen their association. Applying the biofertilizers in their own fields, they are maintaining soil fertility in a healthy manner. Selling these products at modest cost to other farmers has not only been about income but also about sharing their experience with alternative production approaches and therefore promoting more sustainable approaches to agriculture. There were also challenges, notably in the collection of raw material for biocomposting and marketing the finished product. Plans to diversify production to include vermiculture seemed to divert raw material away from the main focus of biofertilizer production.

What lessons can we learn about the success of this endeavor? One factor was certainly the "buy in" by local partners. The Pillaro women's group was proactive from the beginning of discussions of a biofertilizer factory, during the preparation and submission of the proposal, and in the excitement of funding being awarded. This was a powerful incentive to continue involvement to ensure the success of the enterprise. A second factor was the social integration and homogeneity of the group: a tightly linked group of women from the local community. They provided a powerful example of women's involvement in agriculture.[67]

FARM HOUSEHOLD HEALTH

Issue

Globally, poor rural and peri-urban farmers face multiple deprivations such as inadequate shelter and lack of clean water and sanitation, in addition to the hazards of agricultural work.[68] Often poor farmers sell rather than consume what they produce, weighing off income contributions versus food contributions to food security.[69] Food insecurity also has livelihood implications. As a FAO report noted, "Hunger, nutrition and health are strong determining factors on a person's ability to work, their productivity and their cognitive development."[70] Reflecting the "double nutrition burden" faced by these households, multitasking in peri-urban contexts and consequent lack of time can lead to the consumption of simpler, faster, "urban" foods (noodles, pasta, fried and processed foodstuffs) resulting in peri-urban farm families' diets becoming more obesigenic.[71,72]

Among smallholder farmers we surveyed in three Andean MR, musculoskeletal problems were the most common health problem (28 to 43 percent respondents), which they linked to the heavy physical work in which they engaged[73] as well as cold and wet conditions they endured, including foot immersion in irrigation water. Yet pesticides were the hazards that farmers linked to deaths. The daughter of an artichoke farmer in the Mantaro valley shared the story of how her teenage daughter had swallowed readily available hazardous pesticides on their farm, echoing similar experiences worldwide.[74]

Among 98 vegetable farmers surveyed around Huancayo (44 percent women), most were aware that pesticides presented risks to their health, but they were unaware of routes of exposure and high exposure practices, for example, mixing pesticides with bare hands in irrigation canals or backpack sprayers leaking onto the back during application, both observed during farm visits.[75] Among these, 89 farmers, 74 of whom applied pesticides (only five with personal protective equipment), underwent clinical assessments.[76] A majority of farmers showed a range of health problems, including alterations in touch and low concentrations of red cell cholinesterase that indicated chronic neurotoxic effects of highly hazardous pesticide use, consistent with other observations in the Andes.[77,78] In other words, by using pesticides, many smallholder farmers are significantly harming their health, which can lead to decreases in productivity and increased vulnerability.

While pesticide use can be the most severe challenge to smallholders' health, food security also presents important concerns. Food security challenges among smallholders, with their adverse consequences for health and well-being, can be both ongoing and triggered by adverse climatic conditions such as drought.[79] In an examination of the relationships between household food access and livelihood assets across the three metropolitan regions, we found 59 percent of 507 households had encountered some difficulties in obtaining food during certain months of the year.[80] Key livelihood assets indicators associated with better household food access were the age of household survey respondents, participation in agricultural associations, church membership, area of irrigated land, housing material, space within the household residence, and satisfaction with health status. The range of indicators associated with household food access shows the complexity of food security in challenging LMIC contexts.

Adequate consumption of healthy food is compromised by food security deficiencies. Current best estimates are that mean (SD) intake of both fruits and vegetables for working-age adults in low- and middle-income Latin American countries ranges from a low of 287(221) grams per person-day for women aged 45–59 to a high of 408(225) grams per person-day for men aged 30–44 years. Both of these numbers are less than the optimal mean intake of 600 grams per person-day.[81] In HortiSana, Institute for Nutritional Research (IIN) colleagues used qualitative (free list of foods, pile sorts to prioritize top 25 foods, observations in local stores and on farms) and quantitative (semi-quantitative food frequency in seven food groups) methods to assess dietary diversity around Huancayo. They assembled a list of 158 foods, including vegetables, meat products, aromatic herbs, pastas, tubers, milk products, fruits, and grains, which were reduced to 116 different foods through focus groups with FFS participants. Fifty-one persons across all ages provided food frequencies (days in the last week) and provided their perceptions of different foods.[82] Animal foods most frequently consumed included milk or cheese and eggs (each 2–3x/week, milk 4–5x/week, and eggs 4x/week among children) with chicken a distant fourth (approximately one day per week). Among vegetables, tomatoes and carrots were both consumed (about 5x/week, mostly in soups), followed by squash (2 days/week for adults, 3-4 days/week among children). Most other foods in these groups were 1-2x/week or less, indicating relatively limited dietary diversity. The observed gaps in consumption of healthy foods indicate the difficulties in achieving food security with potential negative impacts on health indicators.

Responses

Both reducing harms and increasing benefits for smallholders are key responses for equity concerns. In relation to global health risks from conventional agriculture, a wide range of approaches have been suggested and demonstrated effective in moving toward a more sustainable agriculture with less pesticide use[83] and shifting toward "ecoagriculture" approaches to "nourishing the planet."[84] In particular, the Worldwatch report cites the example of farmers in the Horn of Africa and in East Africa who were able to insulate themselves from the worst effects of drought and increase yields in a rainy year by mulching, reducing tillage, and planting cover crops. Participatory research on six experimental farms produced yield gains of 20–120 percent for maize and 35–100 percent for tef (a staple grain of the Ethiopian diet) compared to farms where conventional methods were used.[85]

To reduce health risks in the Andes, the HortiSana team used a number of different strategies following best practice health promotion approaches to reduction in use of highly hazardous pesticides (red labels) and healthier crop management.[86,87] Strategies included radio spots and classes in schools in Cochabamba, public theatre presentations in Pillaro, and pesticide health and safety training in FFS in all metropolitan regions. Following these interventions, most of the "environmentally conscious" farmers[88] (67 percent in Ecuador, 84 percent in Peru) had stopped using red label pesticides. Compared to environmentally conscious producers, changes were considerably higher among FFS participants and members of the organic producer associations in Ecuador (88 percent and 85 percent, respectively) and marginally greater in Peru (88 percent and 86 percent, respectively). The "risk-averse" producers reduced the use of red label to a much lesser extent (42 percent Peru and 48 percent Ecuador). Parallel changes were observed in the number of plots with no use of agrochemicals and the number of vegetable types planted, with "environmentally conscious" farmers showing the largest improvements.[89] Such changes, when associated with improved pesticide handling practices, have been linked to better neurobehavioural performance (+0.7 SD in overall Z-score) among smallholder potato farmers.[90]

Global responses to the need to increase food security have included programs emphasizing vegetable production in home gardens,[91] expanded to involve widespread transformation of crop choices to improve soil and farm household health.[92] Improvement in food security is recognized as an important rationale for promoting research into more efficient and sustainable horticultural production.[93] Agriculture-based research efforts to increase intake of vegetables include "Globalhort," a worldwide, not-for-profit program intended to foster more effective partnerships among stakeholders for increased research and collective action on increased use of horticultural products to improve household health, especially of mothers and young children. It is sponsored by the Asian-based World Vegetable Centre, ISHS, and other international organizations.[94]

In the Andes, HortiSana team members promoted vegetable and animal source food consumption within a diverse diet around Huancayo through various mechanisms. A recipe book was elaborated with nutritional composition calculations included, based on detailed information gathered on dietary practices in the area and then 15 piloted adaptations of local women's food preparation practices. Five hundred copies were distributed via direct connections, to health centers, among civil society organizations, at workshops, and via green markets. Workshops on healthy diets and nutrition, including hands-on food preparation and special sessions on infant diets and feeding, were conducted with 41 farm families. In follow-up interviews in farm households with preteen children, mothers demonstrated improved knowledge on a varied and balanced diet and increments in consumption of certain foods (some vegetables and chicken, for example) were documented. They particularly valued food they produced themselves for its taste and quality but noted that there were seasons in which they could not produce or consume as many vegetables as they would like, indicating that despite the use of irrigation much of the year, farming conditions still impeded their desired changes toward healthier consumption patterns. Nutrition interventions were also undertaken with 28 health professionals (nurses, midwives, doctors, technicians) at two district health centers in the Huancayo area on the upgrading and/or incorporation of anthropometry, nutrition counseling during consultations, and use of recipes to strengthen the nutritional component of their clinical practice. Small improvements in knowledge were demonstrated on postsurveys compared to prescores.[95]

MARKET INFLUENCES AND OPPORTUNITIES

Issue

Trade expansion and value chain integration have been identified as two of the most important global drivers of change in agriculture.[96] Despite significant growth in agricultural exports from LMICs, exports are a still a fraction of total trade, and domestic markets continue to be of major importance for the vast majority of producers. On the other hand, the expansion in the international trading of agricultural inputs—which perhaps receives less attention—is having a much wider impact. Apart from the year-on-year growth in national imports of agrochemicals in LMICs—a 50 percent increase in Argentina, for example, between 2009 and 2010—one of the major issues is the aggressive, extensive, and long-term marketing system supporting the sales of these products. In many countries these are the new agricultural extension services, the principal source of technical information for smallholder farmers. How can knowledge and information systems relating to an alternative type of agriculture described earlier compete with the global agrochemical business?

A second issue highlighted by Hazell and Wood concerns value chain integration. The growth of urban populations, increases in disposable income, and lifestyle changes lead to changes in the volume, types, and qualities of food products in demand.[97] These changes, in turn, require more integrated value chains to ensure volume, preferences, and food quality. A remarkable indicator of these changes is the growth of supermarkets across the South.[98] However, issues of access and fairness for smallholder producers in LMICs remain of major concern, especially if they remain isolated and unorganized and cannot access the new supply chains to market their products.[99]

While smallholder "peasant" producers in the Andes face significant challenges as a result of the market changes outlined earlier,[100,101] there are also new opportunities for more sustainable agriculture. Overall organic production, with its opportunities to reach new markets and related health benefits, is increasing (see Fig. 9.3).

In HortiSana, initial stakeholder consultations indicated that markets were a key bottleneck to be addressed in promoting healthier, more sustainable agriculture among small producers.[102] There are two sides to this issue. One

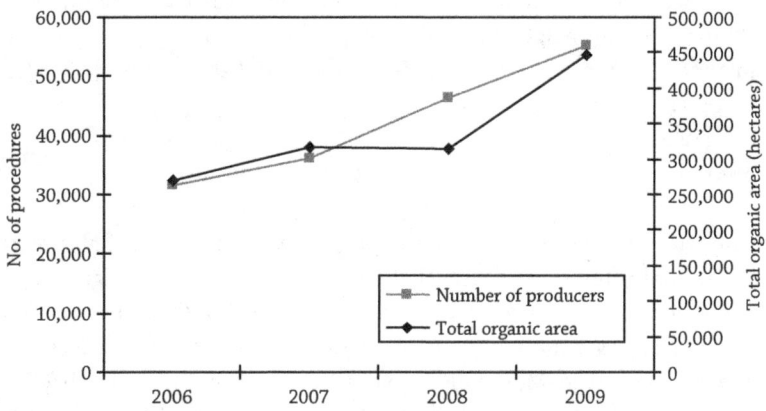

Figure 9.3:
Number of organic producers and total organic area in Peru from 2006 to 2009. (From the SENASA database, http://www.senasa.gob.pe/0/modulos/JER/JER_Interna.aspx? ARE=0&PFL=3&JER=85)

side needs to address producers and their "market readiness,"[103] including the organization of producers, their knowledge, and their networks (see later discusssion). In the HortiSana baseline survey, the majority of farmers were producing crops for local or regional markets (96 percent of vegetable production was sold). The crops mostly produced for home consumption were the traditional potato and maize (14 percent and 12 percent of producers, respectively) and only 1 percent of farmers were producing just for self-consumption. The other side concerns "market opportunities" and market chain analysis,[104] and this led to market studies in the Huancayo and Pillaro metropolitan regions.

In Huancayo, the market study found that prices in organic markets were no different from those in conventional markets. Furthermore, only 5 percent of survey respondents considered organic produce expensive. Most did not consider the price of organic produce a disincentive to buying them. On the other hand, the lack of a price differential with conventional products was a disincentive for farmers to increase production or make investments in switching to organic production, resulting in limited offerings of organic produce and a small buyer base or a "low-equilibrium" poverty trap.[105] Recommendations included increasing the quantity, variety, and quality of organic vegetables through promotion, quality control, and increased relationships between consumers and producers. Establishing or strengthening enterprise associations for organic producers were noted to be particularly important, as the presence of social and human capital among organic producers differentiated those who were successful from those who failed.

Near Pillaro, members of primarily women farmers' associations sought more information on product flows to different, segmented markets. As a result, this became an axis of research for the project.[106] Current and potential consumers of organic produce were found to be in middle- to upper-income groups (according to Instituto Nacional de Estadísticas y Censos categories) and living in urban neighbourhoods. They sought quality produce, available on an almost daily basis in small stores or supermarkets close to their homes.

Responses

Globally, there is an urgent need for appropriate management of global trade in agricultural commodities, especially food. There is need for vigilance over dumping of HIC (high-income countries) goods in LMICs and for supporting LMIC farmers without resort to massive subsidies (see IAASTD 2009 section on Trade and Markets).[107] Avoidance of dumping and subsidies is particularly important in relation to agricultural inputs, so that alternative, more sustainable agricultural practices have a chance to develop. In responding to the marginalization of smallholder farmers, considerable innovation has occurred around the development of fair and alternative trade networks to more equitably link farmers in LMICs with HIC markets, with lessons for building fairer alternative trade domestically.[108]

Linking fairer trade with the introduction of internationally recognized organic certification for HIC or domestic markets is a complex and costly process. Although the costs of certification can be reduced by forming a producer group or association, the annual fee of about $1,200 for a group of 20 farmers still represents a significant investment for smallholder farmers. High costs put organic certification beyond the capacity of most smallholder farmer organizations unless they are supported by nongovernmental or private organizations willing to assist in the process.

A number of international research organizations (FAO, CIAT, CIMMYT, and CIP) have found success in incorporating small-scale farmers in more profitable markets through the organization of farmers that participated in training and are willing to take "risks" in a new business.[109,110] To more effectively involve larger number of these farmers in domestic markets, either organic or otherwise, building producer organizations has been of paramount importance.[111] In the Andes, HortiSana team members worked hard with smallholder producers to form new associations or strengthen existing ones.

In the Huancayo MR, this involved working with FFS groups in different locales to formalize as a legal entity—Agroecological Producer Association TAMIA (*Tamia* is a Quechua word that means "rain"). HortiSana helped TAMIA formulate internal norms and regulations, register in a broader organic producer association, and undergo training in management functions, including planning, budgeting, and participatory guarantees of quality, all essential to accessing higher value markets.[112] Organic produce fairs or "bioferias" were strengthened through the use of promotional materials (posters, street banners, customer leafleting) and provision of an increased diversity of products, for example, in the El Tambo market in Huancayo. In four small towns around Huancayo, new biofairs were organized by the producers' associations in conjunction with municipal authorities and local nongovernmental organizations (NGO)s. The number of farmers selling at these fairs increased, primarily by sharing marketing among producers in each association. Other distribution channels explored were direct marketing to restaurants and health clinics.

The income per TAMIA member was generally low: monthly income per active member from sales in the biofairs during 2010 averaged US$13.8, range US$1.1 to US$52.7. In other words, overall financial benefits were modest, with some members benefiting economically from their sales in the organic markets, but others earning very little. However, detailed interviewing of members found that the greatest benefits they obtained from participation were better health for them and their families and pride in building and participating in their own organization. Building human and social capital proved to be just as important to members as building financial capital. A visit in early 2011 showed that the organization was still solid, as a result of greater

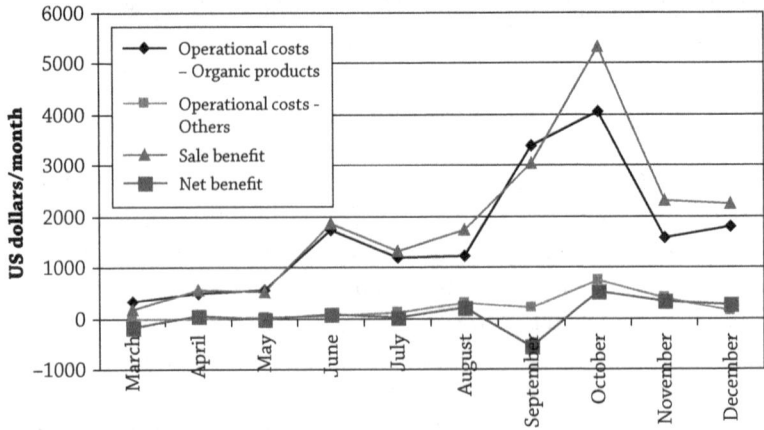

Figure 9.4:
Cost–benefit analysis of the sales point in Ambato from March to December 2010, Ambato, Ecuador. (From internal reports of the Association of Agricultural and Animal Goods of Pillaro.)

confidence in the functioning of the group, their own sense of membership, and their relationship with local institutions.

Near Pillaro, farmers' associations and HortiSana staff put together proposals for a plant to clean and pack crops in Pillaro. As a result of this collaboration, 11 farmers' associations worked together with stakeholders and funders to establish a store for sale of organic produce in a middle-class area of Ambato. The store provided a valuable outlet for sale of the farmers' produce, the final step in the value chain from compost production through to marketing. The business grew steadily from March to October 2010 with a dropoff in production and therefore supply by members in November and December 2010 (see Fig. 9.4). Some costs were subsidized, especially the sales women's salary and the rental of space. Overall profits of around US$750 came from the difference between produce sales and costs. Some challenges still need to be solved, including gradual weaning of the subsidies, better marketing to reach a wider clientele, and providing a larger quantity and greater diversity of produce. In 2011, the outlet was experimenting with diversifying into non-vegetable products (tinned goods, dairy, and handicrafts) to attract more and different customers. This appeared to be a useful strategy in creating a wider customer base and therefore increasing profits for the participating farmers.

APPROPRIATE GOVERNANCE

Issue

Globally, governance can play a role in tackling persistent inequalities in wealth and power between countries and blocks of countries through global governance institutions such as the FAO as well as international NGOs such as OXFAM, as well as within countries in terms of state duties to deal with environments and health and state–civil society relationships.[113] On the negative side, some of the fiercest debates surrounding agriculture, environment, health, and equity have centered on the World Trade Organization and its role in discouraging equitable and sustainable trade.[114,115]

In the Andes, historically governments have been highly centralized, with little allocation of tax or other resources to the provincial-state or municipal levels. This may explain why only a minority of smallholder households in the metropolitan regions where HortiSana worked indicated that the "municipality works in [their] favor" (39 percent around Cochabamba, 44 percent around Pillaro, and 45 percent around Huancayo) and even fewer agreed that the "municipality helps with production matters" (12 percent around Huancayo, 15 percent around Cochabamba, and 25 percent around Pillaro). Lack of support by local government is therefore a significant challenge faced by smallholder farmers in these regions.

Responses

Globally, Hoffman (2011) has argued that governments should strengthen producer organizations and local communities, pointing out that producer organizations are essential for smallholders to become competitive while local communities can contribute local knowledge to agricultural technology.[116]

In the Andes, to seek more equitable and sustainable governance, we designed interventions that worked both "from the bottom up," through strengthening local actions, and "top-down," through working directly with government, while supporting multiagency platforms, which reinforced synergies among different levels of government and civil society.[117] For bottom-up interventions, we drew on earlier experiences in peri-urban Lima involving support to the formation of organic producer organizations.[118,119] HortiSana encouraged the formation of farmer organizations in the Huancayo area and supported them to play active roles in proposal development and presentation and discussion of alternative policies. Taking advantage of the *presupuesto participativo* or "participatory budget," a fast-growing, innovative decentralization of budgeting and increase in democratic accountability in resource allocation being implemented by the Peruvian Government, one farmers' organization prepared a proposal for increasing the production and marketing of organic vegetables and presented it to local government in early 2009. Though not approved on this occasion, the proposal opened up the discussion around the health risks associated with current agricultural practices and the need to develop alternative ways of farming. One indicator that the municipality was listening was its approval of the establishment of a weekly "green market" in the main square to sell organic products later in 2009.

The "top-down" approach to more equitable, sustainable governance involved the sensitization of municipal and regional leaders to the issues of pesticide use, health risks, and the need for an alternative type of agriculture, through roundtable discussions, forums, and special events. One municipality that had participated in these events passed an ordinance in January 2009 promoting organic agriculture and the reduction in use of highly hazardous pesticides 1a and 1b.[120] The following year the municipality worked through the participatory budgeting process to implement a project to promote home gardens and the production of organic vegetables. The latter was the first concrete evidence of the implementation of the municipal ordinance and an example of the potential of participatory budgeting processes to bring greater attention to the food security and livelihood needs of lower income segments of the population.

At the regional level in Peru, HortiSana worked with a platform of both public sector and civil society organizations committed to sustainable agriculture to help pass an accord within the Vision and Plan for Integrated Economic Development of the Region of Junin for 2011–2014. The Accord establishes: "Development of sustainable agriculture, in which sections of government and organizations working with them will promote organic production, productivity, income, security, food sovereignty and organization of smallholder producers of the region." In Ecuador, HortiSana worked through alliances to sponsor a train-the-trainers course, six FFS, three field days, and to develop several proposals, of which two were successful: the biofertilizer plant and the joint marketing effort. In the latter, ABAPP raised US$30,000 from its own members, HortiSana provided US$7,000, the municipality US$5,000, and a local NGO, CESA, another US$5,000, in order to leverage US$50,000 from a fund set up by the Ministry of Economic and Social Inclusion.[121] The group of organizations also worked with the provincial government to develop a Good Agricultural Practice Guide into a legal instrument (*normativa*), to help ensure clean and safe agriculture in the province of Tungurahua. The *normativa* is intended to protect farmers, the environment, and consumers through reduction of hazardous pesticide use and, eventually, a regional certification scheme for organic production.

As experienced in other contexts,[122] mutual efforts to maintain a network of decentralized stakeholders present challenges, particularly across levels (community, municipal, regional). However, the ability to maintain the network as an informal group facilitated the mobilization of local support when opportunities arose. This bore fruit in both obtaining additional financing for alternative approaches to agricultural and food systems as described earlier, as well as the success in policy change, as per the *normativa* earlier. It is not possible to precisely quantify the economic and health benefits achieved through these innovative approaches to governance. However, these actions on governance help create a more enabling environment for achieving the economic benefits producers can gain from the sale of organic produce; they also increase the sustainability of actions on nutrition and healthier consumption by making a concern for healthy food production and consumption more mainstream.[123,124]

CONCLUSION

We have described the current landscape of agricultural and food systems and their implications for environmental sustainability, food security, and human health, particularly highlighting work we have been part of in the Andes. We have woven into our discussion examples of others' and our own efforts to make changes that we think present relevant options for policy makers and people working to improve environmental sustainability, equity, livelihoods, and household food security. The breadth of potential policy and program recommendations to change food systems is far broader than can be encompassed in this one short chapter. Fortunately some recommendations involving tackling climate change, promoting water conservation, working with squatter populations in urban settings, and promoting greater access among low-income communities, all relevant to agricultural and food systems, are described in other chapters in this volume.

Consideration should be given to different levels of drivers of change—global, national, and local—and arenas for response.[125]

As an example of the obligations of *global* organizations, the World Trade Organization must assume the responsibility to actively tackle the distorting subsidies for fertilizer and pesticide use (taking its responsibilities to "improve human welfare" seriously), while at the same time respecting national efforts to support lower external input, "organic" production through research, information, and programs (avoid doing harm). An example from international global governance organizations is the World Bank providing loans and grants to support agricultural development and enhance food security but formally conditioning these loans to exclude highly hazardous pesticide purchase and distribution.[126] We recognize that formal auditing supported by international NGOs is likely needed to ensure that these provisions are met, for example, Pesticide Action Network support of an examination of pest management policy implementation in China.[127] Similar is the need to support researchers, farm organizations, and NGOs in the monitoring of implementation of international best practice guidelines, such as FAO's Code of Conduct on the Distribution and Use of Pesticides,[128] in keeping with writings on transparency and public participation.[129]

At the *national* level, promotion of public goods would include more widespread adoption in other countries of policies such as the concerted efforts in Brazil to realize a Right to Food.[130] Recognizing the challenges faced by LICs in accessing resources for such efforts internally, international donors could prioritize these efforts over those solely aimed at increasing food exports from countries struggling to feed the poor in their own populations. Particularly urgent in Andean countries is the implementation of policies and incentives to increase production and consumption of fruit and vegetables, in keeping with best current understanding of nutritional intake guidelines. Among these would be adequate supports to public health services to more fully implement existing nutritional assessment and education programs.

Ensuring adequate access to land is a policy issue that spans national, provincial, and municipal levels. Land reform usually is a national responsibility, as should be judicious oversight of land leasing or sale to international companies and governments primarily interested in producing food for populations external to the leasing or selling country. Provincial plans can affect urban and rural development poles, and could make intentional decisions to keep fertile areas in agricultural production. Municipal authorities often have more direct oversight or influence over land use, and so they can make food production one of their priorities in land use allocation.[131]

With more active participatory budgeting processes, the provincial and municipal levels are those at which empowerment of traditionally disenfranchised groups can be most fruitful, for example, poor farmers or squatters.[132] Increasing knowledge and skills through action research and participatory learning about production, marketing, health protection and promotion, and policy influence are crucial activities to foster social innovation.

NOTES

1. B. D. McIntyre et al., eds., *International Assessment of Agricultural Knowledge, Science and Technology for Development* (IAASTD) (Washington, DC: Island Press, 2009), accessed June 8, 2011, http://www.agassessment.org/reports/IAASTD/EN/Agriculture%20at%20a%20Crossroads_Global%20Report%20%28English%29.pdf

2. C. Corvalan, S. Hales, and A. McMichael, *Ecosystems and Human Well-Being: Health Synthesis: A Report of the Millennium Ecosystem Assessment* (Geneva, Switzerland: World Health Organization, 2005).

3. C. Hawkes, M. Ruel, and S. Babu "Agriculture and Health: Overview, Themes and Moving Forward," *Food and Nutrition Bulletin* 28, supp 2 (2007): S221–6.

4. McIntyre et al., *International Assessment of Agricultural Knowledge...*

5. M. J. Cohen and J. Garrett, *The Food Price Crisis and Urban Food (In)Security* (Human Settlements Working Paper Series, Urbanization and Emerging Population Issues—2, International Institute for Environment and Development (IIED) and United Nations Population Fund (UNFPA), London, England, 2009).

6. C. Nellemann et al., eds., *The Environmental Food Crisis—The Environment's Role in Averting Future Food Crises. A UNEP Rapid Response Assessment*, accessed April 28, 2011, http://www.grida.no/publications/rr/food-crisis/

7. M. Adata and R. Meinzen-Dick, eds., *Agricultural Research, Livelihoods, and Poverty. Studies of economic and social impacts in six countries* (Washington, DC: IFPRI and Baltimore, MD: The Johns Hopkins University Press, 2007).

8. K. A. Dahlberg, "Regenerative Food Systems: Broadening the Scope and Agenda of Sustainability," in *Food for the Future: Conditions and Contradictions of Sustainability*, ed. P. Allen (New York, NY: Wiley, 1993), 75–102.

9. P. J. Ericksen, "Conceptualizing Food Systems for Global Environmental Change Research," *Global Environmental Change*, accessed June 9, 2011, http://www.eci.ox.ac.uk/publications/downloads/ericksen07-foodsystems.pdf

10. C. Hawkes, M.Chopra, and S. Friel, "Globalization, Trade and the Nutrition Transition," chap. 10 in *Globalization and Health: Pathways, Evidence and Policy*, eds. R. Labonté et al. (New York, NY: Routledge, 2009), 235–62.

11. United Nations Development Programme (UNDP). *Human Development Report 2010, 20th Anniversary Edition. The Real Wealth of Nations: Pathways to Human Development* (Basingstoke, England and New York, NY: Palgrave Macmillan, 2010).

12. S. Daniel, *The Food Crisis and Latin America: Framing a New Policy Approach*, The Oakland Institute, accessed May 26, 2013, http://www.essex.ac.uk/armedcon/themes/food_security/Latin_America-Food_Prices_Brief.pdf

13. *Sustainable Livelihood Guidance Sheets*, Department for International Development (DFID), accessed August 7, 2001, http://www.ennonline.net/resources/667

14. G. Prain and D. Lee-Smith, "Urban Agriculture in Africa: What Has Been Learned?" chap. 2 in *African Urban Harvest: Agriculture in the Cities of Cameroon, Kenya and Uganda*, eds. G. Prain, N. Karanja, and D. Lee-Smith D (Ottawa, Canada: International Development Research Centre and Springer and International Potato Centre, 2010), 13–35.

15. C. C. Crissman, K. Antle, and S. Capalbo, eds., *Economic, Environmental and Health Tradeoffs in Agriculture: Pesticides and the Sustainability of Andean Potato Production* (Dordrecht, The Netherlands: Kluwer Academic Publishers, 1998).

16. J. M. Antle, D. C. Cole, and C. C. Crissman, "Further Evidence on Pesticides, Productivity and Farmer Health: Potato Production in Ecuador," *Agriculture Economics* 18 (1998): 199–207.

17. V. Barrera et al., "Encontrando Salidas para Reducir los Costos y la Exposición a Plaguicidas: Experiencias con ECAs en el Norte del Ecuador," *LEISA* 19, no. 1 (2003): 46–8.

18. D. C. Cole, C. C. Crissman, and A. F. Orozco, "Canada's International Development Research Centre's Eco-Health projects with Latin Americans: Origins, Development and Challenges," *Canadian Journal of Public Health* 97, no. 6 (2004): I8–I14.

19. T. F. Orozco et al., "Health Promotion Outcomes Associated with a Community Based Project on Pesticide Use and Handling among Small Farm Households," *Health Promotion International* 26, no. 4 (2011): 432–46.

20. T. F. Orozco et al., "Monitoring Adherence to the International FAO Code of Conduct on the Distribution and Use of Pesticides—Highly Hazardous Pesticides in Central Andean Agriculture and Farmers' Rights to Health," *International Journal of Occupational and Environmental Health* 15, no. 3 (2009): 255–68.

21. S. Sherwood, "Agricultural Modernisation and the Production of Decline," PhD diss., Wageninngen University, The Netherlands, 2009.

22. G. Adell, *Theories and Models of the Peri-Urban Interface: A Changing Conceptual Landscape,* (literature review, Peri-Urban Research Project, Development Planning Unit (DPU), London, England, 1999).

23. C. Tacoli, *Bridging the Divide: Rural–urban Interactions and Livelihood Strategies.* (Gatekeeper series no. 77, IIED, London, England, 1998), 3–20.

24. G. Prain et al., *Proyecto HortiSana—Horticultura Sana y Sustentable en la Región Andina Central (Ecuador, Perú y Bolivia). Informe Técnico Final para IDRC* (project # 104317-001, Centro Internacional de la Papa (CIP), Lima, Peru, 2011).

25. International Fund for Agricultural Development (IFAD). *Improving access to land and tenure security* (policy paper, IFAD, Rome, Italy, 2008), accessed June 8, 2011 http://www.ifad.org/pub/policy/land/e.pdf

26. J. V. Murra, "'El Archipelago Vertical' Revisited," in *Andean Ecology and Civilization: An Interdisciplinary Perspective on Ecological Complementarity,* eds. S. Masuda, I. Shimada, and C. Morris (Tokyo, Japan: Tokyo University Press, 1985), 3–19.

27. S. Sherwood and J. Bentley, "Katalysis: Helping Andean Farmers Adapt to Climate Change," in "Community-Based Adaptation to Climate Change," special issue, *Participatory Learning and Action* 60 (2009): 65–75.

28. D. Satterthwaite and C. Tacoli, "Seeking an Understanding of Poverty That Recognizes Rural-Urban Differences and Rural-Urban Linkages," in *Urban Livelihoods: A People-Centred Approach to Reducing Poverty,* eds. C. Rakodi and T. Lloyd-Jones (London, England: Earthscan, 2002), 52–70.

29. IFAD, *Improving Access to Land...*

30. C. Tacoli and D. Satterthwaite, *The Urban Part of Rural Development: The Role of Small and Intermediate Urban Centres in Rural and Regional Development and Poverty Reduction. Rural-Urban Interactions and Livelihood Strategies* (working paper 9, International Institute for Environment and Development, London, England, 2004).

31. M. Castro and H. Juarez, "Propuesta Metodológica de Protección de Zonas Agrícolas en Zonas Peri-Urbanas de Lima Metropolitana," (memo to the 10th Congreso Nacional de Arquitectos Arequipa, September 26–28, 2007, Arequipa, Peru: TEMA 2: La Planificación Estratégica: Una Visión del Desarrollo).

32. N. G. Romero and V. U. Rime, *El Suelo,* (technical guide, Urban Harvest/ International Potato Center, Lima, Peru, 2009).

33. P. Smith et al., "Policy and Technological Constraints to Implementation of Greenhouse Gas Mitigation Options in Agriculture," *Agriculture, Ecosystems and Environment* 118 (2007): 6–28.

34. W. Cosgrove and H. Tropp, "Water for Development: Investing in Health and Economic Well-Being Globally" in *Ensuring a Sustainable Future: Making Progress on Environment and Equity,* Heymann J. and Barrera M. eds. (New York: Oxford University Press, 2013).

35. C. de Fraturier et al., "Looking Ahead to 2050: Scenarios of Alternative Investment Approaches," chap. 3 in *Water for Food, Water for Life: A Comprehensive Assessment of Water Management in Agriculture,* ed. D. Molden (London, England: Earthscan, 2007), 91–145.

36. U. Hoffmann, *Assuring Food Security in Developing Countries under the Challenges of Climate Change: Key Trade and Development Issues of a Fundamental Transformation of Agriculture* (United Nations Conference on Trade and Development Discussion Paper No. 201, February 2011), accessed June 8, 2011 http://www.unctad.org/en/docs/osgdp20111_en.pdf

37. M. Mulligan et al., "Andes Basin Focal Project (Andes BFP)," (project no. 63 in, *Final Report to the Challenge Program for Water and Food Project,* December 18, 2009), accessed May 12, 2013 http://www.ambiotek.com/BFPANDES/reports/ BFPANDES_CPWF_Final_Report.pdf
38. Ibid.
39. C. Trivelli and S. Boucher, "Vulnerabilidad y Shocks Climáticos: El Costo de la Sequía para los Productores Agropecuarios de Piura y el Valle del Mantaro" [Vulnerability and Climatic Shocks: The Cost of the Drought Among Agricultural Producers of Piura and the Montaro Valley], *Economía y Sociedad* 61 (2006): 46–56, accessed April 20, 2011 http://cies.org.pe/files/ES/Bol61/06-trivelli.pdf
40. McIntyre et al., eds., International Assessment of Agricultural Knowledge...
41. P. Drechsel et al., eds., *Wastewater Irrigation and Health. Assessing and Mitigating Risk in Low-Income Countries* (London, England and Sterling, VA: International Water Management Institute and International Development Research Centre with Earthscan, 2010), accessed June 8, 2011, http://www.iwmi.cgiar.org/ Publications/books/pdf/Wastewater_Irrigation_and_Health_book.pdf
42. Sherwood and Bentley, "Katalysis: Helping Andean Farmers..."
43. J. Moscoso, T. Alfaro and T. Juarez, "The Use of Reservoirs to Improve the Quality of Urban Irrigation Water," *Urban Agriculture Magazine* 20 (2008): 10.
44. C. Nellemann et al., eds., *The Environmental Food Crisis—The Environment's Role in Averting Future Food Crises. A UNEP Rapid Response Assessment,* United Nations Environment Program (UNEP) & GRID-Arendal, accessed April 28, 2011, http://www.grida.no/publications/rr/food-crisis/
45. J. Pretty, ed., *The Pesticide Detox: Towards a More Sustainable Agriculture* (London, England and Sterling, VA: Earthscan, 2005).
46. Sherwood, *Agricultural Modernisation...*
47. Crissman et al., *Economic, Environmental and Health Tradeoffs...*
48. M. Paredes, *Peasants, Potatoes and Pesticides. Heterogeneity in the Context of Agricultural Modernization in the Highland Andes of Ecuador,* PhD diss., Wageninngen University, The Netherlands, 2010.
49. T. F. Orozco et al., "Relationship Among Production Systems, Pre-School Nutritional Status and Pesticide—Related Toxicity in Seven Ecuadorian Communities—A Multi-Case Study Approach," *Food Nutrition Bulletin* 28, no. 2, supp. (2007): S247–57.
50. Orozco et al., "Monitoring Adherence to the International FAO Code..."
51. Prain et al., *Proyecto HortiSana...*
52. M. A. Altieri, "Agroecology: The Science of Natural Resource Management 5 for Poor Farmers in Marginal Environments," *Agriculture, Ecosystems and Environment* 1971 (2002): 1–24.
53. McIntyre et al., eds., *International Assessment of Agricultural Knowledge...*
54. J. Pretty, "Agricultural Sustainability: Concepts, Principles and Evidence," *Philosophical Transactions of the Royal Society B: Biological Sciences* 363, no. 1491 (2008): 447–65.
55. U. Hoffmann, *Assuring Food Security in Developing Countries...*
56. H. Van der Wulp and J. Pretty, "Policies and Trends," chap. 15 in *The Pesticide Detox: Towards a More Sustainable Agriculture,* ed. J. Pretty (London, England and Sterling, VA: Earthscan, 2005).
57. *AGP- Integrated Pest Management,* Food and Agriculture Organization of the United Nations, accessed May 3, 2013, http://www.fao.org/agriculture/crops/ core-themes/theme/pests/ipm/en/

58. D. C. Cole et al., "An Agriculture and Health Inter-Sectorial Research Process to Reduce Hazardous Pesticide Health Impacts Among Smallholder Farmers in the Andes," *BMC International Health and Human Rights* 11, supp. 2 (2011): S6.
59. Prain et al. *Proyecto HortiSana...*
60. P. Kromann et al., "Use of the Environmental Impact Quotient to Estimate Health and Environmental Impacts of Pesticide usage in Peruvian and Ecuadorian Potato Production," *Journal of Environmental Protection* 2 (2011): 581–91.
61. Prain et al. *Proyecto HortiSana...*
62. A. Taipe, G. Forbes, and S. Bastidas, *Evaluación de la Eficiencia de Tres Dosis de Fosfitos Para el Control del Tizón Tardío en Tres Variedades de Papa,* (Quito, Ecuador: Centro Internacional de la Papa, Estación Experimental Quito, 2009).
63. Barrera et al., "Encontrando Salidas para Reducir..."
64. E. Godtland et al., "The Impact of Farmer-Field-Schools on Knowledge and Productivity: A Study of Potato Farmers in the Peruvian Andes," *Economic Development and Cultural Change* 53, no 1 (2004): 63–92.
65. World Health Organization (WHO), *The WHO Recommended Classification of Pesticides by Hazard and Guidelines to Classification,* (Geneva, Switzerland: WHO, 2009).
66. Prain et al. *Proyecto HortiSana...,* 50, 51
67. *State of Food and Agriculture 2010-11: Women in Agriculture: closing the gender gap for development,* Food and Agriculture Organization of the United Nations, accessed April 20, 2011, http://www.fao.org/publications/sofa/en/
68. D. C. Cole, D. Lee-Smith, and G. W. Nasinyama, eds. *Healthy City Harvests: Generating Evidence to Guide Policy on Urban Agriculture* (Lima Peru: International Potato Center/ Urban Harvest and Makerere University Press, 2008).
69. L. McIntyre and K. Rondeau, "Food Security and Global Health," chap. 22 in *Global Health and Global Health Ethics,* eds. S. Benatar and G. Brock (Cambridge, England: Cambridge University Press, 2011).
70. *State of Food and Agriculture 2010-11...*
71. B. M. Popkin, "The Nutrition Transition and Obesity in the Developing World," *Journal of Nutrition* 131 (2001): 871S–3S.
72. R. Paarlberg, "Governing the Dietary Transition: Linking Agriculture, Nutrition, and Health," (paper, *Leveraging Agriculture for Improving Nutrition and Health,* 2020 Conference, Washington DC, and Delhi, India: International Food Policy Research Institute), accessed February 20, 2011, http://www.ifpri.org/2 020-agriculture-nutrition-health
73. K. Walker-Bone and K. Palmer, "Musculoskeletal Disorders in Farmers and Farm Workers," *Occupational Medicine* 52, no. 8 (2002): 441–50.
74. D. Gunnell and M. Eddleston, "Suicide by Intentional Ingestion of Pesticides: A Continuing Tragedy in Developing Countries," *International Journal of Epidemiology* 32, no. 6 (2003): 902–9.
75. M. L. Solorzano, "Percepciones Respecto al Manejo de Pesticidas Agricolas y su Implicancia en la Salud de los Productores de Hortalizas en Pucara y Chupaca" [Perceptions Regarding the Management of Agricultural Pesticides and Their Implication for Vegetables Producers' Health in Pucara and Chupaca], (masters' thesis, Unidad De Postgrado De La Facultad De Agronomía, Universidad Nacional Del Centro Del Peru, 2011).
76. Clinical assessments consisted of physical examinations by physicians, neurobehavioral testing for visuospatial (Benton) and psychomotor (Purdue Pegboard)

performance, and blood testing for red cell cholinesterase (Ellman method), which declines with organophosphorus and carbamate insecticide exposure (Schmidt 2011). Schmidt Álvarez LCE. *Manifestaciones de Neurotoxicidad Subclínica en Agricultores Que Manipulan Plaguicidas: Estudio en Cinco Comunidades De Huancayo.* Magister Scientiae En Salud Ocupacional Y Ambiental. Facultad De Medicina De San Fernando, Universidad Nacional Mayor De San Marcos. 2011. [Manifestations of Subclinical Neurotoxicity among Farmers exposed to Pesticides. Study in five communities of Huancayo. Masters in Occupational and Environmental Health.]

77. Sixty-nine (77 percent) demonstrated cogwheel rigidity (Ford Manoevre, Nojka sign) consistent with manganese exposure in the fungicide Maneb, 70 (79 percent) showed alterations in fine touch, and 46 (52 percent) in gross touch on clinical examination. Forty-eight (53 percent) showed moderate or severe deficits on the Benton test (scores <9/15) and 59 (66 percent) showed deficits in both hands while using the Purdue Pegboard (scores <10/20), difficulties only partially attributable to low levels of education (9 unable to read or write and 25 with primary school). Furthermore, 38/89 (44 percent) had low concentrations of red cell cholinesterase.

78. Crissman et al., *Economic, Environmental and Health Tradeoffs...*

79. Trivelli and Boucher, "Vulnerabilidad y Shocks Climáticos..."

80. J. Leah et al., "Determinants of Food Security Among Small Farmers in the Andes: Examining the Path," *Public Health Nutrition* 16, no. 1 (2013): 136–45.

81. K. Lock et al., "Global Burden of Disease Due to Low Consumption of Fruits and Vegetables: Implications for the Global Strategy on Diet," *Bulletin of the World Health Organization* 83 (2005): 100–8.

82. Prain et al., *Proyecto HortiSana...*, 45.

83. Pretty, *The Pesticide Detox...*

84. *State of the World 2011: Innovations that Nourish the Planet* The Worldwatch Institute, accessed April 27, 2011, http://www.worldwatch.org/sow11

85. Ibid.

86. S. Sherwood et al., "From Pesticides to People: Improving Ecosystem Health in the Northern Andes," chap. 9 in *The Pesticide Detox: Towards a More Sustainable Agriculture*, ed. J. Pretty (London, England and Sterling, VA: Earthscan, 2005).

87. T. F. Orozco et al., "Health Promotion Outcomes Associated..."

88. A special component of the follow-up survey identified three distinct referent groups of farmers based on their responses to carefully selected statements about their agriculture: "environmentally conscious"; risk averse; and "low social capital" producers (see Pradel et al., in press).

89. W. Pradel, D. C. Cole, and G. Prain, "Evaluating Change in Complex Project Interventions: Mixed Methods Assessments of Health and Environment-Related Outcomes in an Agricultural Project in the Central Andes," in press.

90. D. C. Cole et al., "Reducing Pesticide Neurotoxic Effects in Farm Households," *International Journal of Occupational and Environmental Health* 13 (2007): 281–9.

91. P. R. Berti, J. Krasevec, and S. FitzGerald, "A Review of the Effectiveness of Agriculture Interventions in Improving Nutrition Outcomes," *Public Health and Nutrition* 7, no. 5 (2004): 599–609.

92. R. Bezner Kerr et al., "Growing Healthy Communities: Farmer Participatory Research to Improve Child Nutrition, Food Security, and Soils in Ekwendeni, Malawi," chap. 2 in *Ecohealth Research in Practice: Innovative Applications of*

an *Ecosystem Approach to Health*, ed. D. Charron (New York, NY: Springer and Ottawa, Canada: International Development Research Centre, forthcoming).

93. T. A. Lumpkin, K. Weinberger, and S. Moore, *Increasing Income through Fruit and Vegetable Production Opportunities and Challenges* (draft paper, Consultative Group on International Agricultural Research Science Forum on CGIAR Priorities: Science for the Poor, Marrakech, Morocco, December 6, 2005).

94. Global Horticulture Initiative, official website, accessed May 3, 2013, http://www.globalhort.org/

95. Prain et al. *Proyecto HortiSana...*, 45

96. P. Hazell and S. Wood, "Drivers of Change in Global Agriculture," *Philosophical Transactions of the Royal Society B, Biological Sciences* 363 (2008): 495–515.

97. A. W. Shepherd, *Approaches to Linking Producers to Markets,* (paper 13, Agricultural Management, Marketing and Finance, Food and Agricultural Organizaion of the United Nations, Rome, 2007).

98. T. Reardon and J. Berdegué, "The Rapid Rise of Supermarkets in Latin America: Challenges and Opportunities for Development," *Development Policy Review* 20, no. 4 (2002): 371–88.

99. Shepherd, *Approaches to Linking...*, 23ff.

100. M. Chiriboga and J. F. Arellano, *Diagnóstico de la Comercialización Agropecuaria en Ecuador - Implicaciones para la Pequeña Economía Campesina y Propuesta para una Agenda Nacional de Comercialización Agropecuaria,* accessed June 6, 2011, http://veco.org.ec/fileadmin/CENDOC/Sistemat,%20Consult,%20Dx%20y%20Tesis/Diagn%F3sticos/Diagnostico%20Manuel%20Chiriboga.pdf

101. Ruralter and Alianza de Aprendizaje Peru, *Mecanismos de Articulación de Pequeños Productores Rurales con Empresas Privadas en el Perú* [Mechanisms of Articulation of Small Rural Producers with Private Companies in Peru] (Lima, Peru: Case Studies, 2007).

102. D. C. Cole et al., "Andean Indigenous-Mestizo Peoples, Agro-Ecosystems & Human Health: Horticulture in Peru's Montaro Valley," in *Global Indigenous Health Research Symposium Report. Papers and Presentations: Directions and Themes in International Indigenous Health Research*, eds. J. Reading et al. (Victoria, Canada: Centre for Aboriginal Health Research, University of Victoria, 2008), 27–32.

103. Africa Team, *Linking Farmers to Markets: Participatory Agro-enterprise Development* (Cali, Colombia: CIAT, 2007).

104. T. Bernet, G. Thiele, and T. Zschocke, eds., *Participatory Market Chain Approach (PMCA). User Guide* (Lima, Peru: International Potato Center (CIP), 2006), accessed May 3, 2013, http://www.rfpp.ethz.ch/fellowships/concluded_fellowships/Bernet_Participatory_market_chain_approach-Bernet_2006

105. J. C. Loomis, "No Como Veneno: Strengthening Local Organic Markets in the Peruvian Andes," (master's thesis, Department of Sociology, Colorado State University, Fort Collins, Colorado, 2010).

106. C. P. Pilataxi Guairacaja, *Identificación De Flujos Productivos Y Caracterización De Los Principales Segmentos De Mercado Potencial Para Productos Agroecológicos Del Cantón Píllaro* [Product Flow Identification and Characterization of the Main Segments of Market Potential for Agro-Ecological Products in Pillaro Canton] (Riobamba, Ecuador: Escuela Superior Politécnica De Chimborazo Facultad De Recursos Naturales, Escuela De Ingeniería Agronómica, 2010).

107. McIntyre et al., *International Assessment of Agricultural Knowledge* [reference #1]

108. L. T. Raynolds, D. Murray, and J. Wilkinson, eds., *Fair Trade: The Challenge of Transforming Globalization* (New York, NY: Routledge, 2007).

109. R. Stringfellow et al., *Improving the Access of Smallholders to Agricultural Services in Sub-Saharan Africa: Farmer Cooperation and the Role of the Donor Community* (Natural Resource Perspectives, no. 20., Overseas Development Institute (ODI), London, England, 1997).

110. J. Hellin, M. Lundi, and M. Meijer, "Farmer Organization and Market Access," *LEISA Magazine* 23, no.1 (2007), accessed http://www. agriculturesnetwork.org/magazines/global/how-farmers-organise/ farmer-organisation-and-market-access/at_download/article_pdf

111. M. Lundy et al., *Territorial Approach to Rural Agro-enterprise Development. Manual 1: A Guide to Developing Partnerships, Territorial Analysis and Planning Together* (Cali, Colombia: CIAT, 2005).

112. G. Prain et al., "Organic Vegetables on the Peri-Urban Interface: Helping Low Income Producers Access High Value Markets in Lima, Peru," *Acta Hortica* 881 (2010): 117–23.

113. A. Buchanan and M. DeCamp, "Responsibility for Global Health," chap. 10 in *Global Health and Global Health Ethics*, eds. S. Benatar and G. Brock (Cambridge, England: Cambridge University Press, 2011).

114. Hazell and Wood, "Drivers of Change..."

115. Hoffmann, *Assuring Food Security in Developing Countries...*

116. Ibid.

117. M. Woolcock, "Social Capital and Economic Development: Toward a Theoretical Synthesis and Policy Framework," *Theory and Society* 27, no. 2 (1998): 151–208.

118. B. Arce et al., "Vegetable Production Systems as Livelihood Strategies in Lima-Peru: Opportunities and Risks for Households and Local Governments," *Acta Hortica* 762 (2007): 291–302.

119. Prain et al., "Organic Vegetables on the Peri-Urban..."

120. WHO, *The WHO Recommended Classification...*

121. Prain et al. *Proyecto HortiSana...*, 17

122. G. Thiele, A. Braun, and E. Gandarillas. "Farmer Field Schools and CIALS as Complementary Platforms: New Challenges and Opportunities," in *Participatory Research and Development for Sustainable Agriculture and Natural Resource Management: A Sourcebook*, eds. J. Gonsalves et al. (Laguna, Philippines: CIP-UPWARD, IDRC, IFAD, 2005).

123. G. Thiele et al., "Multi-Stakeholder Platforms for Linking Small Farmers to Value Chains: Evidence from the Andes," *International Journal of Agricultural Sustainability* 9, no. 3 (2011): 423–433.

124. R. Cavatassi et al., "Linking Smallholders to the New Agricultural Economy: The Case of the Plataformas de Concertación in Ecuador," *Journal of Development Studies* 47, no. 10 (2011): 1545–1573.

125. Hazell and Wood, "Drivers of Change"

126. *Kyrgyz Republic Agricultural Productivity Assistance Project Environmental Management Plan,* The World Bank, accessed June 13, 2011 http://www-wds.world-bank.org/external/default/WDSContentServer/WDSP/IB/2011/05/04/000356161 _20110504014847/Rendered/PDF/E27730EA0ECA1E101public10BOX358346B. pdf

127. L. Caizhen, *Monitoring Pest Management in the World Bank-Funded Anning Valley Project, Sichuan Province, China by the Center for Community Development Studies (CDS), Part of Partnerships to Improve Implementation of the World Bank's Pest*

Management Policy, accessed June 13, 2011, http://campus.iss.nl/~caizhen/WORLDB~1.PDF

128. Orozco et al., "Monitoring Adherence to the International FAO Code..."
129. J. Foti and L. de Silva, *A Seat at the Table: Including the Poor in Decisions for Development and Environment* (Washington, DC: World Resources Institute, 2010).
130. Food and Agriculture Organization of the United Nations, *Right To Food Lessons Learned in Brazil* (Rome, Italy: FAO, 2007), accessed May 3, 2013, ftp://ftp.fao.org/docrep/fao/010/a1331e/a1331e.pdf
131. Cole et al., "Andean Indigenous-Mestizo Peoples..."
132. D. Satterthwaite, "Community Action in Informal Settlements: Strategies for Improved Environmental Health and Equity in Low- and Middle-Income Countries" in *Ensuring a Sustainable Future: Making Progress on Environment and Equity,* Heymann J. and Barrera M. eds. (New York: Oxford University Press, 2013).

CHAPTER 10

Access to Healthy Foods in Urban Settings

A Comprehensive Strategy for Low-Income Communities in Montreal

LISE BERTRAND

It is widely recognized that food is a major determinant of health.[1,2,3] In the last decade, numerous studies have been published showing various degrees of relationship between food access, food consumption, and health outcomes.[4,5,6,7,8] Among studies related to the food environment effect, Moore et al report that 22 to 35 percent of people living in areas with the worst-ranked food environments are less likely to have a healthy diet than those in best-ranked food environments.[9] Access to healthy foods reflects existing social and economic inequalities as low-income neighborhoods tend to experience poor food environments.[10,11,12,13,14] Lower income neighborhoods tend to have fewer supermarkets that sell a variety of foods, including fresh fruits and vegetables, and a higher number of convenience stores selling prepared, "empty calorie" foods.[15] Lack of affordable transportation options can complicate access to supermarkets located outside the neighborhood.[16] In addition to geographic distance to large grocery stores, it is important to consider issues of safety and poor walkability that might make access to stores difficult even when they are within geographic proximity. A study conducted in Boston found that perceived supermarket access rather than geographical proximity was associated with increased consumption of fruits and vegetables.[17] In addition to a lack of stores selling healthy foods, low-income neighborhoods often face higher food costs. Studies in the United States and Canada have found that prices for food, including fruits and vegetables, tend to be higher in lower income neighborhoods.[18] Reasons for the price differential might be the lack of larger grocery stores and supermarkets that tend to have lower prices, while small stores charge higher prices.[19]

There is a general consensus about the effects of a low availability of healthy foods upon the prevalence of health problems such as obesity in poor areas.[20] This awareness has led to an increasing focus on improving access to healthy foods. Studies have identified alternative sources of fruits and vegetables such as farmers' markets as one potential avenue to both increase access and lower costs.[21,22] An in-depth study of two farmers' markets in Los Angeles found that costumers felt the market improved access to fruits and vegetables and contributed to healthy eating habits. However, concerns about the costs of fruits and vegetables remained.[23]

Social inequities are thus reflected in such basic needs as food, which are largely conditioned by the food system and by the multiple dimensions of governance.[24] In countries like Switzerland, the food system is even now considered "a prism of present and future challenges for health promotion and sustainable development."[25] This chapter examines healthy food access and equity in Montreal, a high-income North American city, and provides examples of government and community initiatives. The chapter describes how food and food access research have led to new regional targets, with innovative implementation at the community level. Though specific to Montreal, the lessons learned from these community initiatives can be adapted to other settings. This chapter shows:

- an innovative way to integrate food security issues into built environment and urban planning at the local and regional levels;
- how to cast public health evidence in a wider conceptual framework of sustainable development;
- how to ensure that all relevant stakeholders are committed to improving the food system locally and regionally; and
- how unusual public health issues, such as urban food-related interventions (urban agriculture, transportation, neighborhood revitalization, etc.) can be put on the political agenda.

REGION OF MONTREAL AT A GLANCE

The identity of the region of Montreal comes from a number of factors, including its geographic position as an island, its governance structure as a central city with 19 boroughs and 10 other municipalities, its mix of densely populated as well as suburb-like neighborhoods, and its diversity of cultures. A dynamic community network emerges from 29 local, collaborative, intersectoral committees (tables locales de développement social) that focus on improving each aspect of their community life. These actors frequently undertake urban revitalization projects in relation with urban planning, economic development, and transportation, as well as for social housing or other local priorities.

THE MANDATE OF PUBLIC HEALTH DEPARTMENTS

In Quebec, 18 regional public health departments are legally mandated to identify any situation that may put the population at risk of a health problem and to promote preventive interventions. Surveillance of the population's health status, health promotion, evaluation of policies, and strategic programs support that mandate, all of which are informed by appropriate research. In addition, the public health departments must widely disseminate information that is used to influence policies to citizens, elected officials, and decision makers from all sectors.

In Montreal, the public health department (DSP) focuses on reducing inequalities in health and contributing to sustainable development. A large spectrum of disciplines is represented through the six orientations that comprise the public health action plan for the metropolitan region:

- Children's healthy birth and development
- Healthy youth with successful educational outcomes
- Healthy workplaces
- A vaccinated population that is protected from infections and chemical and physical risks
- A healthy urban environment
- A health care system focused on prevention

A specific team is active in the Urban Environment and Health sector, where research, planning, and action focus on the built environment and the following elements:

- Healthy housing conditions
- Access to healthy food
- Transportation, urban planning, and health
- The health impact of heat waves and climate change
- Air quality (outdoor)
- Residential wood burning
- Ragweed

PUBLIC HEALTH AND THE FOOD SYSTEM IN MONTREAL

Analysis of the food system in Montreal has become a necessary task over the years, with an increasing focus on health determinants, social inequalities, and poor access to healthy foods.[26,27] This focus on healthy foods and inequalities is in line with the 2010–2015 Action Plan for Montreal's public health department (Département de santé publique, DSP), which designates the reduction of social health inequalities as the first priority.[28] The 2011 annual report from the director of public health on social inequalities in Montreal reinforces this orientation as it examines the positive effects of Québec's social policies and investments. Health disparities between rich and poor and between neighborhoods are nonetheless persistent on the island of Montreal.[29] For example, "in 2006–2008, the life expectancy of residents in the CLSC [centre local de services communautaires, local community service centre] Hochelaga-Maisonneuve territory was 74.2 years while residents of Saint-Laurent could expect to live 85.0 years, a difference of almost 11 years."[30] These observations emphasize the need for public health actors to orient their actions toward the most vulnerable groups and neighborhoods of Montreal. Research and program planning on food issues have been developed with these priorities in mind, and they are detailed in a specific section of the Action Plan.

Whether it is designed for planning or for influencing policy makers, research is a fundamental component of the DSP's activities; an extensive knowledge of problems specific to its mandated population produces much greater impact on decisions than using commonly believed assumptions or referring to studies from elsewhere.[31] Research on food issues specific to Montreal has been conducted with the intention of establishing partnerships with other initiatives in order to improve the local food environment and healthy food consumption.

Four food issues have been analyzed in depth by the DSP with a focus on inequalities:

1. Incidence of food insecurity
2. Minimum cost of a nutritious food basket
3. Consumption of healthy foods
4. Access to healthy foods in neighborhoods

A General Conclusion Applies to the Four Topics

Depending on their revenue and sometimes on their residence area in the region, Montrealers may pay more for food, cannot purchase their food at the same types of stores, do not have access to an adequate supply of fresh fruits and vegetables within walking distance, or do not consume adequate amounts of healthy foods. The following sections summarize these observations.

Food Insecurity

In a poll conducted by the DSP in 2010, 17 percent of respondents reported at least one of the following: they worried about lack of food, actually did not have enough food, or could not get the quality and diversity of food they desired because of a lack of money.[32] Food insecurity has consequences on people's diets. For example, results from the 2004 Canadian Community Health Survey, Cycle 2.2 Nutrition state that children living in Québec in food-insecure families eat one portion less of fruits and vegetables per day compared to children from food-secure families.[33]

Minimum Cost of a Nutritious Food Basket

The Montreal Diet Dispensary (MDD) monitors food cost based on the nutritional needs of a family for three daily homemade meals. In 2006, the DSP funded a study by the MDD to determine whether food prices vary between sectors of residence. Variation was observed in two neighborhoods with low socioeconomic status, both between sectors and between the highest and the lowest costs of the nutritious food basket.[34] The MDD also estimated that a family on welfare lacked 21 percent of the revenue required to be able to afford the established minimum food cost once other expenses, such as housing, were covered. In September 2011, the cost of a nutritious food basket for a family of four was estimated at $7.42 per person per day. Because any increase in prices occurring in transportation, housing, and electricity directly affects the food budget, social initiatives or public policy interventions must focus on an equitable revenue for people receiving social assistance or working for minimum wage.

Consumption of Healthy Foods

Since 2002, the DSP has conducted a telephone poll twice a year with a representative sample of the regional population about different health behaviors.[35] Nine questions deal with the daily consumption frequency of four specific food categories: whole grain bread, milk and cheese, fruits and vegetables, and legumes. As shown in Figure 10.1, there is very little improvement over a 6-year period in the proportion of the population consuming fruits and vegetables at least 5 times a day.[36] In 2007, 33 percent of the population reported this minimum frequency, compared to 29 percent in 2002.

A significant relationship is observed between fruit and vegetable consumption and revenue. There is a 5 percent gap between the proportion of the population in the lowest category of revenue (<$20,000) who eat fruits and vegetables at least 5 times a day (29 percent) and the proportion earning $60,000 or more who do so (34 percent). This difference is greater among women; 31 percent of women with low revenue and 40 percent of women with the highest revenue eat fruits and vegetables at the minimal frequency. Monitoring food consumption provides a useful tool to relate food habits to social or health trends. It will be important to analyze the impact of rising food prices on fruit and vegetable consumption.

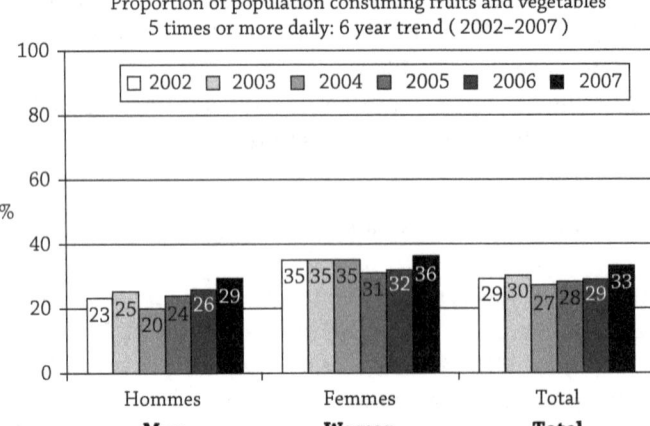

Proportion of population consuming fruits and vegetables
5 times or more daily: 6 year trend (2002–2007)

□ 2002 □ 2003 ▨ 2004 ▨ 2005 ■ 2006 ■ 2007

Figure 10.1:
Proportion of population consuming fruits and vegetables five times or more daily: 6-year trend (2002–2007).

Access to Healthy Foods

As early as 1987, following the Ottawa Health Promotion Charter that prioritized actions to reduce health inequalities,[37] attention was given to food environments to determine whether inequalities were observable at the neighborhood level in Montreal. A study examined, for the first time, prices and availability of basic foods in two neighborhoods differentiated by their socioeconomic status.[38] Results showed that living in a poor sector disadvantaged residents in terms of healthy food choices in both quantity and variety. Healthy choices were limited or not at all available, prices were consistently 3 percent higher, and the poor neighborhood had fewer supermarkets and twice as many corner stores compared to the community with a higher socioeconomic level.

After the publication of the 1987 study, many of the DSP's local community partners reported a lack of adequate food stores in poor communities and asked for more information on the food resources available in Montreal.[39] With their collaboration, food retail mapping was performed throughout the region of Montreal from 1999 to 2002, in order to capture food distribution disparities between local health center territories. Results showed that food distribution was uneven from one territory to another and even within the same territory. Although the overall picture did not show that retail services were lacking mostly in low socioeconomic areas, we nonetheless observed large numbers of corner stores compared to groceries or supermarkets in many underprivileged neighborhoods. An example is shown in Figure 10.2.

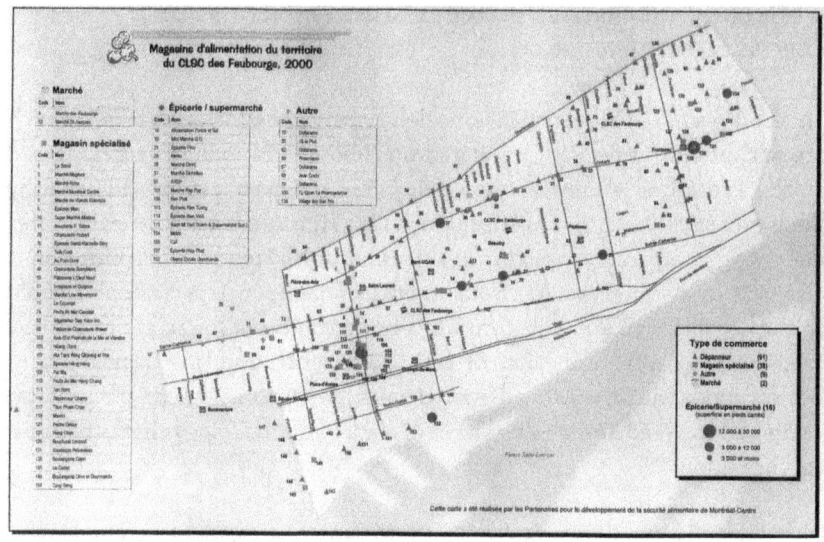

Figure 10.2:
Example of food retail serving a local health center territory.

Figure 10.2 illustrates a neighborhood characterized by a diversity of socioeconomic groups, including university students, single-occupancy residences, and single-parent families, among others. Circles represent groceries and supermarkets, squares are specialty or ethnic food stores, and triangles indicate corner stores. The latter are easily seen in greater number on the right of the map, where the poorest segment of the population is concentrated.

These observations raised concern among health planners about the nutritional quality of foods available in poor areas, which are largely serviced through numerous corner stores whose purpose is to accommodate customers with ready-to-use goods. While the model of "food deserts," defined by UK food policy advocates as "areas of relative exclusion where people experience physical and economic barriers to accessing healthy foods" within neighborhoods in central cities,[40,41,42] does not mean lack of stores in Montreal, access to healthy foods nonetheless remains a concern.

Public health objectives do indeed target foods that will promote health and prevent the most prevalent chronic diseases, such as obesity, cancer, cardiovascular diseases, and diabetes.[43,44,45,46] However, research, mainly conducted in the United States, has focused more on food retailing than on specific food availability in different commercial outlets and its effect on healthy food consumption.[47,48,49,50,51] Supermarkets are almost exclusively considered in research measuring food accessibility.[52]

The food system in Montreal is not solely dependent on supermarkets, which are not present in densely populated neighborhoods. Public markets, green stores, and ethnic stores, as shown on previous maps, can provide healthy foods on a small scale. However, looking only at the number and types of stores does not give an accurate picture of access to healthy foods. Transportation is also part of the food system; from an environmental perspective, one would like to see a city where motorization is not a condition for access to healthy foods. Along with promotion of active transportation, the availability of healthy foods within walking distances must also be considered.

These facts guided the elaboration of a study methodology that is relevant for the region.

- Fresh fruits and vegetables (F/V) as a proxy for healthy foods in general
  A large number of studies have been published on the preventive role of fruits and vegetables in regard to several chronic diseases, such as cancers, cardiovascular diseases, or obesity.[53,54,55,56] The 2004 Canadian Community Health Survey, Cycle 2.2 Nutrition established significant relationships between fruit and vegetable consumption and other health behaviors such as physical activity and smoking.[57] The Quebec National Public Health program specifies objectives related to F/V promotion.[58] Measuring the availability of fruits and vegetables in neighborhoods gives an indication of the quality of the food environment in general.
- Availability measured by total selling area of fresh F/V over a given territory
  We measured fruit and vegetable selling area in all food stores, including public markets, offering more than 75 sq. feet F/V (this measure was adopted after pretests were conducted to estimate the minimal surface offering an appropriate variety of fruits and vegetables in a store). These measures were calculated at Dissemination Area (DA) level, the smallest territorial unit for which Statistics Canada provides Census data.
- Proximity: 500 m and 3 km buffer zones around DA centroid
  The proximity concept differs according to the type of transportation available to carry grocery bags. In this study, proximity was established for two buffer zones, taking into account whether individuals owned a car. A walking distance of 500 m is suggested for pedestrians, including parents with children, or older people.[59] Other studies suggest that consumers owning a car consider 3 km as proximal for grocery shopping.[60] We first created an index combining F/V measures on the two buffer zones. Figure 10.3 shows that even with a 98 percent rate of motorization, people living in the West Island sector, to the left of the map, do not have access to fresh fruits and vegetables at proximity to their residence, this fact being explained by the suburb-like geography of municipalities

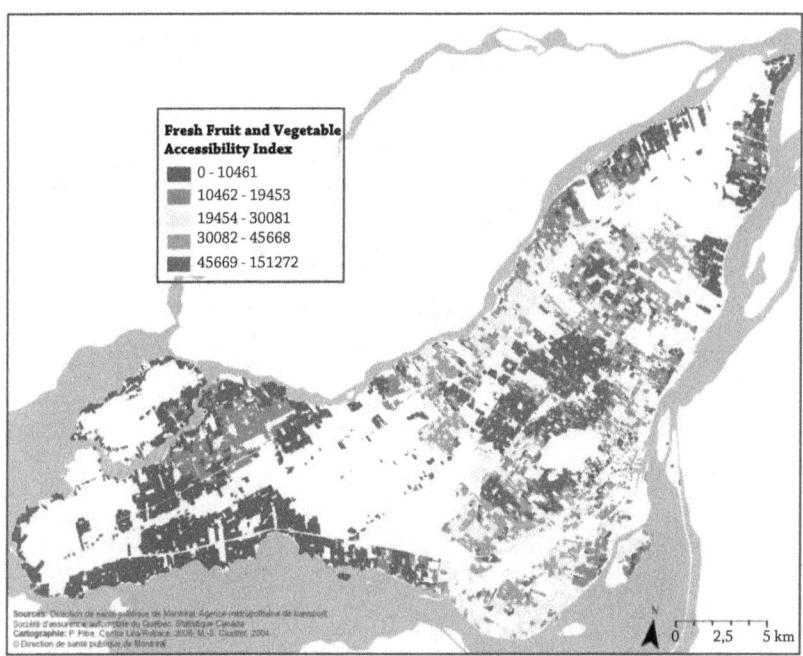

Figure 10.3:
Fresh fruit and vegetable accessibility.

in the sector; however, people in the more densely populated center of the island have access to an excellent supply, taking into account both the two buffer zones and the motorization rates at the DA level.

Figure 10.4 excludes the West Island subregion and focuses on more densely populated boroughs of Montreal, where fresh fruit and vegetable availability was analyzed solely on the basis of walking distance. We thus estimated that if all citizens had to walk for their food purchases, 34 percent of them would not have access to any supply of fresh F/V. If we add the population with access to the lowest range of recorded F/V surfaces in the stores, that is, between 75 and 640 square feet, we estimate that 40 percent of Montrealers live in sectors where fresh fruit and vegetable availability is low.

Disparities Not Linked to Socioeconomic Status

The main focus of this research was to determine whether there are disparities in fresh F/V availability among Montreal neighborhoods and, if so, who is the most exposed to inequities and where. Statistical comparisons were performed for different socioeconomic strata. No relationship was found between socioeconomic status of DAs and their respective F/V supply, whether measured in terms of walking distance or taking into account the motorization rate. This

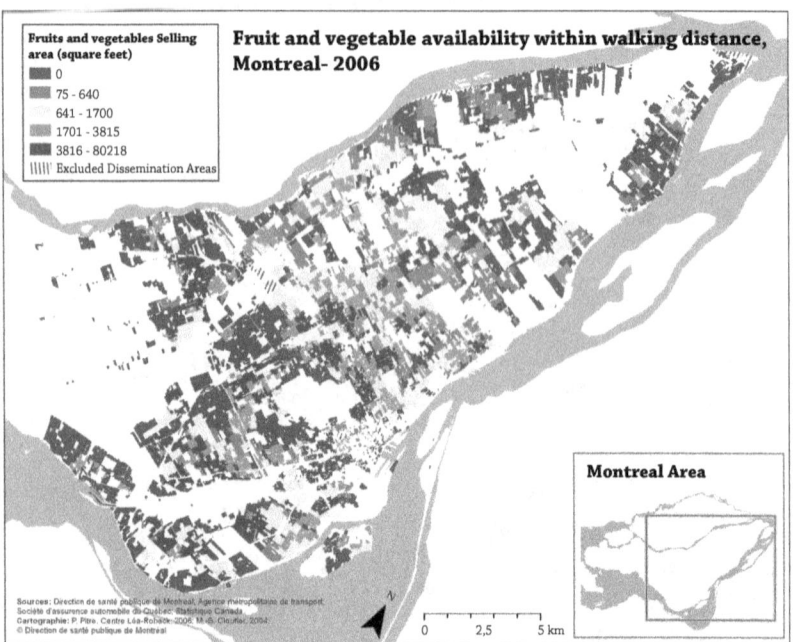

Figure 10.4:
Fruit and vegetable availability within walking distance.

observation does not confirm the results of US studies, which report associations between race, poverty, and lack of food stores.[61,62] The difference might be explained by more heterogeneity in Montreal neighborhoods; homogenous racial and economic communities are not predominant in Montreal to the extent that they are observed in the United States.[63] Multiethnicity in Montreal, similar to many European cities, seems to present a more complex social and physical context.[64] It is also important to recall that presence of stores is not the variable of interest in the Montreal study, but rather the total availability of fresh fruits and vegetables in residential neighborhoods.

However, if we consider the population with low revenue as a whole, more than 35 percent of low-income people do not have access to an adequate supply of fruits and vegetables within walking distance. Many of them also live in neighborhoods with low motorization rates and where public transportation is lacking.

The Montreal Strategy to Improve Food Environment and Reduce Inequalities

Knowledge of the food issues described herein prompted action by the Montreal DSP to raise interest among key community partners to address healthy food accessibility problems. In addition to communicating the results of the studies and their negative effects on population well-being, MDSP took up a leadership role with a grant program (1M$) designed for local communities. A framework was elaborated from data gathered on the population health and food needs, and from actual community dynamics related to food security in the region.[65] The framing document gives specific objectives directed toward improving healthy food access, mainly fresh fruits and vegetables; the strategy enacted is based on local community participation in all decisions to determine the best solutions to meet people's needs. Priority is given to poor and underserved communities (Fig. 10.5).

This funding program is managed by the Urban Environment and Health sector of MDSP, which is responsible for the built environment and to sustainable development. Working on food access calls for actions that need to be linked with urban planning, economic vitality, social development, and environmental factors, which together lead to sustainable development.

The model shown in Figure 10.6, presented as a framework for the funding program, summarizes types of actions that can be carried out to reduce food inequities and support sustainable development.

Several actions undertaken as part of the MDSP's initiative are favorable to both the food system and sustainable development. For example:

- Partnering with local merchants or food producers and advocating for revenue improvement are actions associated with economic development.

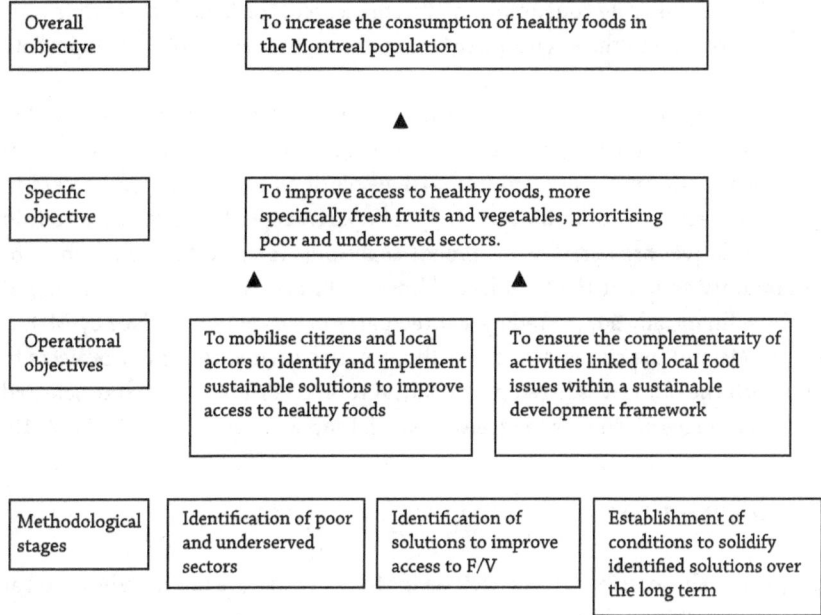

Figure 10.5:
Schematic summary of the framework for the Program to Support the Development of Food Security.

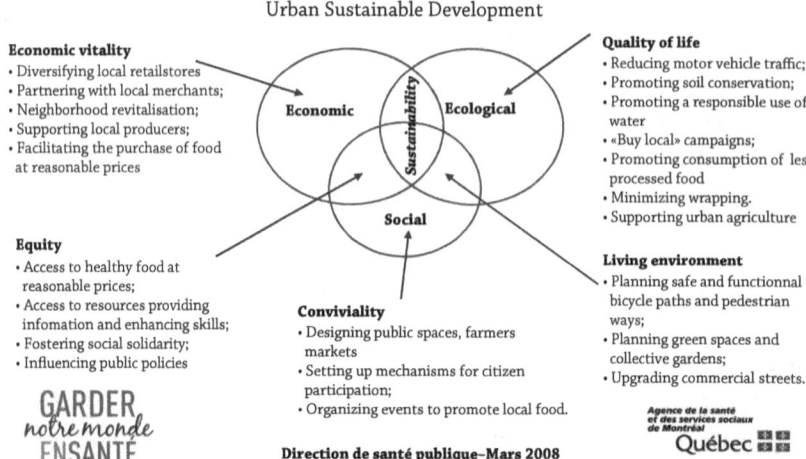

Food Security in the Perspective of
Urban Sustainable Development

Economic vitality
• Diversifying local retailstores
• Partnering with local merchants;
• Neighborhood revitalisation;
• Supporting local producers;
• Facilitating the purchase of food
  at reasonable prices

Quality of life
• Reducing motor vehicle traffic;
• Promoting soil conservation;
• Promoting a responsible use of
  water
• «Buy local» campaigns;
• Promoting consumption of less
  processed food
• Minimizing wrapping.
• Supporting urban agriculture

Economic **Sustainability** **Ecological**

Social

Equity
• Access to healthy food at
  reasonable prices;
• Access to resources providing
  infomation and enhancing skills;
• Fostering social solidarity;
• Influencing public policies

Living environment
• Planning safe and functionnal
  bicycle paths and pedestrian
  ways;
• Planning green spaces and
  collective gardens;
• Upgrading commercial streets.

Conviviality
• Designing public spaces, farmers
  markets
• Setting up mechanisms for citizen
  participation;
• Organizing events to promote local food.

GARDER
notre monde
ENSANTÉ

Direction de santé publique–Mars 2008

Agence de la santé
et des services sociaux
de Montréal
Québec

Figure 10.6:
Food security and sustainable development

- Green public spaces, collective gardens, and citizens' mobilization in
  their neighborhood's food improvement plan are promising strategies for social development.
- Reducing motorized transportation for grocery shopping and
  encouraging consumption of unprocessed, fresh, and local foods contribute to the environmental dimension of sustainable development.

Our strategy promotes a collaborative process involving citizens and stakeholders from municipal, commercial, social, and private sectors; their common goal is to find long-term innovative solutions to healthy food access in
poor, underserved communities. The main partners with the capacity to lead
such initiatives are social development coalitions, referred to as the center of
community action at the local level. These coalitions are already multisectoral
and are financially supported by a three-party program put in place by MDSP,
Centraide and the city of Montreal. They were all invited to submit projects in
line with the objectives listed previously. A total of 17 initiatives were selected
by a committee of experts to receive financial support between 2008 and 2012.

A Process That Takes Time

As previously described, the activities in this program are not merely aimed at
providing additional commercial food services. They are first based on social
development approaches, with and by the community. Because food environment improvement involves the whole community in defining where, what,

and how solutions are needed, leaders of initiatives must first take time to mobilize citizens and other stakeholders. Analysis of sites where healthy foods are not offered should guide leaders in planning which actions to undertake. For example, they will need to know how the local borough administration rules the commercial permits, zoning, public spaces, and various policies dealing with urban planning. Leaders are also encouraged to approach merchants, if present, to build cooperation, rather than competition, on healthy food supply. Each initiative then adjusts to its own rhythm. So far, actions have mainly focused on urban agriculture or local producers' markets, as initiating and sustaining this process takes time. Figure 10.7 provides an example of organizational phases. Indicated periods run from April to March.

Mercier-Ouest is part of an eastern borough of Montreal (Mercier/Hochelaga Maisonneuve), where large tracts of land are occupied by industries, institutions, the Canadian army, and the port of Montreal. The Guybourg

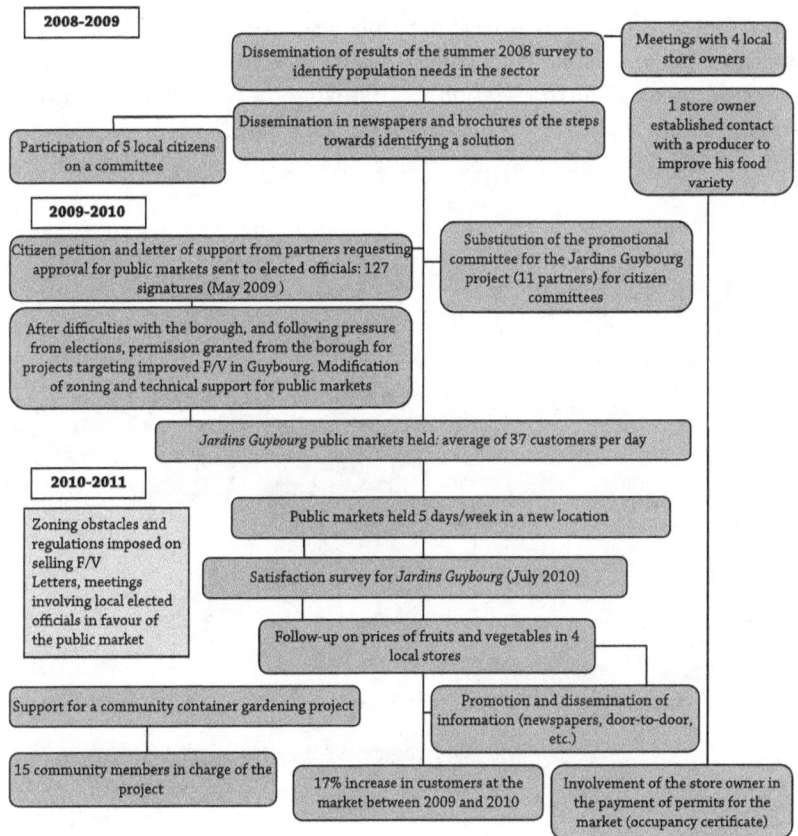

Figure 10.7:
Mobilization for better access to healthy foods in Guybourg district, Mercier-Ouest (Montreal), 2008–2011.

neighborhood is about five blocks wide, surrounded by nonresidential areas where services like schools, banks, and retail have gradually closed over the years. Figure 10.8 shows a circle around this area where availability of fresh fruits and vegetables is either 0 or low according to the MDSP study.

Although several other zones also appear neglected, the coalition "Mercier-Ouest Quartier en Santé" opted to focus on Guybourg mainly because of the presence of a community organization in this district that showed readiness to join an experimental approach. The Coalition of 70 individuals has a diverse membership, with representatives from nongovernmental organizations, institutions such as Local Health Services Center, citizens, and elected officials.

Before submitting a project in line with the funding program, in the summer of 2008 "Mercier-Ouest Quartier en santé" validated the MDSP study findings against the Guybourg community's perceptions of its food environment[66] and found significant interest in greater access to fresh foods in the surrounding area. Having to purchase their foods in other neighborhoods, 60 percent of Guybourg residents indicated that they would improve their F/V consumption if fruits and vegetables were available near their home. The survey was publicized in the community and local merchants who own corner stores were consulted to get their cooperation in improving the quality and quantity of healthy foods available in the neighborhood. One merchant was instrumental in the implementation of a public market in Guybourg. While this merchant

CSSS Lucille-Teasdale
Fruit and Vegetable selling area within 500 m radius

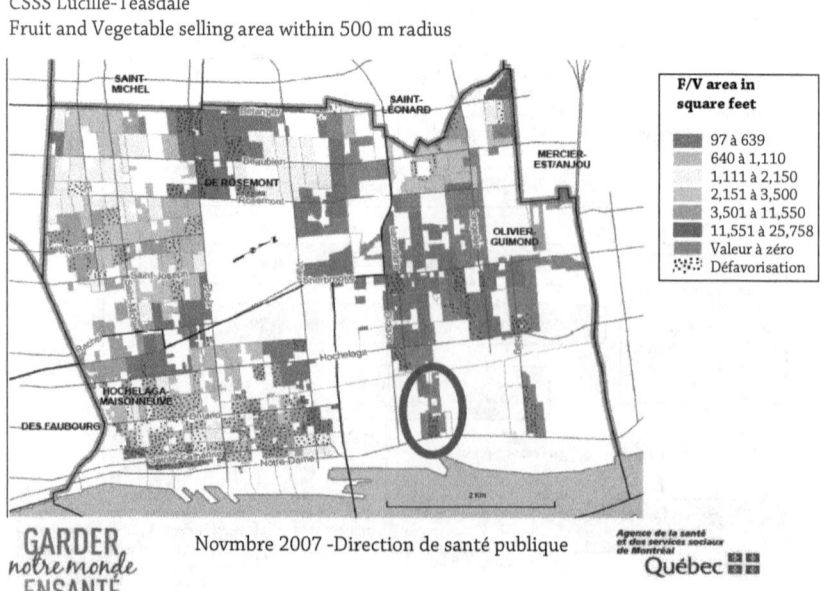

Figure 10.8:
Availability of fruits and vegetables in the CSSS Lucille-Teasdale area.

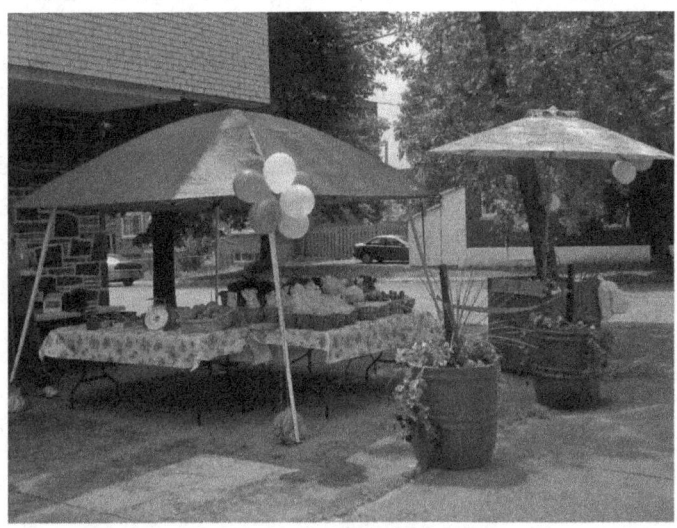

Figure 10.9:
Picture of community vegetable market. From: Gestion Cléhas, *Étude de Préfaisabilité. Offre d'un Point de Service de Fruits et Légumes Frais*. La Table de Concertation pour la Sécurité Alimentaire de Mercier-Ouest (2008).

did not modify his own store, he partnered with his food producer uncle to create an outdoor market. As early as May 2009, people living in Guybourg were encouraged to sign a petition addressed to the borough administration, requesting permission to sell F/V on the grounds of a community organiza-tion located in a former school. Even though the project funding came from a public health institution focusing on improving population living conditions, it was still regarded as a commercial activity by the borough's administration. Letters were sent by MDSP to support the petition, explaining the need for the healthy food project in the district, from both the perspective of community health benefit and also as an instrument of district revitalization. The corner store owner paid for the necessary permits for the producer to operate a stall all summer; he gained immediate support from Guybourg residents. Initiative leaders also mobilized community organizations to offer educational activities along with the seasonal project.

Although the borough's administration allowed the public market in the summer of 2009, the coalition had to start its process all over again when it chose another site for the second season in 2010. Letters and meetings with elected officials were once more on the initiative agenda. The long pro-cess ended with the adoption of a zoning modification in favor of a public space where fresh foods could be sold by the producer. A satisfaction sur-vey conducted at midsummer reported a faithful and satisfied clientele.[67] Seventy-three percent of respondents were regular customers; 75 percent of residents indicated a satisfactory variety of fresh F/V; and 93 percent of them praised the products' freshness. A 17 percent increase was observed in the market frequentation from 2009 to 2010. In the initiative's third year, another project was started to foster access to fresh fruits and vegetables in Guybourg. Two community organizations, Y'a quelqu'un l'aut'bord du mur (YQQ) et l'Éco-quartier Maisonneuve-Longue-Pointe, worked with Guybourg citizens on an urban agriculture project, which not only beautified a disused school yard but also provided knowledge, skills and self-esteem to garden-ers who participated in food production (see Fig. 10.10). Partnerships have been extended through local media participation with regular reports on the initiative.[68,69]

WILL THE PROGRAM OBJECTIVES BE MET?

In this case, increasing fruit and vegetable consumption is a relatively easy goal to measure.[70] One could survey fresh fruit and vegetable consumption within a community at the beginning and at the end of an initiative. However, simple measures cannot be applied to a context of complexity, even if the final objective is clear. Complex processes involving multiple partnerships at multiple levels need to be taken into account in the final analysis of the initiatives' outcomes. A few evaluations have been published on the effect of increasing healthy food availability in different types of stores or other outlets on food choices or consumption, but there is a paucity of evidence

Urban agriculture potential: low tech, low cost

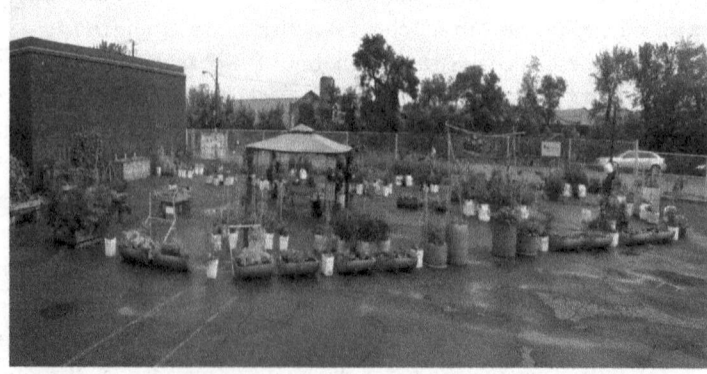

GARDER
notre monde
ENSANTÉ

Agence de la santé
et des services sociaux
de Montréal
Québec

Figure 10.10:
Table de concertation de Mercier-Ouest Quartier en santé, 2008.

on the effect of complex social development approaches.[71,72] Authors from the social development field emphasize the fact that community empowerment is as important as health objectives to ensuring the long-term effects of any intervention.[73,74,75,76] The influence of life context on health comes from the rapport established between the community and its environmental life conditions, whether these are material or social. Neighborhood characteristics such as urban planning, attractiveness, population composition, socioeconomic level, socialization opportunities, and services, are part of an individual and collective sense of control, which is strongly linked with health conditions.[77] The MDSP program planning agents devised a tool that would allow a follow-up of the 17 local initiatives and a transversal analysis of the 4-year program application. The main questions underlying the analysis are as follows:

1. What strategies were used to mobilize citizens and local actors? To what extent did they participate? What were the obstacles or the facilitating factors?
2. To what extent were complementary actions linked with the three dimensions of sustainable development? Were the actions on food availability integrated with other development approaches being conducted in the community?
3. What stage of development have the initiatives attained in reference to methodological phases?
4. To what extent do solutions to improve healthy food access present permanent conditions?
5. To what extent does the program improve access to healthy foods, namely fresh fruits and vegetables, in poor and underserved communities?

Indicators for Analysis of the Program's Effects

Table 10.1 summarizes a set of indicators associated with both the operational objectives of the program and the main strategies proposed in the framework. Validation of the indicators to be measured was ensured through three meetings with respondents from the community initiatives. Their input is the most important since the overall analysis is based on each initiative's actions. Qualitative and quantitative data were extracted from information provided in each initiative's annual report, for a total of three reports per initiative. NVivo9 software was chosen to perform qualitative data analysis because it facilitates comparative analysis and cross tabulations between qualitative and quantitative parameters. MDSP contracted an external expert in evaluation for this final work.

The overall analysis of the program's implementation through the 17 initiatives carried out between 2008 and 2011 was presented and discussed in

Table 10.1. INCREASING ACCESS TO HEALTHY FOODS

Results (what?) Operational results (how?)	Sector targeted Consensus decision	Solution identified Three dimensions of sustainable development taken into account in selecting a solution Integration of the solution identified in the development process	Set in place conditions to ensure the permanence of the identified solutions Partnership agreements Community engagement
Ensuring the complementarity of actions from a sustainable development perspective	• Issues identified along the three dimensions of sustainable development • Aligning the development initiatives in place in the sector	• Taking into account issues that are important for the three dimensions of SD when selecting solutions • Integrating the solutions with development initiatives currently in place • Involvement of intersectoral partners in selecting a solution	• Setting in place conditions linked to the three dimensions of SD • Setting in place conditions linked to current development initiatives • Involvement of intersectoral partners in maintaining the solution
Mobilizing community members and local actors	Participation mechanisms: 1. community members: • actions • name/characteristics 1. level of participation 2. local actors • actions • name/characteristics • contribution/ engagement Types of actions set in place to mobilize community: 1. community members • actions • name/characteristics • level of participation 2. local actors • actions • name/characteristics • contribution/ engagement	Participation mechanisms: • community members: • actions • name/characteristics 1. l evel of participation 2. local actors • actions • name/characteristics • contribution/ engagement Types of actions set in place to mobilize community: 1.community members • actions • name/characteristics • level of participation 2.local actors • actions • name/characteristics • contribution/ engagement	Participation mechanisms: • community members: • actions • name/characteristics 1. level of participation 2. local actors • actions • name/characteristics • contribution/engagement Types of actions set in place to mobilize community: 1.community members • actions • name/characteristics 1. level of participation 2. local actors • actions • name/characteristics • contribution/engagement

winter 2012. The main observations from the final report are summarized in the sections that follow.[78]

Mobilization

All initiatives have approached citizens at one stage or another. The most active strategies that involved citizens were the organization of public assemblies, particularly the creation of decisional committees. In 15 out of 17 initiatives, citizens participated in some form of fresh fruit and vegetable promotion in their community (the number varies between 3 and 38) or took part in committees such as administrative boards. However, citizens in precarious economic situations are less likely to participate actively on working groups. As an example of citizen participation, citizens in the Petite Bourgogne neighborhood involved the community in a petition asking the *Office municipal d'habitation* (municipal housing office) for a physical space where residents from a large housing complex—les ilôts St-Jacques—could have access to low-cost fresh foods. They launched "Le café citoyen" in the third year of their initiative.

Initiatives have partnerships with various actors who are present at the local level; community organizations and the municipal sector are the most frequently mentioned, followed by health and economic sectors. Although common grounds of partnership are observed throughout the 17 initiatives, partnerships vary depending on community dynamics. From annual reports and regular meetings organized by the MDSP with leaders from the local initiatives, one can easily observe the importance of support from the boroughs' administration in the success of initiatives focusing on improving the availability of healthy food in specific neighborhoods. Complementary inputs through collaboration with other programs and policies are essential, including integrated urban revitalization, family policy, master plans, or sustainable development plans since commercial licenses, zoning, public spaces, and walkable streets must be included in the food landscape.

Economic and community development corporations mainly acting on social economy are also useful partners in estimating the feasibility and long-term self-sustainability of different food access solutions. They are present in at least eight initiative committees.

INTEGRATION OF FOOD INITIATIVE WITH OTHER DEVELOPMENT APPROACHES

Six initiatives show their strong partnership with other development approaches focused on local issues, such as urban planning, lodging, transportation, or commercial revitalization. This occurs most often when key local actors analyze the community problems as part of an overall plan of action. While a holistic approach is the goal for many initiatives, the participation of actors representing the three dimensions of sustainable development appears to be uneven. Environmental actors are absent most frequently from actions targeting food improvement; however, references to environmental issues such as emphasis on local foods, packaging reduction, and consumers' proximity is consistent in the initiatives' annual reports.

VIABILITY OF SOLUTIONS IDENTIFIED FOR BETTER FOOD ACCESS

In 2011, seven initiatives out of 17 come out of the analysis as fulfilling some conditions of a viable solution. Integration within another development approach, a history of community mobilization, and structure of governance appear to be important conditions in place for these seven initiatives. Out of the other initiatives, seven are still experimenting with different models of solutions within the community and two are at a first stage where mobilization and decision about the process are not yet complete. These results confirm the need to allow time for projects to mature, especially in a complex process of mobilization requiring community engagement and change.

CONCLUSION

The planning process for food access improvement described in this chapter illustrates the importance of providing an overarching direction to functions performed at a regional level. Reducing health inequalities and chronic diseases are not objectives pertaining solely to the region of Montreal. However, strategies adopted in the city have to be closely linked to Montreal population needs. From research to program management and evaluation, a good knowledge of social problems, existing actors, effective strategies, and political issues are well recognized as essential, but mobilizing such knowledge is rarely applied because of the significant time investments required.

As demonstrated in this chapter, the planning cycle of an important health component, from research to program evaluation, facilitated the financial management of activities that were given specific objectives. Food interests are so numerous and involve so many sectors that it is easy to lose sight of what one wants to accomplish. The MDSP used research to support appropriate food programs that add value to what is already being done by other actors.

Moreover, our data do not support only the importance of the planning process; they serve as arguments to raise the interest of urban planners, merchants, and other authorities in the process of revitalization. We realize that a diversity of municipal policies can be linked to health objectives such as improving healthy food consumption. For example, in one borough the family policy was facilitated through the implementation of fresh foods services.

Another important lesson drawn from the 3-year exercise relates to longer term financial support. Although important stakeholders such as the city of Montreal administration, Centraide, Québec en Forme, Conférence régionale des élus, and others adopted MDSP objectives for improving access to healthy foods through their programs, local communities need time to adjust their specific needs to these initiatives. Viable solutions can be implemented, but most of them need support during more than a 3-year term.

The lessons learned from this chapter can be applied beyond the city of Montreal, or the region of Quebec. In any context, future planning should identify food access (F/V) as a health and urban social development issue and integrate food system planning into the overall strategies. Through a process involving multiple stakeholders, and with objectives established at the regional level designed to support local communities, the healthy food needs of all residents can be met.

NOTES

1. World Cancer Research Fund/American Institute for Cancer Research, *Food, Nutrition and the Prevention of Cancer: A Global Perspective* (Washington, DC: American Institute for Cancer Research, 1997).
2. World Health Organization, *Obesity: Preventing and Managing the Global Epidemic* (report, WHO consultation on obesity, WHO/NUT/NCD/98.1, Geneva, Switzerland, 1998).
3. European Heart Network, *Food, Nutrition and Cardiovascular Disease Prevention in Europe* (Brussels, Belgium: European Heart Network, 1998).
4. M. A. Franco et al., "Neighborhood Characteristics and Availability of Healthy Foods in Baltimore," *American Journal of Preventive Medicine* 35, no. 6 (2008): 561–567.
5. K. Morland et al., "Neighborhood Characteristics Associated With the Location of Food Stores and Food Service Places," *American Journal of Preventive Medicine* 22, no. 1 (2002): 23–29.
6. N. Wrigley, D. L. Warm, and B. M. Margetts, "Deprivation, Diet and Food Retail Access: Findings From the Leeds 'Food Deserts' Study," *Environment and Planning A* 35 (2003): 151–188.
7. L. Moore and A. Diez Roux, "Associations of Neighborhood Characteristics With the Location and Type of Food Stores," *American Journal of Public Health* 96, no. 2 (2006): 325–331.
8. N. I. Larson, M. T. Story, and M. C. Nelson, "Neighborhood Environments: Disparities in Access to Healthy Foods in the U.S.," *American Journal of Preventive Medicine* 36, no. 1 (2009): 74–81.
9. Moore and Diez Roux, "Associations of Neighborhood Characteristics…"
10. S. J. Algert, A. Agrawal, and D. S. Lewis, "Disparities in Access to Fresh Produce in Low-Income Neighborhoods in Los Angeles," *American Journal of Preventive Medicine* 30, no. 5 (2006): 365–370.

11. S. Cummins and S. MacIntyre, "Food Environments and Obesity-Neighborhood or Nation?" *International Journal of Epidemiology* 35 (2006): 100–104.
12. J. Gittelsohn and S. Sharma, "Physical, Consumer, and Social Aspects of Measuring the Food Environment Among Diverse Low-Income Populations," *American Journal of Preventive Medicine* 36, no. 4, supp. (2009): S161–S165.
13. M. Story et al., "Creating Healthy Food and Eating Environments: Policy and Environmental Approaches," *Annual Review of Public Health* 29 (2008): 253–272.
14. R. E. Walker, C. R. Keane, and J. G. Burke, "Disparities and Access to Healthy Food in the United States: A Review of Food Desert Literature," *Health and Place* 16 (2010): 876–884.
15. K. Photokuchi, "Attracting Supermarkets to Inner-City Neighborhoods: Economic Development Outside the Box," *Economic Development Quarterly* 19, no. 3 (2005): 232–244.
16. Walker et al., "Disparities and Access to Healthy Food…"
17. C. E. Caspi et al., "The Relationship Between Diet and Perceived and Objective Access to Supermarkets Among Low-Income Housing Residents," *Social Science and Medicine* 75 (2010): 1254–1262.
18. Cummins and MacIntyre, "Food Environments and Obesity…"
19. C. Chung and S. L. Myers, "Do the Poor Pay More for Food? An Analysis of Grocery Store Availability and Food Price Disparities," *Journal of Consumer Affairs* 33, no. 2 (1999): 276–296.
20. Cummins and MacIntyre, "Food Environments and Obesity…"
21. Institute of Medicine, *Local Government Actions to Prevent Childhood Obesity*, (Washington, DC: The National Academies Press, 2009).
22. V. Ruelas et al., "The Role of Farmers' Markets in Two Low Income, Urban Communities," *Journal of Community Health* 37 (2012): 554–562.
23. Ibid.
24. "Making Waves—Cultiver l'espoir," special issue, *Canada's Community Economic Development Magazine*, 17, no. 2 (2006).
25. Health Promotion Switzerland, *Triggering Debate—White Paper. The Food System* (2010), accessed May 13, 2013, http://www.scp-knowledge.eu/sites/default/files/knowledge/attachments/WhitePaper.KickbuschIlona.HPS_.pdf
26. *Plan régional de santé publique 2010–2015. Garder Notre Monde en Santé* (Montreal, Canada: Direction de Santé Publique, Agence de la Santé et des Services Sociaux de Montréal, 2010).
27. *Les Inégalités Sociales de la Santé à Montréal* (rapport du Directeur de Santé Publique, Agence de la Santé et des Services Sociaux de Montréal, Canada, 2011), accessed May 5, 2013, http://www.dsp.santemontreal.qc.ca/media/dossiers_de_presse/inegalites_sociales_de_sante.html
28. Ibid.
29. J. Leduc-Gauvin, *Alimenvi: L'environnement Alimentaire dans le Quartier St-René-Goupil* (Montreal, Canada: Département de Santé Communautaire, Hôpital du Sacré-Cœur de Montréal, 1988).
30. *Les Inégalités Sociales de la Santé…*
31. Ibid.
32. *Sondage Régional sur la Santé, Données Sur l'Insécurité Alimentaire dans la Population Montréalaise* (Montreal, Canada: Direction de Santé Publique, Agence de la Santé et des Services Sociaux de Montréal, 2010).
33. C. Blanchet and L. Rochette, *Sécurité et insécurité alimentaire chez les Québécois: une analyse de la situation en lien avec leurs habitudes alimentaires* (Direction de l'analyse

et de l'évaluation des systèmes de soins et services, Institut national de santé publique du Québec, Canada, 2011), accessed May 13, 2013, http://www.inspq. qc.ca/pdf/publications/1333_SecurtieAlimentQucAnalSituationHabAliment.pdf

34. *Étude sur le Coût du Panier à Provisions Nutritif dans les Divers Quartiers de Montréal— Rapport Synthèse* (Montreal, Canada: Dispensaire diététique de Montréal, 2006).

35. *Espace Montréalais d'Information sur la Santé, Suivi des Habitudes Alimentaires,* Agence de la Santé et des Services Sociaux de Montréal, Sondage Biannuel de la DSP, accessed May 5, 2013, http://emis.santemontreal.qc.ca/ sante-des-montrealais/axes-dintervention/environnement-urbain-et-sante/ habitudes-alimentaires/

36. N. Pouliot and L. Bertrand, *La Santé est-elle au Menu des Montréalais?* (Montreal, Canada: Direction de Santé Publique. Agence de la Santé et des Services Sociaux de Montréal, 2009).

37. Ibid.

38. N. Drolet, *Des gestes plus grands que la panse. Le monitoring de la sécurité alimentaire: Comment? Pourquoi?,* accessed May 5, 2013, http://www.dsp. santemontreal.qc.ca/index.php?id=523&tx_wfqbe_pi1[uid]=881

39. Ibid.

40. Wrigley et al., "Deprivation, Diet and Food Retail..."

41. Low Income Project Team, *Low Income, Food, Nutrition and Health: Strategies for Improvement* (London, England: Nutrition Task Force, UK Department of Health, 1996).

42. Policy Action Team 13, National Strategy for Neighbourhood Renewal, *Improving Shopping Access for People Living in Deprived Neighbourhoods. A Paper for Discussion* (London, England: Department of Health, 1999).

43. World Cancer Research Fund/American Institute for Cancer Research, *Food, Nutrition and the Prevention...*

44. World Health Organization, *Obesity: Preventing and Managing...*

45. European Heart Network, *Food, Nutrition and Cardiovascular...*

46. *Programme National de Santé Publique 2003-2012* (Quebec, Canada: Ministère de la Santé et des Services Sociaux du Québec, Gouvernement du Québec, 2008).

47. K. Morland, S. Wing, and A. Diez Roux, "The Contextual Effect of the Local Food Environment on Residents' Diets: The Atherosclerosis Risk in Communities Study," *American Journal of Public Health* 92, no. 11 (2002): 1761–1767.

48. Morland et al., "Neighborhood Characteristics Associated..."

49. S. N. Zenk et al., "Neighborhood Racial Composition, Neighborhood Poverty, and the Spatial Accessibility of Supermarkets in Metropolitan Detroit," *American Journal of Public Health* 95, no. 4 (2005): 660.

50. S. Cummins et al., "Healthy Cities: The Impact of Food Retail-led Regeneration on Food Access, Choice and Retail Structure," *Built Environments* 31, no. 4 (2005): 288–301.

51. Cummins and MacIntyre, "Food Environments and Obesity..."

52. Morland et al., "Neighborhood Characteristics Associated..."

53. A. R. Ness and J. W. Powles, "Fruit and Vegetable and Cardiovascular Disease: A Review," *International Journal of Epidemiology* 21, no. 1 (1997): 1–13.

54. E. B. Rimmi, A. Aschiero, and E. Giovanucci, "Vegetable, Fruit and Cereal Fiber Intake and Risk of Coronary Heart Disease Among Men," *Journal of the American Medical Association* 275, no. 6 (1998): 447–451.

55. B. D. Cox, M. J. Whichelow, and F. T. Prevost, "Seasonal Consumption of Salad Vegetable and Fresh Fruit in Relation to the Development of Cardiovascular Disease and Cancer," *Public Health and Nutrition* 3, no. 1 (2009): 19–29.

56. P. VanVeer, M. C. Jansen, and M. Klerk, "Fruit and Vegetable in the Prevention of Cancer and Cardiovascular Disease," *Public Health and Nutrition* 3, no. 1 (200): 103–107.

57. *Canadian Community Health Survey Cycle 2.2, Nutrition (2004). Nutrient Intakes from Food,* Health Canada and Statistics Canada, accessed May 5, 2013, http://www.hc-sc.gc.ca/fn-an/surveill/nutrition/commun/cchs_guide_escc-eng.php

58. *Programme National de Santé Publique...*

59. H. J. Shaw, "Food Deserts: Towards the Development of a Classification," *Geographic Annals* 88B, no. 2 (2006): 231–247.

60. J. J. Hubert, "À l'écoute des tendances," *L'Alimentation* Janvier-Février (2004): p.4.

61. M. P. Galvez et al., "Race and Foodstore Availability in an Inner-City Neighborhood," *Public Health and Nutrition* 11, no. 6 (2008): 624–631.

62. Franco et al., "Neighborhood Characteristics and Availability..."

63. J. Pearce et al., "A National Study of the Association Between Neighbhourhood Access to Fast-Food Outlets and the Diet and Weight of Local Residents," *Health and Place* 15, no. 1 (2009): 193–7.

64. Cummins and MacIntyre, "Food Environments and Obesity..."

65. *Cadre de Référence pour le Soutien au Développement de la Sécurité Alimentaire dans la Région de Montréal 2008-2012* (Montreal, Canada: Agence de la santé et des services sociaux de Montréal. Direction de santé publique, 2008).

66. Gestion Cléhas, *Étude de Préfaisabilité. Offre d'un Point de Service de Fruits et Légumes Frais. La Table de Concertation pour la Sécurité Alimentaire de Mercier-Ouest* (2008)

67. Ibid.

68. «Des fruits et légumes frais à portée de main». Le Flambeau de l'Est. 23 juillet 2010. accessed May 13, 2013, http://www.flambeaudelest.com/Actualites/2010-07-23/article-1604095/Des-fruits-et-legumes-frais-a-portee-de-main/1

69. «Fête des récoltes dans les projets d'agriculture urbaine» Le Flambeau de l'Est. 24 septembre 2010. accessed May 13, 2013, http://www.flambeaudelest.com/Actualites/Vos-nouvelles/2010-09-24/article-1790773/Fete-des-recoltes-dans-les-projets-d%26rsquo%3Bagriculture-urbaine/1

70. Pouliot and L. Bertrand, *La Santé est-elle...*

71. P. Tarnapol Whitacre, P. Tsai, and J. Mulligan, *The Public Health Effects of Food Deserts: Workshop Summary* (Washington, DC: Institute of Medicine and National Research Council, The National Academies Press, 2009).

72. *The CDC Guide to Fruit and Vegetable. Strategies to Increase Access, Availability and Consumption,* Centers for Disease Control and Prevention, accessed May 5, 2013, http://www.cdph.ca.gov/SiteCollectionDocuments/StratstoIncreaseFruitVegConsumption.pdf

73. G. Laverack and R. Labonté, "A Planning Framework for Community Empowerment Goals within Health Promotion," *Health Policy and Planning* 15, no. 3 (2000): 255–62.

74. B. Ninacs et al., *La Santé des Communautés: Perspectives pour la Contribution de la Santé Publique au Développement Social et au Développement des Communautés, Revue de Littérature* (Institute National de Santé Publique, Montreal, 2002).

75. "Soutenir le Développement des Communautés" and "Soutenir l'Action Intersectorielle Favorable a la Santé et au Bien-Être," in *Programme National de Santé Publique* (Quebec, Canada: Ministère de la Santé et des Services Sociaux, Gouvernement du Québec, 2008), 61–70.

76. M. De Koninck, *Inégalités de Santé et Milieux de Vie* (Carnet synthèse, Réseau de recherche en santé des populations du Québec, Canada, 2007).

77. Ibid.

78. J. Gaudet et al., *Bilan d'Implantation du Programme de Soutien au Développement de la Sécurité Alimentaire dans la Région de Montréal 2008-2011.* (Montreal, Canada: Agence de la Santé et des Services Sociaux de Montréal, 2012).

CHAPTER 11

Water for Development

Investing in Health and Economic Well-Being Globally

WILLIAM COSGROVE AND HÅKAN TROPP

In 1776, in his monumental work *Wealth of Nations,* Adam Smith noted how diamonds are worthless in use yet invaluable in exchange, while the opposite was true for water.[1] This paradox still persists. Water has for too long been treated as a free good that can be wasted by overabstraction and as a recipient of pollutants. Unlike diamonds, water is a basic requirement for human development. It is essential for human health and the survival of the ecosystems upon which people, especially the poor, depend. Water is essential for sustainable economic and social development and is one of the most important inputs for a wide array of economic sectors, including health, food production, industry, energy, and tourism.

The distribution of water and related services and benefits varies greatly between different socioeconomic strata in society and across regions. A slum dweller in a city may only have 5–10 liters of water at her disposal per day, while a middle-class person in the same city may use 100–200 liters per day.[2] Many countries, particularly in low-income regions, face both physically and socially related water challenges,[3] limiting economic activity and leaving people with inadequate drinking water and vulnerable to poor sanitation. In some cases, even if fresh water is naturally available, without adequate infrastructure and management, this water may not reach a significant percentage of the population. In 2001, 189 nations of the United Nations General Assembly committed to achieving the Millennium Development Goals (MDGs), and through them to reduce the proportion of those living in absolute poverty by half by 2015. Recognizing the central role played by water in connection with poverty, the MDGs committed to halving the proportion of people without access to clean water and basic sanitation by 2015.

This chapter looks at how increased investments in water can make major contributions to human health and economic and social development, and promote greater socioeconomic equity with a focus on the economic benefits and costs of increasing access to water and sanitation services and improving water resource management. Increased investments in water are instrumental to realizing a wide range of development benefits. Improved water and sanitation will keep people, the poor in particular, more healthy and productive. More sustainable water resources management will have positive impacts on ecosystem services and can also lead to better water productivity in agriculture and industry.

Conventional wisdom holds that countries need considerable economic growth before they can start to invest in improved water resources management and water supply and sanitation services. But the relation between development and investment is much more dynamic than suggested by conventional knowledge. Increased investment priority to improved water resources management and water services provides economic and social boosts to development. In other words, the absence of improved water resources management and water services puts limitations on development, since large segments of the population find it increasingly difficult to live healthy and productive lives without access to clean water. Moreover, without proper water stewardship it will become increasingly difficult to meet increased water demands for production of food, industrial goods, and biofuels, as well as to maintain the ecosystems on which all of these activities depend. Looming climate change impacts on rainfall and other weather patterns and on water demand make the challenge for increased water investments even more urgent.

CURRENT STATE OF WATER RESOURCES AND EQUITY

Globally, over 1 billion people lack access to a reliable source of safe drinking water, while 2.4 billion people have no access to hygienic sanitation facilities and 1.2 billion people lack any sanitation facility at all. Each day, on average 5,000 children die due to preventable water- and sanitation-related diseases. Figure 11.1 presents the progress in sanitation and whether countries are on track to meet the MDG of halving the number of people without basic sanitation by 2015. Overall many countries will miss the target and at the current rate of improvement the MDG on sanitation will be missed by 1 billion people.[4] Many of the most off-track countries are found in sub-Saharan Africa and South Asia.

Countries are doing slightly better on the target related to water supply, but here also many sub-Saharan African countries are off track. Many developing countries are facing increasingly severe shortages of water resources and services. In 2007, one-third of the world population was estimated to be suffering from physical or economic water stress.[5] Climate change will make this worse. According to projections, the number of people at risk from

Sanitation: most countries in Sub-Saharan Africa and in Asia are not on track to meet the MDG target

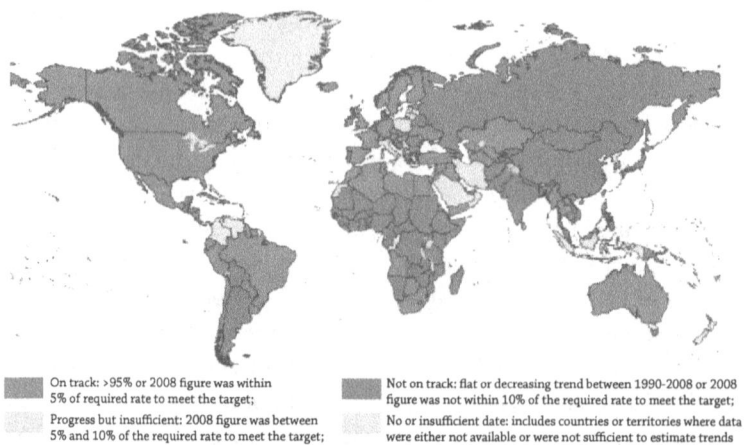

On track: >95% or 2008 figure was within 5% of required rate to meet the target;

Progress but insufficient: 2008 figure was between 5% and 10% of the required rate to meet the target;

Not on track: flat or decreasing trend between 1990-2008 or 2008 figure was not within 10% of the required rate to meet the target;

No or insufficient date: includes countries or territories where data were either not available or were not sufficient to estimate trends

Figure 11.1:
Sanitation: Most countries in sub-Saharan Africa and Asia are not on track to meet the Millenium Development Goal target on sanitation by 2015. (From: WHO and UNICEF Joint Monitoring Programme. 2010. *Progress on Sanitation and Drinking-water: 2010 Update*, WHO and UNICEF, Paris.)

physical water stress will be between 0.4 billion and 1.7 billion by the 2020s, between 1.0 billion and 2.0 billion by the 2050s, and between 1.1 billion and 3.2 billion by the 2080s.[6] Water stress is considered severe when the ratio of total water use to renewable water supply exceeds 40 percent.[7] Using this measure, it is estimated that by 2030 close to half the world's population, or 3.9 billion people, will be living under conditions of severe water stress under the assumption of a business-as-usual scenario.[8]

Figure 11.2 shows that the majority of people living in water-stressed areas are found in the so called BRIC-countries,[9] especially India and China, and in other countries outside of the Organisation for Economic Cooperation and Development (OECD). The category Rest of the World (ROW) contains a large portion of least developed countries, economies in transition, and emerging economies. Growing water stress will be particularly felt in those countries that cannot afford or decide to downplay required investments in water (economic stress). Moreover, the stress on water use that is an effect of population growth will mainly affect countries that are already impoverished.

Similarly, poor countries will also have a much harder time coping with climate change impacts such as increased rainfall variability, which exacerbate the problems of water shortages.[10] Consider, for example, the Netherlands and Bangladesh, two low-lying countries close to the sea where agriculture plays important economic roles. The Netherlands invested heavily in infrastructure to keep seawater at bay to prevent flooding and have been working with integrated water decision-making approaches for more than 30 years. They

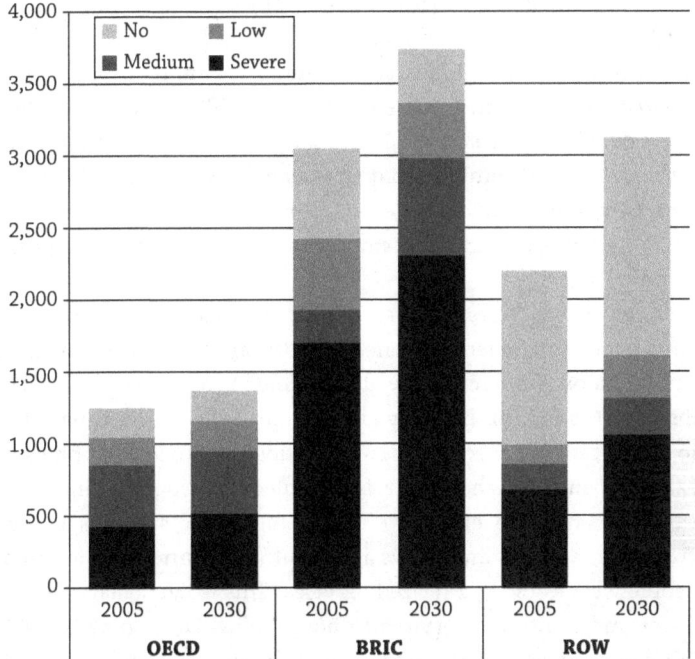

Projections, by stress level (in millions)

Legend:
- No
- Low
- Medium
- Severe

Y-axis: 0 to 4,000 (in increments of 500)

X-axis: 2005, 2030 (OECD); 2005, 2030 (BRIC); 2005, 2030 (ROW)

Figure 11.2:
Water stress projections. (From OECD, *Managing Water for All: An OECD Perspective on Pricing and Financing* [Paris: OECD, 2009].)

continue to invest significantly in planning and management as well as infra-structure to withstand potential sealevel rise over the next 70–100 years.[11] Bangladesh, with a gross domestic product (GDP) per capita in 2009 of 87 times less than the Netherlands, can hardly afford to make similar types of investments, although they are much needed.[12] Consequently, many farmers in Bangladesh live with very high risks of flooding which prevent them from long-term investments in increased agricultural productivity.

The gap between available and demanded water is expected to be particularly significant for China and India. While all sectors are demanding more water, the industrial sector in China is expected to make up the lion's share of new domes-tic water demands over the next 20 years. Other regions are also expected to experience increased demand. Water demand in sub-Saharan Africa agriculture is expected to increase close to three times compared to today's levels.[13]

Dwindling water resources availability and increasing water demands are driven by a number of factors:

- *Low investments in water.* In the water sector of developing countries there has been chronic underinvestment in infrastructure and the development of human and institutional capacity. In sub-Saharan Africa the median government spending for water and sanitation is 0.48 percent of GDP.[14] In contrast, the OECD has estimated that for low-income countries the government spending should be around 6 percent of GDP, since there is a need to make up for previous investment deficits in the sector. The levels of expenditure on water services for high-income countries that already have water and sanitation infrastructure should on average be approximately 0.75 percent of GDP (ranging between 0.35 percent and 1.2 percent depending on OECD country).[15]

- *Poor governance.* Water is often used in inefficient and unplanned ways. The water use efficiency in the agricultural sector, which globally consumes almost 70 percent of water, is only in the range of 30–40 percent for many countries. In many cities around the world some 40 percent to 50 percent of piped water supply is lost due to leaking pipes.[16] These examples indicate that there is considerable scope for improving the existing water use efficiency. Increasing water stress is many times grounded in governance flaws and insufficient infrastructure to provide people with water and related services. This is particularly the case for water and sanitation services to households. Only some 5–10 percent of total available water is used by households, and in most cases the lack of water and sanitation is not due to lack of water per se but lack of increased and sustained investment in governance, management systems, and infrastructure development.[17] In addition, discretionary decision making and corruption are rampant in many countries, leading to misappropriation and misuse of water as well, which can drive up prices and siphon off public water budgets.

- *Growing populations and economies, and increasing living standards.* By 2030 the world's population will have increased by 2.4 billion people.[18] All of these people can be expected to demand access to water for basic human consumption, as well as water for agriculture, energy, and industry to produce food and other goods. As countries develop, people tend to consume more water- and energy-intensive products, such as meat, as compared to grains. The rise in the consumption of meat, milk, and eggs in fast-growing developing countries has no precedent. Annual growth in world grain consumption increased from an average of 21 million tons per year from 1990 to 2005 to 41 million tons per year from 2005 to 2010.[19] There are now about 3 billion people eating greater quantities of grain-intensive livestock and poultry products than in earlier decades.

- *Climate change impacts.* It is evident that the impacts of climate change will seriously affect the availability and quality of water resources. Climate change is expected to seriously increase rainfall variability, which can lead to dramatic changes in water availability and increase intensity and frequency of extreme events, such as floods and droughts. Moreover, it can lead to significant changes in viability of agriculture and other economic sectors as well as having negative health impacts. For example, in South Asia, agricultural yield is expected to decline and child malnutrition is expected to increase by 20 percent due to climate change.[20] Extreme climatic events will take a toll on economic growth, and in many low-income countries poor people—many times already living in drought- or flood-prone areas—will be hardest hit. For example, Malawi loses 1.7 percent of its GDP on average every year due to the combined effects of droughts and floods. It is smaller scale farmers and those in the flood-prone southern regions of Malawi who are worst affected.[21] Floods and droughts often lead to loss of life, homes, infrastructure, and basic services such as water and health care. In addition, floods also heighten the risk of waterborne diseases, and create breeding grounds for disease-carrying insects such as mosquitoes, causing increased incidents of malaria.[22]

- *Overexploitation and pollution of water resources.* The combination of poor governance, growing populations, and expanding economies drives an ever-increasing demand for and exploitation of water. In many river basins and lakes around the world, water resource uses are already over-committed. For example, 15 percent of India's total agricultural production is done through groundwater depletion.[23] In addition, an increasing proportion of water sources are becoming polluted, sometimes in irreversible ways. For example, increasing levels of pollutions are widespread in China. Many of its major rivers are seriously polluted, which will have significant consequences for people's health as well as ecosystems. The total cost of air and water pollution in China in 2003 alone was estimated at 5.78 percent of the GDP.[24]

IMPORTANCE OF WATER FOR DEVELOPMENT

Social and economic development relies on the availability of water resources and people being able to access water services in efficient and equitable ways. The costs of inadequate sanitation and water supply, through increased health costs, lost working and education days, and loss of productivity will be greatest in some of the poorest countries. Sub-Saharan Africa loses 5 percent of GDP or some US$28.4 billion annually due to inadequate water and sanitation, exceeding the total aid flows and debt relief to the region in 2003.[25] Gains from improved water supply, sanitation, and water resources management benefit poor people most since they are typically those that are most affected by low-quality water and sanitation services.

Human Health

The lack of access to safe water, basic sanitation, and good hygiene practices is a significant risk factor to poor health in developing countries. In 1997 it was reported that waterborne illnesses or "dirty-water" diseases—those caused by water that has been contaminated by human, animal, or chemical wastes, are to blame for over 12 million deaths a year.[26] According to the World Health Organization (WHO), more than 1.6 million children die each year due to lack of sanitation and access to safe and clean water, and half of the hospital patients in the developing world are suffering from sanitation- and water-related diseases.[27] Approximately 1.8 million people die every year from diarrheal diseases, of which almost 90 percent are children under the age of 5 years.[28] About 133 million people annually suffer from high-intensity intestinal worm diseases that are linked to poor sanitation, including ascariasis, trichuriasis, and hookworm disease, which often lead to severe consequences such as cognitive impairment, massive dysentery, or anemia.[29]

Malaria is a risk for 50 percent of the world's population. In 2008, it was estimated that there were 243 million cases, leading to 863,000 deaths, 89 percent of which were in Africa.[30] The poorest children are still less likely to receive antimalarial medicines and to have access to insecticidal nets. The underlying cause of malaria is failure to drain stagnant water, which is the breeding ground for mosquitoes.

In Africa and Asia especially, development efforts of all kinds are being undermined by the rapid spread of HIV and AIDS. The problem is so serious in parts of sub-Saharan Africa that life expectancy of a person born between 1995 and 2000 is as low as 49 years. Without the effects of AIDS, the figure would be 62 years. HIV/AIDS increases an individual's susceptibility to diseases related to water, sanitation, and hygiene. Once infected, the person is also much more likely to die from these diseases. Health care services in poor countries are increasingly finding their limited facilities and resources overwhelmed by the volume of patients. This has led to an increasing trend toward home-based care, which brings new urgency to the need for adequate water and sanitation facilities in homes.

The evidence is overwhelming that improved water supply and sanitation facilities and better hygiene behavior radically improve people's health (see Table 11.1). As just one example, improved water supply can reduce diarrhea by up to 25 percent. Hygiene interventions, including hygiene education and the promotion of hand washing, can reduce the number of diarrhea cases by up to 37 percent, and sanitation interventions can reduce diarrhea by 32 percent. Additional improvements to household drinking water quality, such as point-of-use water treatment, can reduce diarrhea episodes by 31 percent.[31]

Table 11.1. IMPACTS ON DIARRHEAL DISEASE REDUCTION BY TYPE OF INTERVENTION

Type of Intervention	Reduction in Diarrhea Frequency (%)
Hugiene	37
Sanitation	32
Water supply	25
Water quality	31
Multiple	33

Source: A. Prüss-Üstün, R. Bos, F. Gore, and J. Bartram, *Safer Water, Better Health: Costs, Benefits and Sustainability of Interventions to Protect and Promote Health* (Geneva: World Health Organization, 2008).

A Cost–Benefit Approach to Improved Water Services

To bridge the world's water resources gap between water supply and demand by 2030 requires massive investment. According to one estimate, if only supply measures are considered, it will require annual investments of US$200 billion, but if a more balanced supply and demand approach is used, it will require investments around US$50–60 billion per year.[32]

One of the most recent cost estimates suggests that required annual spending in developing countries on new coverage to meet the MDG targets for sanitation and drinking water is US$14.2 billion for sanitation and US$4.2 billion for drinking water. New capital investment needs for sanitation are higher than for drinking water because of the larger number of people without access to improved sanitation, and because of the higher estimated cost per capita for sanitation interventions for both piped and nonpiped options. In addition, the cost of maintaining existing services was estimated at a further US$21.6 billion annually for sanitation and US$32.2 billion annually for drinking water.[33] This example only includes investment requirements to meet the MDGs on drinking water supply and sanitation, and it does not take into account investment requirements for universal water and sanitation coverage. Moreover, it neglects the direct and indirect cost of governance inefficiencies, such as corruption and mismanagement, suggesting that required investments may be much higher.

While the resources required for adequate water management are considerable, the benefits far outweigh investments. Meeting the MDG target implies an annual health sector cost saving of US$7 billion globally. An additional US$340 million is saved annually due to avoidance of costs of drugs, treatment, and time lost. Meeting the MDG target for safe water supply and sanitation would gain 322 million working days per year and bring about economic yields of close to US$12 billion a year from productivity gains from income earned by those saved from premature death, gains in health care services in treating fewer patients, and the direct costs to patients of medication and transportation.[34] More benefits will come from illness avoided and days lost in terms of formal or informal employment, productive activities in the household and/or school attendance. Potential improvements to school attendance reach a staggering 270 million days and imply enormous long-term benefits for economic development. The WHO estimates that the overall economic benefits of halving the proportion of people without sustainable access to safe drinking water and sanitation by 2015 would outweigh the investment cost by a ratio of 8:1.[35]

WHO cost estimates are the most sophisticated currently available, as they take into account existing levels of service and incremental improvements. Their evaluation estimates the costs and benefits of a range of interventions to achieve the MDG target, from using basic technologies to providing universal access to in-house piped water and sewer connections. The costs of providing access to safe water and adequate sanitation will vary from relatively expensive when high standards are applied and sophisticated technology used, to substantially less expensive when simple technology that demands low maintenance is used. Costs of water improvement vary from US$0.33 per person served per year in Africa for household water treatment using chlorine, to US$12.75 for household water connection, including both hardware and software components. For sanitation the costs range from a cheap small pit latrine at US$4.88 per year per person served to a more expensive option with household sewer connection and partial treatment of wastewaters at US$10.03.[36]

Similarly, a World Bank review examining how much it would cost to avoid 1 year of healthy life lost provides empirical evidence of the effectiveness of simple measures that bring substantial health improvements and prevent the loss of DALYs.[37] For various interventions, the review estimated the following costs per DALY saved:

- Hygiene behavior change: US$20 per DALY saved
- Water connections in rural areas: US$35 per DALY saved
- Malaria control: US$35–70 per DALY saved
- Improving indoor air quality with better stoves: US$50–100 per DALY saved

The benefits of preventive action provide another way to consider the immediate economic impacts of water supply and sanitation. Consider the cholera epidemic that swept Peru in 1991 and cost US$1 billion to treat. It is estimated that US$100 million, or a tenth of what was actually spent treating the disease, could have prevented the epidemic. In such circumstances the cost–benefit ratio of preventative investments in water and sanitation is very high.[38]

Improving health through investments in water supply and sanitation services has several immediate benefits for the economy, but it also delivers important long-term economic growth benefits. Human capital theory and endogenous growth theory suggest that there are substantial economic benefits for education. A person without basic literacy and numeracy skills is not able to participate as effectively in political processes and higher levels of societal organization. Investing in water management and services provides people with the chance to spend more time in school, and to do so more effectively. With less time ill and less time spent fetching water, women and girls in particular are able to devote more time to learning. Furthermore, better health strengthens cognitive ability.[39]

Some of the aggregate gains that can be made in the area of sanitation are presented in Box 11.1. Due to insufficient sanitation alone, Cambodia, Indonesia, the Philippines, and Vietnam lose 1.3–7.2 percent of their GDP annually (see Box 11.1).

The biggest potential gain for increased productivity and production within both households and economic sectors amounts to US$64 billion per year globally. For example, the relocation of a well or borehole to a site closer to user communities, the installation of piped water supply to households, and closer access to latrines can save each individual many hours each day, translating into increased economic production and higher school attendance rates.

As seen in Table 11.2, achieving the MDG target for both water supply and sanitation would bring substantial economic benefits. The economic benefits would be greater in regions where the number of those without access is high and where the diarrheal disease burden is significant. The total global economic benefits of reaching MDG targets for water supply and sanitation accrue to more than US$84 billion, with an estimated cost of US$11 billion with each US$1 invested on average bringing an economic return of US$8.

Box 11.1: ECONOMIC IMPACTS OF POOR SANITATION

Cambodia, Indonesia, the Philippines, and Vietnam lose an estimated US$9 billion a year because of poor sanitation (based on 2005 prices). That is approximately 2 percent of their combined gross domestic product, varying from 1.3 percent in Vietnam, 1.5 percent in the Philippines, 2.3 percent in Indonesia, and 7.2 percent in Cambodia. The annual economic impact is approximately US$6.3 billion in Indonesia, US$1.4 billion in the Philippines, US$780 million in Vietnam, and US$450 million in Cambodia. The universal implementation of improved sanitation and hygiene would mitigate these impacts, including 45 percent of the losses attributed to health. This would lead to an annual gain of US$6.3 billion in the four countries.

Source: World Bank—Water and Sanitation Program. Economic Impacts of Sanitation in Southeast Asia. Jakarta. (2008).

Access for all could translate into US$263 billion in economic benefits with annualized costs of only roughly US$26 billion.

Choosing more advanced types of technologies such as provision of regulated in-house piped water and sewer connections would lead to large overall gains, including an average global reduction of diarrheal episodes of around 70 percent, but this type of intervention is also the most expensive.[40] Implementing universal access to in-house piped water and sewer connection would cost more than US$130 billion annually. Though clearly more expensive, such infrastructure is still estimated to provide a cost–benefit ratio of US$4 (see Table 11.2).

Many studies confirm these considerable economic benefits. The OECD has prepared a cost–benefit analysis looking specifically at what is needed in order to meet the MDG sanitation target alone. The analysis provides figures in terms of the net present value (NPV).[41] With a discount rate of 5 percent and 10 percent, the NPV of meeting the MDG sanitation target is US$400 and US$412 billion, respectively. The results confirm again that the benefits of investment in water and sanitation far outweigh the costs.[42]

Social Development

Water and sanitation also have an impact on key development areas such as child development, gender equity, and education. Before they reach school age,

Table 11.2. BENEFIT–COST RATIO OF WATER AND SANITATION COVERAGE SCENARIOS IN DEVELOPING COUNTRIES AND EURASIA

Water and Sanitation Coverage Scenario	Annual Benefits in US$ millions	Benefit–Cost Ratio by Intervention
Halving the proportion of people without access to improved water sources by 2015	18,143	9
Halving the proportion of people without access to improved water sources and improved sanitation by 2015	84,400	8
Universal access to improved water and sanitation services by 2015	262,879	10
Universal access to improved water and improved sanitation and water disinfected at the point of use by 2015	344,106	12
Universal access to a regulated piped water supply and sewage connection by 2015	555,901	4

Source: A. Prüss-Üstün, R. Bos, F. Gore, and J. Bartram, *Safer Water, Better Health: Costs, Benefits and Sustainability of Interventions to Protect and Promote Health* (Geneva: World Health Organization, 2008).

infants and young children suffer the consequences of lack of access to safe drinking water and basic sanitation services. Children under 5 years of age in particular are exposed to a multitude of health threats, while their families lack the physical or economic means to combat them. Malnutrition—particularly protein-energy malnutrition—stunts growth, impairs cognitive development, and, crucially, lowers children's resistance to a wide range of infections. The eye infection trachoma, which can lead to severe visual impairment and blindness, also spreads more rapidly when there is lack of safe water and good hygiene.

In rural areas in sub-Saharan Africa, girls and women can spend several hours per day collecting water. People also spend considerable time queuing for public toilets or finding a safe place to defecate. This is productive time lost—time that could be spent on a wide range of more productive activities such as child care and food harvesting. For mothers and daughters who are mainly responsible for fetching the water that their families need for drinking, bathing, cooking, and other household uses, the penalties of inadequate water and sanitation services are much more severe. The burden borne by women of hauling water from distant sources is often shared by their young daughters, leaving girls with neither the time nor the energy for schooling. Women also face the challenge of maintaining basic household hygiene and keeping their own and their infants' hands and bodies clean, without contaminating the stored water they need for drinking and cooking. Sick children consume a considerable part of their time, which otherwise could be used for other crucial activities. Pregnant women require access to enough water of good quality to protect them from serious diseases such as hepatitis. When women are living with HIV/AIDS, their suffering has a double impact on their families' water supply. Not only may they face increasing difficulty to fetch and carry water or fulfil their roles as home carers, but their daughters, who would normally share the water-hauling burden, have to bear the entire load while tending to their sick parents.

Improving access to safe water and sanitation has been shown to improve education outcomes; piped water supplies allow girls to attend school instead of fetching water, and sanitation services encourage higher female enrollment and improve the working environment for female teachers. In addition, new data suggest that levels of infectious diseases may directly affect cognitive ability.[43]

ECONOMIC GROWTH AND POVERTY REDUCTION

Water is critical for a number of economic activities such as agriculture, energy, industry, and tourism. As demonstrated earlier, investing in improved water and sanitation has high cost–benefit ratios. In addition, there is a strong correlation between increased national income and the proportion of population with access to improved water supply. As an illustration, the poorest countries with per capita annual income below US$750 in purchasing power parity

(PPP)-adjusted 1990 currency that enjoyed annual average growth of 3.7 percent had improved access to clean water and sanitation services. Similarly, poor countries (i.e., with the same per capita income) without improved access had average annual per capita GDP growth of only 0.1 percent.[44] The interaction between improved water resources management and services and economic growth is mutually reinforcing and has the potential to start a virtuous cycle that improves the lives of poor people. A 0.3 percent increase in investment in household access to safe water is associated with a 1 percent increase in GDP.[45] Economic growth itself can also drive increased investments in improved water management and services. As recently acknowledged by the UN Environment Programme (UNEP) Green Economy Report: "early investment in water is a necessary precondition to progress."[46] At the household level this will imply significant new livelihood opportunities, especially for poor people.

Cycles of floods and droughts can cause reduction of the annual GDP of a country by 14 percent in countries with per capita GDP of less than $2.00 PPP adjusted.[47] Two recent examples illustrate this. In 2010, a heat wave and associated drought and fire in Russia caused the loss of standing forests with an economic value of $300 billion and a reduction in grain harvested from 100 million to 60 million tons. In Pakistan, torrential rains in northern Pakistan resulted in floods that damaged or destroyed 2 million homes, displaced 20 million people, damaged or destroyed 2.5 million hectares of cropland, and drowned over 1 million livestock.[48] Reduction of an economy's dependence on rainfall variability promotes gains in GDP. In Kenya, the 1997–1998 floods and the 1999–2000 droughts provide examples. The floods cost the country at least US$870 million, or 11 percent of GDP; the drought, at least US$1.4 billion a year, or 16 percent of GDP. On average the country experiences a flood that costs 5.5 percent of GDP every 7 years and a drought that costs it about 8 percent of GDP every 5 years. This translates to a direct long-term fiscal liability of about 2.4 percent GDP per annum. This means that Kenya's GDP annually should grow at a rate of at least 5–6 percent in order to start reducing poverty if no changes are made to manage rainfall variability. In 1996, a good year in Kenya, real GDP growth was 4.1 percent.[49] Climate change will have significant impact on rainfall variability and intensity. The effects of climate change will require economic safeguards for poor people and the development of a capacity to adapt for climate change as they are the most vulnerable and also those least able to pay for safeguards, such as insurance systems for lost yields. One conclusion from the Stern Report (2007) is that if a business-as-usual approach persists, the effects of climate change can equal to a 5 percent annual reduction of global GDP. The costs of taking immediate action to avoid worst-case scenarios can be limited to 1 percent of global GDP on an annual basis. The Intergovernmental Panel on Climate Change states that "water and its availability and quality will be the main pressures on, and issues for, societies and the environment under climate change."[50]

Agriculture and food production are by far the largest users of water, particularly in developing countries.[51] Increases in the demand for food over the next 25 years will be met mainly by increasing the yield from land already under cultivation. Irrigated land currently produces 40 percent of the world's food on 17 percent of the world's agricultural land.[52] Investments to expand and improve the efficiency of irrigation and rain-fed agriculture, including water storage, water distribution, drainage, and management, will be necessary to meet the world's growing demand for food. It will be key for many developing countries to become less dependent on rainfall variability. In addition, threats to the availability of water for agriculture will make it impossible for many countries to produce enough food to feed their population, in some cases even with significant changes in water management. In the past 40 years the low cost of mechanized pumping, which is often subsidized, has led increasingly to over-pumping water from aquifers to provide water for irrigation. As rapidly growing cities and industry claim more water, they compete with the same sources that are already being used for agriculture. Melting of glaciers endangers the sustainability of flows in rivers in plains adjacent to the mountains that provide water during periods of low precipitation. Physical scarcity of water already exists in Northern Africa and the Middle East,[53] and economic water scarcity[54] in much of sub-Saharan Africa, South Asia, and parts of South America. Reduced production because of water scarcity will cause even greater price increases and volatility.

For the majority of people living in low-income countries, agriculture is the most important sector in terms of employment but lags in terms of productivity, contributing only 23 percent to GDP.[55] Any poverty reduction investment strategy must therefore consider food production together with water management if it is to be effective. Reducing the strain on water systems will require matching what is farmed to what water resources can provide on a sustainable basis.

Poor people's self-employment and wage employment opportunities in urban and especially rural areas depend on water. The dependence on water is most evident for smallholders, in many countries the largest group of poor people. As the land resources of poor smallholders are typically scarce, a major income-generating strategy is to improve the agricultural output of their holdings through intensification. Among the many factors that enable intensification, increasing water productivity is crucial. Water in the form of year-round irrigation, supplementary irrigation, and water harvested and conserved with a range of water management techniques improves yields, allows for better-yielding varieties, enables continuing production during the otherwise slack season, and, last but not least, reduces risks due to erratic rainfall. Harvests used for household consumption and sale directly contribute to food security and fulfillment of monetary needs.[56]

Water is also indispensable for other rural income sources for both smallholders and landless people, such as raising livestock. Trees and shrubs for fuel wood, timber, fruits, and medications need water. Catching fish for family consumption can provide a major source of protein for poor households and provides incomes for small artisan fishermen and -women. Water is also needed for various small industries and crafts, like brick making, pottery, or beer making. Given the multiple and increasing demands on water, and its important role in poverty alleviation, global action is needed not only to ensure that water is available for drinking and sanitation but for all of the economic activities on which the poor depend.

POLICY APPROACHES FOR WATER EQUITY

Need for Global Action

The preceding analysis has shown that sustainable economic and social development depends on the availability of water resources and their good management. While there is scope for improved management almost everywhere, there are basins and countries where even with optimum resource management there will not be enough water to meet all of the needs of the inhabitants.[57] In situations where this happens, the poor are once again those who are likely to be affected most.

Water is a global resource that is distributed according to global climatic and hydrological patterns. Its distribution may vary, but it is part of a global cycle. This cycle can be interrupted by human interventions at multiple levels. For example, the impacts of climate change on a water resource may have regional and global, or direct and indirect sources that are far removed.

Water usage on a national level cannot be isolated from global drivers such as the demand for agricultural produce and other water-intensive products through trade. The global dimensions of water are also closely related to global equity—only 3 percent of the planet's water is fresh water and it is a finite resource. Nevertheless, there is enough accessible water on the planet to meet the needs of the global population if access to the benefits of water is treated as a global issue. Greater recognition of the fact that water is not solely a local or regional issue that can be governed at the basin level alone is essential.

International boundaries fail to divide water resources neatly. Almost 40 percent of the world's people live in river basins shared by more than two countries. This represents almost half the world's land (excluding Antarctica), and 60 percent of the world's fresh water. In addition, about 2 billion people worldwide depend on groundwater supplies, which include approximately 300 transboundary aquifer systems.[58] The unavoidable reality that water resources do not respect political boundaries demonstrates the supranational dimensions of water and represents a compelling case for international cooperation on water management. Our international interdependencies are woven through water, and the decisions relating to water use on a national level cannot be isolated from global drivers and trends. In fact, billions of tons of water every year are exported and imported according to countries' needs and tastes.[59] A range of water-scarce countries have become net importers of water due to their inability to meet the food needs of their populations without importing water through agricultural commodities. Other countries are importers of food due to the consumer tastes and demands of their populations for particular foodstuffs and products that cannot be produced domestically. As a result of importing agricultural products, Japan consumes 4.5 times the water it uses for its own production, and Algeria twice as much as it uses within the country. The virtual water imported by China represents only 9 percent of the amount of water used for domestic agriculture, but because of its large population even small increases in this number would have significant effects on the world market for agricultural produce.[60] Income, food, energy, and human and environmental health all depend on water. Yet these multiple sectors have been managed in silos rather than as part of an overarching and strategic framework across society and the economy. This can ultimately lead to short-term and unsustainable decision making and increase the number of people with water shortages. Climate change exacerbates this problem further.[61] Modern economic thinking and policy making have created an economy that is so out of synch with the ecosystem on which it depends that it is approaching collapse.[62]

Changing this situation will require a water governance framework under which water is managed as a natural resource across sectors and regions, locally and globally, through representative institutions that have the appropriate authority.

The international water community has recognized the need for globally coordinated action, as demonstrated by numerous actions: the Mar del Plata Declaration (1977); the Drinking Water and Sanitation Decade of the 1980s; and the Dublin Principles and Chapter 18 of Agenda 21 from the Earth Summit (1992). However, it has also become clear that greater effort is needed to raise awareness and support among all stakeholders. As one institutional response, the World Water Council was created to promote local and global actions among all stakeholders in order to spread the benefits of water. Another response was the formation of the Global Water Partnership (GWP) to promote the concept of integrated water resources management.

Increasing pressures on transboundary waters require significant effort to either renegotiate existing but inadequate transboundary water management arrangements or to establish new ones where they do not yet exist. According to UN Water, 158 of the world's 263 international river basins lack any type of cooperative management framework.[63] While there is no functioning international convention that regulates international waters, the UN Convention on the Law of the Non-navigational Uses of International Watercourses adopted in 1997 established principles that can still be used as helpful guidelines.

Similarly, in Europe, the UN Economic Commission for Europe Convention on the Protection and Use of Trans-boundary Watercourses and International Lakes has also been used as the basis for adoption of many bilateral and multilateral agreements in other parts of the world.

Together with UNEP and UNDP, GWP undertook a global assessment of integrated water resources management across the world, which was launched in 2012 at the UN Conference on Sustainable Development, commonly referred to as Rio+20. Rio+20 has provided an opportunity to address the need for global institutions and measures to ensure the benefits of water to all. Among issues discussed were the special needs of the least developed countries, especially those that are water poor. The results could provide input to negotiations in the Doha Round of the World Trade Organization. Important measures in moving forward include tariff- and quota-free access for least developed countries' exports that require less water for their production and targeting more generous development assistance and grant funding for water infrastructure for countries committed to poverty reduction.

By paying particular attention to special interest groups, Rio+20 also offered an opportunity to advance discussions on processes at national and regional levels for governing water, and how expertise might be shared in this area to move toward improved water management in all respective countries and regions. A successful example of the success of such an approach is provided by the Montreal Protocol on Substances That Dilute the Ozone Layer.[64]

Setting an Economic Value on Environmental Services

Water, and how it is managed, contributes to the production and consumption of ecosystem services and goods. Ecosystems, including lakes, rivers, forests, and wetlands, generate vast and important economic benefits.[65] Yet there are rarely any assessments made of the value of wider ecosystem services beyond the ability to produce raw materials. This applies not only to the high-profile issues surrounding carbon sequestration and storage but also issues such as, soil erosion control, water purification, maintenance of genetic diversity for crops and medicines, and air pollution control. The reality is that ecosystem services have high economic value, as shown in Figure 11.3. If additional dimensions of ecosystem services, such as their role in regulating climate, minimizing disease, waste management, and recreation, are ignored, decision makers only hear one part of the story.

The economic costs of environmental degradation have been estimated at 4 percent to 8 percent of GDP in many developing countries.[66] How this can play out in a particular locality in a developing country is illustrated by the case of the Waza Logone Floodplain in Cameroon. The decision to build an irrigation system upstream of the floodplain resulted in loss of the annual floods, with devastating ecological and socioeconomic results. In this area the effects of flood loss were significant, incurring livelihood costs of close to $50 million

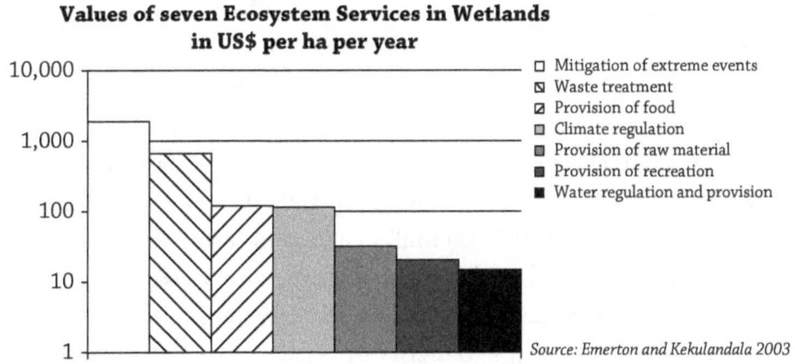

Values of seven Ecosystem Services in Wetlands in US$ per ha per year

Legend:
- □ Mitigation of extreme events
- ◪ Waste treatment
- ▨ Provision of food
- ◻ Climate regulation
- ▦ Provision of raw material
- ■ Provision of recreation
- ■ Water regulation and provision

Source: Emerton and Kekulandala 2003

Figure 11.3:
Values of seven ecosystem services in the wetlands, Muthurajawela Marsh, Sri Lanka, in USD/ha per year. (From L. Emerton and L. D. Kekulandala, *Assessment of the Economic Value of Muthurajawela Wetland* (occasional papers of IUCN, No. 4, Colombo, Sri Lanka, 2004).)

over the last two decades. Up to 8,000 households suffered direct economic losses totaling more than US$2 million per year through reduction in dry season grazing, fishing, natural resource harvesting, and surface water supplies. The affected population, mainly pastoralists, fisherfolk, and dryland farmers, represent some of the poorest and most vulnerable groups in the area. The economic value of floodplain restoration would be immense. The return of waters to these areas has the potential to restore up to 90 percent of the floodplain area, at a capital cost of approximately US$10 million. It could add more than $2.5 million a year to the regional economy, or US$3,000 per km² of flooded area, recovering the initial investment costs in less than 5 years. Ecological and hydrological restoration will also have significant impacts on local poverty alleviation, food security, and financial well-being. Releases of floodwater will rehabilitate vital pasture, fisheries, and farmland areas used by nearly a third of the population, to a value of almost US$250 per capita. The importance of ecosystem services has similarly been recognized in Vientiane, the capital of Lao, where wetlands offer flood control and wastewater treatment services valued at US$2 million per year. It has been estimated that these ecosystem services constitute investment savings of more than US$18 million in damage costs avoided and US$1.5 million in the artificial technologies that would be required to fulfill the same functions.[67]

A study of Muthurajawela Marsh, a coastal wetland in a densely populated area in North Sri Lanka, is another example of the value of ecosystem services. The economic significance of conserving the wetland, which is under increasing pressure from industrial and urban development, was estimated using both direct and indirect benefits.[68] Several direct services (agriculture, fishing, and firewood) contribute to local incomes (total value US$150 per hectare per year), but the most substantial indirect benefits, which accrue to a wider group of the population and to several economic actors, are related to flood relief (US$1,907 per hectare) and industrial and domestic wastewater treatment (US$654 per hectare). The value of carbon sequestration, in this case as in most existing valuation studies, was estimated using conservative assumptions (a damage cost of US$10 per tonne of carbon).[69] In sum, while fewer than 5,000 people live directly on the marsh, it benefits over 30,000 people and plays an important role in poverty alleviation. Similar ecosystem values have been estimated at the country level as well. For example, in Uganda, the use of inland water resources is worth almost US$300 million a year in terms of forest catchment protection, erosion control, and water purification services. Almost 1 million urban dwellers rely on natural wetlands for wastewater purification services.[70]

Recognition of the multiple benefits of ecosystem services is resulting in innovative systems to pay for environmental services in several countries. For example, in New York City, drinking water supply is obtained from watersheds in the Catskill Mountains north of the city. Water quality was traditionally very good, with little or no treatment required for its use. By the end of the 1980s, however, agricultural and other developments in the Catskills threatened the water quality. In response, New York City planners chose to work with upstream land owners in the Catskill watersheds to eliminate water quality problems, instead of constructing a water treatment system. The resultant plan included payments for both on-farm capital costs and pollution-reducing agricultural measures. The implementation cost is estimated to be only 20 percent of the water treatment system approach, with the payments to water providers coming directly from the revenues collected from water users in New York City. This approach protected the watersheds and the other environmental goods and services they provide, including recreation and biodiversity conservation. Similar approaches are being used in other places. In Heredia, Costa Rica, a system to pay for environmental services was established that taxed the connected water users in order to pay farmers in the watershed to undertake improved conservation measures. In Tana River Basin, Kenya, green water credits, which involve a payment and reward mechanism for upstream land and water managers and downstream water users, have been applied successfully. The main activities in the latter program include upstream soil and water conservation techniques applied by farmers that led to more water being available of higher quality downstream.[71]

Governance

Countries that improve governance can increase their national income by two to three times in the long term. Additional long-term effects are evident, including reduced child mortality and illiteracy.[72] The causality between governance and economic growth is complex, as it is true that improved governance can be both a cause of growth and a consequence of growth. In the case of water management, good governance underpins effective investments. A particular case in point of the downside of poor governance is corruption. Corruption raises transaction costs, undermines economic development, and makes it harder to attain development targets. Bribes, kickbacks, collusion, and substandard work can increase the cost of water provision by 20 to 30 percent, raising the cost of meeting the water-related targets of the MDGs by almost US$50 billion.[73] This does not take into account costs in the form of alternative use of funding (or opportunity cost) to increase water provision. It also excludes costs of pollution and the natural resource overuse that can follow in the trail of corrupt behavior.

There are currently an increasing number of examples worldwide to improve transparency and accountability in water decision making. The Berliner Wasserbetriebe (BWB) utility company, which provides Berlin and its surrounding areas with drinking water and sewage services, has developed far-reaching strategies to prevent corruption. Several measures were applied to strengthen consumer influence, accountability, and transparency, including the creation of a multistakeholder Integrity Committee and an external *Ombudsman* to protect whistleblowers. BWB staff received trainings to be more perceptive to corruption risks, and Web-based information was provided to the public on anticorruption measures.[74] Similarly, in Bangalore, India, the quality of water services from a user perspective was benchmarked and assessed by the National Public Affairs Centre (PAC), a civil society organization, through three separate citizen report cards. The citizen report cards triggered reforms in public water utilities in the city, enhancing public sector accountability and responsiveness. Although the first report card in 1994 gave low ratings to all major city service providers, it did not have an immediate impact since only a few service providers acknowledged the problems and took corrective actions. However, the second report card in 1999 indicated partial improvement in some services, while the third report card in 2003 revealed substantial improvements by almost all service providers, as well as perceived decline in corruption. The proportion of people satisfied with the Bangalore Water Supply & Sewerage Board services increased dramatically from 4 percent in 1994 to 73 percent in 2003.[75]

While it is difficult to estimate the economic benefits of improved water governance, or the costs of poor governance, it is clear that investment in governance and management is critical to expand and sustain investments already made. Clear division of roles and responsibilities, well-defined property rights, effective judiciary and enforcement systems, and access to information and stakeholder participation all make significant contributions toward improved quality of water resources management and water services. The application of participatory irrigation management in a number of schemes in India, Mexico, and Turkey has yielded considerable gains. For example, increased participation through water user associations and similar types of organizations can lead to increased collection of water tariffs, improved management and operation of irrigation facilities, and higher agricultural productivity.[76]

When it comes to participatory processes for water management, the process followed in Québec to develop its National Water Strategy is replicable elsewhere.[77] The multiyear process centered on a participatory approach that sought to engage all stakeholders, and it built transparency into government decision making. From March 15, 1999 to May 1, 2000 a commission of the Bureau d'audiences publiques sur l'environnement (BAPE) held 142 public meetings in the 17 administrative regions of Québec.[78] The hearings were divided into two stages. In the first stage, public meetings dealing with the proposed management orientations were first held in Montréal. The commission then toured the regions and went on to organize theme-oriented meetings. A specific consultation was held with the Inuit and Cree nations on the territories of Northern Québec. At the end of the first stage, more than 1,000 documents were made public. In the second stage, the commission heard 379 briefs. The BAPE report entitled *Water: A Resource to Be Protected, Shared and Enhanced* was submitted to the Minister of the Environment on May 1, 2000. In its report, the commission placed special emphasis on three main aspects: improved governance through water management at the river basin level; the preparation of the portrait of each region reflecting the public's expectations concerning the management of water and aquatic ecosystems; and a reform of the legislation and institutions in order to implement an integrated water and aquatic ecosystem policy. In 2002, the Government of Québec released the Québec Water Policy entitled *Water: Our Life, Our Future*. Most of the recommendations of the BAPE commission were adopted in the policy which seeks to:

- manage water in an integrated manner, from a sustainable development perspective;
- ensure the protection of this unique resource of our collective heritage; and
- better protect public health and the health of ecosystems.

The BAPE process could be modified by other regions to take into account different legal and regulatory structures, cultures, and the relevant strength of government institutions at the national and subnational levels. Given the current understanding of global issues, it might even be time for Québec to review its policy using a similar process.

Public and Private Sector Investments

The economic and social benefits of improved water supply, sanitation, and water resources management make a compelling case for decision makers around the world to increase investment in water to make short- and long-term development gains. Investing in the health of people, ecosystems, and more efficient and sustainable water use is an investment that not only provides immediate economic benefit but also safeguards previous and future social and economic gains.

Yet many countries make insufficient investments in water. For example, in 2006 the GDP per capita for sub-Saharan Africa was US$920. With less than a half a percent of GDP being devoted to water, this translated to average per capita spending on water and sanitation of a little less than US$4.50 per person. Countries like Ghana, Tanzania, and Uganda may be required to at least double the spending on water and sanitation to reach the MDG target, and development aid may be necessary in low-income countries.[79]

While many countries neglect water investments, there are exceptions. In its most recent 5-year plan covering 2011–2015, China put a high priority on water conservation and aims to double its level of investments into projects to improve water conservation to more than US$600 billion during the next decade. The government also encourages loans to and private investment in the water sector to ensure funding for conservation. Already, a number of public–private partnerships have materialized in relation to wastewater treatment in the country. Some of the proposed measures by the government will address floods in many regions and droughts in the southwest part of the country. China aims to build effective flood control and drought relief systems by the end of 2020. Moreover, the central government will subsidize the maintenance of water projects with public benefits in western regions and poverty-stricken areas. The government also set ambitious aims to eradicate the problem of unsafe drinking water in rural areas by the end of 2015.[80]

Both the public and private sectors are investing in technology, as it is one of the drivers of change that may bring positive results in the relatively near future. Agricultural production could be greatly increased through expanded use of current water-saving technologies in many regions. Increasing net benefits or value per unit of water has key implications for farming decisions, economic growth, poverty reduction, equity, and the environment. There is much more scope for increasing value per unit of water in agriculture (economic water productivity) than in physical water productivity, which is becoming increasingly constrained. Strategies for increasing the value of water used in agriculture include:

- increasing yield per unit of supply or depletion;
- changing from low- to high-value crops (from wheat to strawberries, for example);
- reallocating water from lower to higher value uses;
- lowering the costs of inputs (e.g., labor efficiency, or appropriate technology);

- increasing the health benefits and the value of ecological services from agriculture;
- decreasing social, health, and environmental costs (e.g., minimizing degradation of other ecosystems);
- obtaining multiple benefits per unit of water (e.g., using treated wastewater for agriculture); and
- achieving more livelihood support per unit of water (e.g., more jobs, nutrition, and income for the same amount of water).[81]

Promising technological innovations currently being explored include continual refinement of Global Information Systems (GIS) with ability for real-time monitoring of agricultural crops and water quality and quantity; information technology permitting a global collective intelligence system; nanotechnology to replace current water sensors; water purification and desalination; biotechnology to grow food plants, biofuels, and trees; using saline or brackish water; disease and drought resistance of crops; seawater-based food; and biomass, including algal production, plant-based meat substitutes, and (in vitro) cultured meat.

Cooperation with the private sector could make technologies available soon after their development. Google provides one example through the manner in which they are cooperating with governments and nongovernmental organizations to upload GIS-based information for easy access onto their platform Google Earth. Originally, the Urban Inequities Survey (UIS) methodology was developed by UN-HABITAT to monitor, assess, and disaggregate urban water and sanitation service coverage by gender and socioeconomic status, and to display the data spatially. GIS can then be used to identify populations that are not served by water and sanitation facilities. UIS has been partnered in dozens of cities around the word. It was carried out in 17 secondary urban centers in Kenya (2006), Uganda (2007), and Tanzania (2007) as part of the UN-HABITAT-supported Lake Victoria Region Water and Sanitation Initiative. This methodology interested Google.org, which recently piloted UIS in seven towns in Zanzibar, Tanzania (2009, 201) and six Lake Victoria towns in Uganda and Tanzania mainland (2010). UN-HABITAT entered into an Agreement of Cooperation with the national statistics office in each participating country to collect UIS data through household surveys and to coordinate this pilot intervention.

UIS not only provides information for monitoring access to infrastructure and basic service coverage before, during, and after intervention, it also provides baseline, midterm, and endline information for evaluating the impact of interventions on living conditions in terms of access to water, sanitation, and other human settlements dimensions measured by the MDG indicators and the UN-HABITAT agenda. The application of UIS methodology has enabled this pilot project to identify the needs of select towns in Zanzibar and the Lake

Victoria region in terms of access to infrastructure and basic services such as water, sanitation, solid waste management, drainage, and other human settlements dimensions.[82]

CONCLUSION

Improved water supply and sanitation and responsible water resources management boost countries' economic development, and, if benefits are shared within society, they contribute greatly to human health and poverty eradication. As has been shown, investing in water is good for economic and social development—improved water resources management and water supply and sanitation contribute significantly to increased production and productivity within economic sectors and increase quality of life, especially for the poorest.

It is critical that the economic benefits are understood and clearly articulated at every level for improved water supply and sanitation, as well as responsible water resources management, and that these benefits are included in strategic macroeconomic decision making. Investments in water must be promoted for the economic benefits they generate, which considerably outweigh investment costs. Hence, for many governments it becomes an issue of refocusing and reprioritizing their investment options to give more attention to the role of water in development. A set of guiding principles to action are suggested next. These can provide a starting point for the development of international, national, and local strategies to target case-specific investment challenges and priorities:

- Donors should increase and refocus their development assistance and better target those poorest low-income countries that are most off track to meet the water and sanitation MDGs and/or those countries with high levels of water stress.
- Governments of middle- and low-income countries should reallocate resources so that they target investments that benefit those without adequate access to water and related services.
- Decision makers must properly plan sound water resources management and infrastructure and apply safeguards for social and environmental impacts. Interventions of improved water management and infrastructure must target those who are poorest. Targeting those with lowest capacities and levels of access to water for various health and productive uses is a sound investment strategy and provides high returns.
- Decision makers should invest more in governance, management systems, and capacities to sustain investments made and to attract new investments. Poor governance constitutes an increased investment risk and can lead to suboptimal investments.

It is vital that governments and other decision makers are aware of the concerted leadership and commitment that must accompany improved water resources management and services. Only then can meaningful priorities be set to bring about the reforms and investments required. In addition to national and local efforts, international collaboration must accelerate improved access to clean water and improved water resources management across international boundaries. Even though there remain many challenges to increased public and private investments in water, the obstacles are small in comparison to the economic and social benefits that such investments will provide both to poor people and to entire national economies.

NOTES

1. A. Smith, *An Inquiry into the Nature and Causes of the Wealth of Nations* (London: Meuthen, 1904).
2. United Nations. *World Water Development Report 2006: Water a Shared Responsibility* (Paris, France: Berghahn Books and UNESCO Publishing, 2006).
3. United Nations. *World Water Development Report 2006: Water a Shared Responsibility* (Paris, France: Berghahn Books and UNESCO Publishing, 2006).
4. World Health Organization/UNICEF *Meeting the MDG drinking water and sanitation target : the urban and rural challenge of the decade* Accessed May 22, 2013 http://www.who.int/water_sanitation_health/monitoring/jmpfinal.pdf
5. D. Molden, ed., *Water for Food, Water for Life: A Comprehensive Assessment of Water Management in Agriculture.* (London, England: Earthscan, (2007).
6. B. C. Bates et al., eds., *Climate Change and Water. Technical Paper of the Intergovernmental Panel on Climate Change* (Geneva, Switzerland: IPCC Secretariat, 2008).
7. OECD, *Managing Water for All: An OECD Perspective on Pricing and Financing* (Paris, France: OECD, 2009).
8. Ibid.
9. BRIC countries consist of Brazil, Russia, India, and China. South Africa has been added as a fifth country to make BRICS. Water is an ever-growing challenge in these countries.
10. A. Steer. From the Pump Room to the Board Room: water's central role in climate change adaptation. World Bank. 2010 accessed May 22, 2013 http://siteresources.worldbank.org/INTSDNET/Resources/COP16_Water_Event_AndrewSteer_Keynote_Presentation.pdf
11. The United Nations World Water Development Report: Water for People, Water for Life, 2009, accessed May 22, 2013 http://unesdoc.unesco.org/images/0018/001819/181993e.pdf
12. See World Bank GDP per capita indicators for 2009: Accessed May 23, 2013 http://data.worldbank.org/indicator/NY.GDP.PCAP.CD http://data.worldbank.org/indicator/NY.GDP.PCAP.CD
13. United Nations Environment Programme, Green Economy Report, 2011. Towards a Green Economy: Pathways to Sustainable Development and Poverty Eradication,accessed May 26, 2013, http://www.unep.org/greeneconomy/greeneconomyreport/tabid/29846/default.aspx

14. J. Joyce et al., *The Impact of the Global Financial Crisis on Financial Flows to the Water Sector in Sub-Saharan Africa. Report No. 28,* (Stockholm, Sweden: Stockholm International Water Institute, 2010).

15. OECD. *Benefits of Investing in Water and Sanitation: An OECD Perspectives.* (Paris, France: OECD Publishing, 2011)

16. United Nations, *World Water Development Report 2006…*

17. Ibid.

18. United Nations Environment Programme, *Green Economy Report 2011…*

19. L. R. Brown, *World on Edge: How to Prevent Environmental and Economic Collapse* (New York, NY: Norton, 2011).

20. United Nations Environment Programme, *Green Economy Report 2011…*

21. K. Pauw, J. Thurlow, and D. van Seventer, *Droughts and Floods in Malawi: Assessing the Economy-Wide Effects* (IFPRI Discussion Paper 00962), accessed May 22, 2013 http://ebrary.ifpri.org/cdm/compoundobject/collection/p15738coll2/id/1370/rec/20

22. See for example: *Climate Change and Health, Fact Sheet No. 266,* World Health Organization, accessed May 1, 2013, http://www.who.int/mediacentre/factsheets/fs266/en/

23. J. Briscoe and R. P. S. Malik, *India's Water Economy: Bracing for a Turbulent Future* (Oxford, England: Oxford University Press and The World Bank, 2006).

24. World Bank and State Environmental Protection Administration, People's Republic of China, *Cost of Pollution in China: Economic Estimates of Physical Damages* (Washington, DC: The World Bank, 2007).

25. United Nations Development Programme, *Human Development Report 2006: Water for Human Development* (New York, NY: UNDP Human Development Report Office, 2006).

26. D. Hinrichsen, B. Robey, and U. D. Upadhyay, *Solutions for a Water-Short World. Population Reports* (Series M, No. 14, Baltimore, Johns Hopkins School of Public Health, Population Information Program, December 1997).

27. *World Water Week,* World Health Organization, access August 30, 2010, http://www.who.int/mediacentre/events/meetings/2010/world_water_week/en/index.html

28. World Health Organization, *Water, Sanitation and Hygiene Links to Health: Facts and Figures* (Geneva, Switzerland: WHO, 2004).

29. World Health Organization, *Prevention and control of Schistosomiasis and Soil-transmitted Helminthiasis* (technical report series no. 912, WHO, Geneva, Switzerland, 2002).

30. C. D. Mather and D. Loncar, *Updated Projections of Global Mortality and Burden of Disease, 2002-2030: Data Sources, Methods and Results,* WHO, accessed December 12, 2012, http://www.who.int/healthinfo/statistics/bod_projections2030_paper.pdf

31. A. Prüss-Üstün et al., *Safer Water, Better Health: Costs, Benefits and Sustainability of Interventions to Protect and Promote Health* (Geneva, Switzerland: World Health Organization, 2008).

32. The 2030 Water Resources Group, 2009. Charting Our Water Future: Economic frameworks to inform decision-making. accessed May 23, 2013, http://www.2030waterresourcesgroup.com/water_full/Charting_Our_Water_Future_Final.pdf

33. Hutton G and J. Bartram. *Regional and Global Costs of Attaining the Water Supply and Sanitation Target (Target 10) of the Millennium Development Goals* (2008)

World Health Organization, accessed May 26, 2013, http://www.who.int/water_sanitation_health/economic/mdg_global_costing.pdf

34. G. Hutton and L. Haller, *Evaluation of the Costs and Benefits of Water and Sanitation Improvements at the Global Level* (Geneva, Switzerland: World Health Organization, 2004).

35. Ibid.

36. Ibid.

37. The disability adjusted life year (DALY) is a summary measure of population health, and 1 DALY represents 1 year of healthy life lost. The DALY is used to estimate the gap between the current health status of a population and the ideal situation, where everyone in that population would live to old age in good health. See K. Lvovsky, *Health and Environment* (environment strategy paper no.1, World Bank, Washington, DC, 2001).

38. World Health Organization, *Water, Sanitation and Hygiene...*

39. K. Michaelowa, *Returns to Education in Low-Income Countries: Evidence for Africa,* (presentation, Committee on Developing Countries of the German Economic Association, Hamburg Institute for International Economics, Hamburg, Germany, June 30, 2000).

40. Hutton and Haller, *Evaluation of the Costs...*

41. Net present value (NPV) is the present value of future cash flows in relation to a particular investment. NPV compares the value of one dollar today with its future value, taking into account inflation and profit margins. If NPV is positive for a particular project, it is considered well worth investing in; if negative, stay away from investing.

42. F. Rijsberman, *The Water Challenge* (Copenhagen Consensus Challenge Paper, International Water Management Institute, Colombo, Sri Lanka, 2004).

43. World Health Organization and UNICEF, *Water for Life. Making it Happen,* (Geneva, Switzerland: World Health Organization, 2005).

44. J. D. Sachs, *Macroeconomics and Health: Investing in Health for Economic Development* (report, Commission on Macroeconomics and Health, WHO, Geneva, 2001).

45. World Bank, *World Development Report 1994 – Infrastructure for Development* (Washington, DC: World Bank, 1994).

46. United Nations Environment Programme, *Green Economy Report...*

47. UNESCO, *The United Nations Development Report 3: Water in a Changing World* (London, England: Earthscan, 2009).

48. Brown, *World on Edge...*

49. Republic of Kenya, *The Aftercare Study on the National Water Master Plan* (Tokyo, Japan: Nippon Koei, 1998).

50. Intergovernmental Panel on Climate Change Technical Paper on Water and Climate Change, p 7, accessed May 23, 2013, http://www.ipcc.ch/pdf/technical-papers/climate-change-water-en.pdf http://www.ipcc.ch/pdf/technical-papers/climate-change-water-en.pdf

51. Worldwide, agriculture uses 69 percent of water, compared with 23 percent by industry and only 8 percent by households. In contrast, agriculture's share of GDP in 2001 was only 5 percent globally, while industry's share was 31 percent and that of services 64 percent. In developing countries, however, the water proportion used by agriculture is much higher, for example, 97 percent in Pakistan, 93 percent in India, 87 percent in China, 86 percent in Egypt, and 76 percent in Indonesia, to list a few of the most populated developing countries. World Bank,

World Development Report 2003: Sustainable Development in a Dynamic World (Washington, DC: World Bank, 2003).

52. S. Hansen and R. Bhatia, *Water and Poverty in a Macro-Economic Context* (Oslo, Norway: Norwegian Ministry of the Environment, 2004).

53. J. Bucknall, *Making the Most of Scarcity: Accountability for Better Water Management Results in the Middle East and North Africa* (Washington, DC: The World Bank, 2007).

54. Economic water scarcity occurs when the investments needed to keep up with growing demand are constrained by financial, human, or institutional capacity.

55. World Bank, *World Development Report 2003...*

56. World Water Vision Unit. *Results of the Gender Mainstreaming Project: A Way Forward* (Marseille, France: World Water Council, 2000).

57. World Water Assessment Programme, *The United Nations World Water Development Report 3: Water in a Changing World* (Paris, France: UNESCO, and London, England: Earthscan, 2009).

58. *Transboundary Waters: Sharing Benefits, Sharing Responsibilities,* United Nations Water Task Force on Transboundary Waters, accessed May 1, 2013, http://www. unwater.org/downloads/UNW_TRANSBOUNDARY.pdf

59. A. Y. Hoekstra, *Proceedings of the International Expert Meeting on Virtual Water Trade* (Value of Water Research Report Series No. 12. IHE, Delft, The Netherlands, 2003).

60. Ibid.

61. A. Steer, *From the Pump Room...*

62. Brown, *World on Edge...*

63. United Nations Taskforce on Water, *Transboundary Waters...*

64. United Nations Environment Programme *The Montreal Protocol on Substances that Deplete the Ozone Layer* (2000), accessed May 26, 2013, http://ozone.unep. org/pdfs/Montreal-Protocol2000.pdf

65. Such benefits can be divided into Use values and Non-use values. Use values refer to direct, indirect, and option values. Direct values: food, fodder, timber, fuel, and so on. Indirect values: various ecological services, such as flood control, water purification, nutrient retention, and so on. Option values: future possible direct and indirect economic gains. Finally, the Non-use values refer to intrinsic moral, cultural, and aesthetic values of ecosystems.

66. World Bank, *Making Sustainable Commitments: An Environment Strategy for the World Bank* (Washington, DC: World Bank, 2000).

67. L. Emerton and E. Bos, *Value: Counting Ecosystems as Water Infrastructure* (Gland, Switzerland and Cambridge, England: IUCN, 2004).

68. L. Emerton and L. D. Kekulandala, *Assessment of the Economic Value of Muthurajawela Wetland* (occasional papers of IUCN, No. 4, Colombo, Sri Lanka, 2004).

69. Ibid.

70. L. Emerton and E. Muramira, *Uganda Biodiversity: Economic Assessment* (Kampala, Uganda: Uganda National Biodiversity Strategy and Action Plan, National Environment Management Authority, 1999).

71. United Nations, *World Water Development Report 2009: Water in a Changing World* (London, England and Paris, France: Earthscan, UNESCO Publishing, 2009).

72. D. Kaufmann, "Myths and Realities of Governance and Corruption," in *Global Competitiveness Report 2005-06,* 81-98, accessed May 26, 2013, http://mpra. ub.uni-muenchen.de/8089/1/MPRA_paper_8089.pdf

73. Transparency International and Water Integrity Network, *Global Corruption Report 2008: Corruption in the Water Sector* (Cambridge, England: University Press, 2008).

74. Water Integrity Network, *Corruption Prevention Strategies of the Berlin Water Utility* (WIN case information sheet, no. 4, Berlin, Germany, 2009).

75. P. Stålgren, *Corruption in the Water Sector: Causes, Consequences and Potential Reform* (Swedish Water House Policy Brief Nr. 4, SIWI, 2006).

76. United Nations, *World Water Development Report 2009...*

77. W. J. Cosgrove, "Public Participation to Promote Water Ethics and Transparency," in *Water and Ethics* Edited by M. Ramón Llamas, Luis Martínez-Cortina and Aditi Mukherji (London, England: Taylor & Francis, 2009).

78. Quebec's Bureau d'audiences publiques sur l'environnement is its environmental public hearings board.

79. UN Millennium Project, *Millennium Development Goals Needs Assessments for Ghana, Tanzania, and Uganda* (background paper, United Nations, New York, NY, 2004).

80. J. Zhu, "China to Invest $608b in Water Projects," *China Daily,* January 31, 2011., accessed May 26, 2013, http://www.chinadaily.com.cn/china/2011-01/31/content_11942365.htm

81. Molden, *Water for Food...*

82. *Urban Inequity Survey,* UN Habitat, accessed December 12, 2012, http://h20initiative.org/index.php/component/content/article/82-methodologies/147-urban-inequity-survey

CHAPTER 12

The Potential of Clean Energy for Equity in Remote Communities in the North

TIM WEIS

Current energy production in remote First Nations is largely dependent upon systems using diesel or other types of fossil fuels. These systems depend upon resources that must be imported from out of the territory, over long distances. Millions of litres of diesel fuel a year are transported by air, barge, and tractor train into remote communities for existing diesel electric power plants. In addition to the air pollution that burning fossil fuels generate, the transportation of such large amounts of fossil fuel into a remote harsh environment presents many opportunities for a major spill. In addition, the cost of purchasing fossil fuels, either directly or passed through the consumers via electricity rates, accounts for a significant drain of cash resources from already cash poor communities.

Mushkegowuk Council and Nishnawbe-Aski Nation press release, February 5, 1997

The cost and limited access to affordable energy in remote Canadian communities is an important inequity that residents in these communities face compared to those living in the rest of the country. Many remote communities in Canada continue to rely on imported diesel fuel to power local generators. The continued use of imported fuel results in higher risks of local air and water pollution as well as economic impacts such as price volatility, and the long-term dependence on resources from outside of the communities. Electricity prices in remote communities can be as much as 10 times those in the rest of the country, and they can present a barrier to economic development as well as consuming significant amounts of local government resources that could otherwise be directed to social and community development and the improvement of health and economic inequalities.

Canada has close to 200,000 citizens in approximately 300 remote communities that are not connected to either territorial or provincial electric grids,[1] many of which rely on diesel-powered electric generators. Remote communities are generally defined as being those that are not connected to the North American electrical grid and have at least 10 permanent residences.[2] Canada has hundreds of remote sites ranging in size and population from unmanned telecom stations to the Territorial capital cities with several thousand people. There are industrial sites, including logging field camps, resource extraction mines, and military outposts, as well as predominantly residential communities, the majority of which are Aboriginal. The number of sites fluctuates as industrial sites are being developed and decommissioned; some remote communities are connected to provincial or territorial power grids, such as the connection of seven remote communities in Northern Manitoba in 1997[3]; and occasionally a new community is started.

Using the aforementioned definition, every community within the three Canadian territories would be considered to be remote, even though there are electrical grids in both Yukon and the Northwest Territories that connect several communities around the capital cities Whitehorse and Yellowknife. Remote communities are not limited to the three territories, however; in fact, six out of the ten Canadian provinces have at least one remote community (only Saskatchewan, New Brunswick, Prince Edward Island, and Nova Scotia do not), with British Columbia having more remote communities than any other Canadian jurisdiction. The social, technical, and economic frameworks in small communities are very different from those in industrial sites or even large communities. This chapter focuses exclusively on the residential communities that rely on diesel generators as their primary source of electricity generation.

There are significant differences within the category of communities that would be broadly described as small and residential. These communities comprise four major Aboriginal groups (First Nations, Inuit, Innu, and Inuvialuit), as well as non-Aboriginal communities. Among the Aboriginal communities, there are varying degrees of self-governance, including the Inuvialuit, who since 1984 have major regional land ownership, to historical treaty zones to communities still undergoing lengthy land claim negotiations. As a result of these variations, electricity services and financial structure can be very different from community to community, even within the same jurisdiction. As an illustration, in 2006 residents of Wapekeka First Nation in Northern Ontario, which is serviced by Hydro One Remote Communities, paid rates that were similar to consumers in southern Ontario for every kilowatt-hour (kWh) of electricity they consumed,[4] while residents of Poplar Hill First Nation, which runs its own microutility, paid a fixed monthly fee regardless of consumption. The actual cost of generating electricity can also vary dramatically within the same region, as in the case of Northern Ontario where average generation costs in 2008 ranged from as low as 0.27 $Cdn/kWh in North Spirit Lake to 1.32 $Cdn/kWh in Wawakapewin.[5] These differences can have major impacts on the viability of alternatives such as wind power, as well as consumption patterns and the social motivation for changes.

The high prices of electricity generation often represent significant costs directly to the remote community's budget or indirectly as a competing cost to the agency that is responsible for supplying energy in the community. The costs of diesel fuel, risks of fuel spill mitigation, local air quality, and long-term sustainability are often cited as reasons for communities to look for alternative solutions that would result in a cleaner, more economically effective energy supply. Meanwhile, the utility companies that are responsible for these juris-dictions either lose money servicing these communities[6] or pass on the high costs of generation to their customers, or a combination of both.[7] The constant import of diesel fuel also results in funds leaving the community that could be used for other community projects and programs. Limited generator sizes can become a cap on local development, which can restrict economic development opportunities such as building tourist lodges, fish processing and refrigeration, or even new community buildings or housing projects.[8]

Given the high costs and environmental impacts of diesel fuel, alternative energy sources provide many benefits to remote communities. Canada has had a range of projects to promote the use of alternative energy sources, par-ticularly wind-diesel projects. While some have been more successful, there remain many obstacles to a widespread switch to alternative energy use. The price of diesel fuel increased significantly since the year 2000, including some major increases just prior to the global economic recession in 2009. This has in part driven an increasing interest in renewable energy projects in remote Canadian communities. In addition to providing price stability and predict-ability, renewable energy resources can provide additional revenue streams for community residents and stimulate community economic development while retaining energy expenditures within the community.

COMMUNITY ENERGY NEEDS

To assess consumption patterns and long-term energy options, many remote communities have undertaken community energy planning processes over the past decade.[9] Community energy planning involves inventorying current energy consumption, costs, and risks, and assessing future needs and supply alternatives, as well as opportunities to educate community members and/or leaders on where and how they are using energy. As part of energy planning, it is common that community members and/or leaders voice their concerns and priorities surrounding energy use. The Pembina Institute has worked with several dozen remote communities on energy demand assessment and plan-ning processes. The goal of these projects included:

- determining where energy is used in the community;
- determining the breakdown of costs—economic and environmental;
- suggesting energy and cost savings opportunities that may exist in the community;
- suggesting energy supply options that may exist in the community; and
- providing a foundation for energy planning in the community.

As part of the studies, meetings were held with local community decision makers such as chief and council, band manager, band employees, and at times surveys of community members. These meetings informed those involved about the purpose of the work but also offered opportunities to gather community input on local energy concerns and their reasons for participating in such studies. The most common responses included concerns with respect to the rising energy costs for community members, reducing energy costs to the community budget that is spent on building heating and electricity, gaining access over the control of the local electricity source, and improving local energy security as opposed to importing fuel from outside of the community. Communities that had had significant diesel fuel spills that contaminated land or water would raise this as a top-level concern. While priorities varied from community to community, there was consistently an interest in exploring alternative energy sources as a means to reduce costs as well as to improve or protect the environment. This can be seen by the number of remote communities who are currently pursuing various alternative energy projects across Canada, ranging from the Oujé-Bougoumou biomass project in Northern Quebec[10] to Community Energy Planning in Wha Ti, Northwest Territories.[11] Given the diffuse nature of these communities, the particular resources available to each one, and the particular challenges they face, there is no standard development path to follow, and costs are unique to individual communities and projects. As such, pursuing an energy alternative is not an easy task. At times, individual projects may be economically beneficial, but the community can face capital cost or financing challenges; at other times the economics may depend on the future price forecasts for imported diesel fuel, which are far from certain, and other times direct support may be required to make an alternative solution viable in the short term, although it may provide long-term price stability while improving energy security and availability.

CONSTRAINTS TO ALTERNATIVE ENERGY IN REMOTE COMMUNITIES

While there has been increasing interest in renewable energy from communities, progress has been slow. This has been particularly striking when it comes to wind energy, which has experienced rapid growth in large-scale facilities while stalling in remote communities.

Harnessing the wind has long been perceived as a potential alternative electricity source to overcome the high costs of diesel power and provide a cleaner and more sustainable approach. Early government research and development in wind power in Canada's north was focused on remote communities; in fact, the first wind-diesel research project began on the Magdalene Islands in Canada in 1978.[12] There have been more than 10 Canadian wind-diesel demonstration or pilot projects by utilities and governments since that time as well as a few commercial ventures where independent power producers have negotiated deals to sell wind power to remote community grids.[13] Most of the projects met with marginal success, some had earlier mechanical problems such as in Sachs Harbour, Northwest Territories and Big Trout Lake, Ontario, which after having overrun initial installation budgets were abandoned. Others, such as Kasabonica Lake, Ontario; Rankin Inlet, Nunavut; and Cambridge Bay, Northwest Territories failed as a result of a lack of ongoing operations and maintenance. Finally, projects such as Kuglutuk, Northwest Territories (NWT) had unusual accidents, including being hit by lightning. In all cases, the diesel savings were not deemed to be significant enough to warrant reconditioning or repairing the projects after the initial pilot or grant money had been spent to build them. While mechanical failures are part of the normal operation of any rotating machinery, including diesel engines, wind generators do not have the same availability of replacement parts or locally trained technicians to troubleshoot and repair equipment. While commercial wind turbines have been operating in the Yukon for over 15 years in extremely harsh icing conditions, no wind-diesel projects in the NWT and Nunavut have lasted 10 years. As a result, by the late 1990s much of the interest in wind-diesel systems had waned. Since the year 2000 only one wind-diesel system has been installed in Canada.

By way of comparison, it is instructive to observe that large-scale wind power has averaged annual growth rates of new installations over 20 percent since the first federal production incentive was introduced in 2002. In 2010, commercial, utility-scale wind power installations had surpassed 4,000 MW of installed capacity, such that approximately 2 percent of Canada's overall national electricity is generated from the wind.[14] Given research and deployment in remote communities began decades earlier in Canada, one might expect they would be well ahead of utility-scale turbines, but in fact this is not the case, and there remains a policy gap to facilitate cleaner options in remote communities.

The relative lack of success of renewable energy projects in remote communities, particularly wind-diesel projects, speaks to the persistence of substantive obstacles. Despite the high prices and other community concerns about a reliance on diesel imports, there remain numerous barriers to the deployment of alternative electricity systems in remote communities that have prevented a generalized switch to alternative energy.

Subsidized or Average Cost Energy Prices

Subsidies to existing electricity costs are a notable barrier in the remote Canadian context. Many jurisdictions in Canada spread the costs of remote power generation across the broader rate base, sheltering inhabitants of remote communities from the full exposure to their electricity costs.[15] Additional subsidies can exist in terms of grants or funds given to building diesel plants as essential community infrastructure, as well as emergency support for price spikes. While this is a barrier to alternatives, it is also difficult to change. Living costs are very high in remote communities, and in many cases income opportunities beyond subsistence hunting are low. As such, while wind energy systems could argue for similar or matching support, it is unlikely that such subsidies would be removed.

Lack of Information

Lack of information can also be a key barrier in remote communities. It is difficult to expect remote communities to be able to devote time and money to staying on top of the most recent technical developments in energy alternatives. Many Aboriginal communities in Canada have election cycles as often as every 2 years, making information continuity an ongoing challenge.[16] Communities often rely on precedents set by other communities,[17] and so a lack of operating projects can produce a self-perpetuating cycle. Community energy planning has often been cited as an opportunity for communities to overcome information gaps and promote renewable energy such as wind-diesel; others have suggested that such efforts are often beneficial in leading to improved energy efficiency, which is laudable but rarely results in renewable energy supply alternatives.[18] Information gaps do not only exist at the community level, however, as utilities are also often not aware of the most recent advances in renewable energy technology.

Transaction Costs

The impact of transaction costs can be amplified in remote communities as a result of high transportation costs both of equipment and of skilled labor to install it. This can be a barrier to a project even before it is started, but ultimately it becomes part of the high upfront costs of clean energy systems.

High Front-End Capital Costs/Lack of Credit

While high capital costs are a common barrier to renewable energy projects in general, the inability to access credit is a challenge for small communities, particularly Aboriginal ones, as lenders can be averse to working with these communities for fear that they will be unable to seize assets to recover a defaulted loan.[19]

Perceived Technology Performance Uncertainty and Risk

The perception of risks remains a barrier to wind-diesel projects in Canada, largely as a result of the legacy of failed projects described earlier. Failed projects can have very long institutional memories, long after the specific reasons for failure have been forgotten. As a result, the perception of risks is as a separate barrier, which can also include concerns that go beyond previous projects.[20]

Institutional Mismatch of Energy Costs and Capital Costs

An institutional mismatch or a lack of a legal framework for developers to be able to either develop or own a project, or sell the energy that is created, either in the form of electricity or in some cases heat, are both examples of regulatory barriers that are often the unintended consequences of rules drafted to deal with other legal issues. They can remain barriers, as any attempt at their removal is either challenging or perceived as insurmountable.

Lack of Legal Framework for Independent Power Production

In the past some provinces and territories have had legal restrictions on who is able to sell electricity.

Lack of Technical or Commercial Skills

The lack of technical skills to develop, construct, and maintain new technologies in remote communities is not unique to wind-diesel projects. A lack of "critical mass for classroom training and the related costs"[21] limits communities' ability to acquire the skills required to develop a wind-diesel project locally. Compounding this problem is the ongoing challenge of retaining skills within a community, as inhabitants are often mobile between communities or leave for larger centers looking for employment.

Lack of Utility Acceptance of Technologies/Prejudice against a Technology Because of Poor Past Performance

Specific to wind-diesel systems, a lack of utility acceptance is often related to either the legacy of failed historic projects to the next barrier identified as the difficulty of dispatching or controlling the output of wind energy systems into the existing utility infrastructure.[22] This can either be a perceived or a real limit due to the availability or cost of technologies such as flywheels or power electronics required to smooth variable power output. These barriers can be combined into the state of the technical maturity of the overall system, including the wind turbines themselves, the control systems, and the integration equipment. As discussed earlier, there have been several unsuccessful remote wind-hybrid projects in Canada that have in part led to a lack of interest in further developments.

Competition for Access to Resources

Competition for access to resources is different in remote communities than when developing renewable energy projects in the "southern" context. The latter typically involves alternate land uses such as agriculture or even preservation of viewscapes, and the most common competition is ensuring sufficient distance from the local airstrip for safe take-off and landing. Competition is therefore very much related to the barrier of restrictions on siting and construction and is in effect a capital cost barrier, as the ability to extend power lines outside of the community would alleviate many of these constraints. This is in essence the same as the barrier identified as the lack of utility grid access to remote sites, which in the case of remote communities or large-scale utility development is constrained by limits to the existing grid infrastructure.

Restrictions on Siting and Construction

One advantage that many Aboriginal communities have is some degree of autonomy over the development of projects on or close to their territories, be it reserve, treaty, or traditional lands. The risks of permitting are therefore typically less of an unknown than it would be to other utility-scale projects.[23]

Lack of Utility Grid Access to Remote Sites

In remote communities, it can be very expensive to build power lines very far outside of the community, and so wind energy projects are restricted to close proximity to existing infrastructure.[24]

Risks of Permit Process

All wind energy projects in Canada require approval from Transport Canada and Navigation Canada as a result of potential interference with airport landing strips. In addition, any project that involves federal government support needs to have a federal environmental assessment, which can require up to a year of monitoring for potentially impacted species.[25]

Institutional Mismatch of Capital Costs and Fuel Price Risks

In the context of remote communities, institutional mismatches between capital costs and fuel prices can be the result of the fact that utilities are responsible to public utility boards that review annual rates based on current costs and whose mandate does not tend to look beyond the current year. Long-term potential savings that result in short-term price increases can be blocked by public utility boards even when a utility is interested in pursuing such alternatives.

Difficulty of Quantifying Environmental Costs

Environmental damage resulting from diesel fuel use is externalized in the form of air emissions, while the remediation of contaminated soils as a result of diesel spills tends to be funded by Indian and Northern Affairs Canada (INAC) and not the local utility or fuel supplier. Although there are real costs that are borne by the community as a result of a spill, including the loss of usable resources and land, they are more difficult to quantify. Emission reductions resulting from small projects are also generally too small to overcome transaction costs that would make them marketable to voluntary or mandated offset markets.

Lack of Detailed Geographic Resource Data

Like almost all wind energy projects, the local wind speeds need to be measured, as the performance of a wind turbine is highly dependent on the characteristics of the local wind regime. One advantage that most remote communities in Canada have is that they frequently have local airports with anemometers. While these data are often not logged over long periods of time, it is not difficult to use the preexisting equipment to start to track wind speeds and obtain a reasonable estimate of the quality of the local wind speeds before investing in additional monitoring equipment.

Lack of Government Support

While there have been government support programs in the past at federal, provincial, and territorial levels in Canada, one of the difficulties with these programs has been the lack of long-term availability or predictability of such support mechanisms. While several pilot projects have been developed, a lack of long-term support has not created a long-term deployment strategy.

Opposition of Existing Interest Groups

In some communities, there is a local fuel supplier who is independent of the electricity provider and stands to lose if an alternative is pursued. These interests can impede the development of renewable systems such as wind power if the fuel supplier is politically connected or is not a part of the new project.

High Costs of Developing New Infrastructure and Market Institutions

New energy technologies are at a disadvantage as they do not have the volume of maintenance infrastructure and institutions as traditional technologies, making it difficult to compete and offer the same level of service; this is particularly true in remote and rural settings. For remote communities in Canada, this essentially becomes an operations and maintenance cost barrier, as well as a barrier due to a lack of local skilled labor that can easily be drawn upon.

Cold Weather

Extreme temperatures are often raised as a potential impediment to wind-diesel systems in Canada. While cold-weather modifications need to be made to the turbines that operate in Northern Canada,[26] they have been demonstrated to be able to function in extreme cold temperatures as exemplified by the numerous turbines operating in Alaska.[27] Blade icing is also frequently cited as a potential danger, and while it is an issue that needs to be considered when planning a project, being in a cold climate does not necessarily predispose a turbine to frequent icing conditions; rather, altitude and humidity and likelihood of freezing rain tend to have more of an impact and are not necessarily correlated with latitude.[28]

STRATEGIES FOR RENEWABLE ENERGY IN REMOTE COMMUNITIES

A common aspect of successful renewable energy policies for large-scale clean energy development is the importance of stability as well as a comprehensive design of a renewable energy policy.[29,30] A government program to encourage clean energy systems in remote communities should therefore not only target this technology but also needs to address multiple barriers to their development and/or be a part of a broader framework of policies that does.

There are numerous policy instruments that can and are being used to foster the deployment of renewable energy technologies around the world. Typically these policies are directed at on-grid applications and may not necessarily be applicable to or address the key barriers to development in a remote context. Nonetheless, it is worth examining what policy instruments are being used to determine how they may be applied to or adapted for off-grid communities and what options could be pursued by the government of Canada to encourage remote wind-diesel systems. Aboriginal Affairs and Northern Development Canada (AANDC), formerly INAC, has the primary responsibility and authority to fulfil the federal government's legal and treaty responsibilities to Aboriginal and First Nation's communities. AANDC provides funding for basic community infrastructure as well as operation and maintenance of this equipment.[31] As such, it is consistent to expect support for developing alternatives to also come from the federal government as the vast majority of remote communities in Canada are either Aboriginal or Northern, or both.

It has been argued that a "policy framed around specific goals and targets is more likely to achieve results than vague support" such as a government or utility goal for "more" renewable energy.[32] This argument is supported by the fact that technology neutral programs such as the Aboriginal and Northern Climate Change Program (ANCCP) and the Northern Community Action Program (ANCAP) programs put in place by INAC between 2001 and 2007 resulted in no wind-diesel projects in Canada.[33,34] This, combined with the fact that wind-diesel systems provide unique technological challenges, suggests that a program specific to remote wind energy is more likely to achieve results.

Incentive options for renewable energy projects in general can be classified in the broad categories of lowering capital costs, providing a production-based incentive, developing capacity or technical training, and mandating minimum generation portfolio mixes. "Polluter pays" options such as a carbon tax are also at the disposal of the federal government. However, such policies are inevitably a much broader national effort and are not specific to remote communities. While "polluter pays" options are often considered to be among the most economically efficient options to make clean energy technologies cost competitive, such policies do not address the already very high energy costs in remote communities. A summary of incentive options, excluding polluter pay options, that are available to the federal government are listed in Table 12.1.

Capital Cost Reductions

Reducing the capital cost for remote communities' projects can be important since equipment such as wind turbines and integration hardware typically make up the largest proportion of the overall project costs.[35] There are multiple ways of accomplishing this task, ranging from simple rebates to tax

Table 12.1. COMMON POLICIES/PROGRAMS GOVERNMENTS USE TO SUPPORT ALTERNATIVE ENERGY SYSTEMS

Instrument	Cost Recovery Source	Policy Requirements
Capital Cost Reductions		
Rebate or Grants	Tax or Rate Base	Establishment of qualifying technologies
Property or Income Tax Credit	Tax Base	Tax rule changes (credit limited to size of tax appetite)
Sales Tax Rebate	Tax Base	None
Financing Support	Tax Base	Agreements with financial institutions
Production Incentives		
Feed-in Tariff	Rate Base	Market system operator regulations
Production Top-Up	Tax Base	Establishing qualifying criteria
Capacity Development		
Community Energy Planning	Tax Base	None. Some jurisdictions are making it a requirement.
Technical Training	Tax Base	None
Mandating Generation Portfolios		
Renewable Portfolio Standard	Rate Base	Provincial legislation to set quotas and rules for trading
Emissions Offsets	Rate Base	Legislation to set market rules

Source: Adapted from Bailie, A., Doukas, A., Weis, T., Beckstead, C., and Haines, G. (2009). Renewable Energy Policies for Remote and Rural Communities, Report prepared for Agriculture and Agri-Food Canada, available online at http://www.rural.gc.ca/RURAL/display-afficher.do?id=1290792790023&lang=eng.

mechanisms to lowering financing costs. Rebates can be a fixed amount or proportional to system costs. Direct monetary contributions can provide the additional benefit of being a "bankable" asset that project developers and/or communities can use to secure financing or leverage complementary fund programs. This can be particularly beneficial for small communities that often have difficulty in accessing capital.

Alaska's Renewable Energy Grant Program was created in Alaska in 2008 and is administered by the Alaska Energy Authority.[36] The program addresses barriers to remote community renewable energy projects, including capital costs. It was designed to provide US\$50 million per year over a 5-year period for assistance to utilities, independent power producers, local governments, and tribal governments toward the development of renewable energy projects. Grants for feasibility studies, energy resource monitoring, and design and construction are all eligible. Additionally, Alaska has undertaken regional scoping and planning to determine the viability of wind projects for across the state.[37] Initial results indicate that it has in part been responsible for at least 20 new wind-diesel projects under development.[38] It is worth noting that the establishment of the fund has also resulted in resource mapping, training programs, and the establishment of new ENGOs and university programs, none of which are funded directly by the fund itself.

As a one-time transaction, capital cost reduction mechanisms can be attractive to policy makers for their relative simplicity and the fact that they tend to take place in a single fiscal year. Rebates are often administered directly from the tax base, and depending on the size or the rebate or the scope of the program objectives, rebates can become expensive for the issuing government if they are not carefully designed. An alternative design can be to set up a fund by charging a rate rider on the bills of consumers, which is pooled into a renewable energy fund which can be used to pay for rebates or loan guarantees or to provide the capital to cover lost tax revenues.

In principle, tax incentives operate in a similar manner to direct grants, although they do not require direct budgeted spending. While this fact can make them attractive to policy makers, in many cases for remote communities, the entity that may benefit from a government program may have little or no tax appetite to be able to take advantage of such programs.

Financing support not only helps to reduce project costs, but it can also enable the access to capital, which can be a challenge for small projects even when the economics are otherwise favorable. Often lending institutions may not be comfortable with small community-based projects, small developers, and/or new technologies that they are unfamiliar with. Financing support on its own is limited to projects that are otherwise viable.

While these types of programs are relatively easy to administer for governments, they do not necessarily result in successful long-term projects, as the funding is geared toward building a project, not ongoing operations. Forced repayments, or "claw-backs," can be built into such programs to try to minimize paying for unsuccessful efforts, but they may be difficult to extract from a failed project proponent.

Production Incentives

Rather than providing one-time incentives to reduce the initial cost of an energy system, support mechanisms and incentives can be linked directly to the energy output or production. There are two common production mechanisms that are used to support renewable energy systems, the simplest being an incentive that is paid as a top-up or a premium on top of the (likely fluctuating) energy price. The second is to set a fixed price (or tariff) for any renewable energy that is "fed" into the electricity grid. This mechanism is known as a feed-in tariff (or FIT) and is credited by many as being the most effective tool at deploying renewable energy.[39] The tariff is not based on the displaced energy cost, but rather the price is set such that if the renewable energy system operates well it will ensure a modest profit for the power producer.[40] An FIT is in essence simply paying the price for the type of energy that is desired, without trying to link it to the price of fossil fuels either directly or indirectly.

Despite their successes for grid-connected renewable power generation, FITs have not been used to target remote communities. In the Canadian context, there are several complicating factors to developing such a policy for remote communities. Each remote community is unique, has limited local grid capacity, and has significantly different quality of local renewable resources. As such, setting standard prices for renewable energy systems is difficult because each community needs to be considered on a case-by-case basis. Additionally, many remote communities in Canada do not belong to larger utilities, including many within provincial boundaries, notably in Ontario and British Columbia. Instead, they operate, and are responsible for their own diesel systems independently, and therefore would not have a broader rate base to absorb price premiums.

In Canada, the ecoENERGY for renewable power program (eERP) and its predecessor, the Wind Power Producer Incentive (WPPI), were both federal incentives that provided a producer with one cent per kilowatt-hour (kWh) for the first 10 years of a project's life. Unlike an FIT, which is supported through the utility rate base, a production incentive is funded through the tax base. This fact means that these programs not only require an initial commitment of government spending, but they also require a continued allocation of annual budgets to sustain them. The WPPI program was successful in supporting most of the first 1,000 MW of wind energy projects in Canada, which was superseded by the eERP, which was successful in helping to support over 4,500 megawatts of renewable power capacity,[41] most of which was wind energy projects. Neither program supported a wind energy project in a remote community.

One distinct advantage that a production incentive has in the context of the Canadian federal government is that it can be offered without interfering with provincial or territorial regulations, and furthermore it can be complementary to programs or incentives offered by the latter within their respective jurisdictions.

The Northwest Territories Power Corporation issued a request for proposals for wind energy projects in 2008, which offered wind energy producers the avoided cost of diesel fuel for any electricity they could sell into selected communities, and it was only open for tenders for a year.[42] There were no successful projects that resulted from this effort, perhaps in part as a result of the uncertainty around future diesel prices, but broader standing offers of this nature would lay the groundwork for a production-based clean energy procurement policy in these communities in the future.

Capacity Development

Two common capacity-building efforts for remote communities include community energy planning and technical training. Community energy planning includes collecting data on current energy demand and costs, and examining alternatives for demand side management and energy supply. Energy planning has been carried out for many remote communities in Canada[43] as a first step in examining energy alternatives. Community energy plans typically involve estimates of economic environmental implications of the current energy choices in the community while examining the implications of other future energy options, and it includes consultations with community members regarding local priorities to help inform decision makers in making choices that best meet the goals of their communities. Communities in the Northwest Territories are required to complete an "Integrated Community Sustainability Plan" that must be submitted to a strategic environmental assessment in order for them to receive federal government gasoline tax transfers. Energy plans can be useful for determining the potential for local renewable energy systems, while gauging the level of local support for such a project. One example of this effort is the Tlingit First Nation community energy planning process, which resulted in a run-of-river hydro project on the Taku River in British Columbia.[44]

Having local skills to properly install and maintain energy equipment can be important to ensure that preventative maintenance occurs and that necessary repairs can be done in a timely fashion. Renewable energy systems such as wind turbines are technologies that local diesel plant operators are not accustomed to operating, and repairs can become extremely expensive, particularly if repair technicians need to travel great distances into the community to service the equipment. An audit of renewable energy systems in remote Australian communities in the year 2000 found that about one-third of the systems installed in these communities were not functional.[45] Ensuring that adequate maintenance training is done locally, as well as training on any specialized integration equipment with the diesel systems, can help to ensure that installed equipment will operate as well as possible. This can be done by ensuring that experts who travel to install the systems also train local technicians, as well as programs that bring community members to centralized training facilities. This training is important to ensure that well projects operate as they are designed to do, and it can significantly reduce ongoing costs. In the case of wind turbines, training can include how to safely climb a tower, when bearings need to be greased, and how to replace rotor breaks. Such training can either be a part of the project itself or a component of another incentive program. Capacity building both in terms of energy planning and local technical training can be an essential step in that it can affect the long-term success of a project, but it does not make an otherwise uneconomic project a viable one on its own.

Australia's Bushlight program has used education and community energy planning to build local capacity. The Bushlight program focuses on solar photovoltaic systems. It was initiated by Australia's federal government in 1999 and was extended for an additional 4 years in July 2007. Bushlight is funded through the Renewable Remote Power Generation Program (RRPGP), which, in 2007 was awarded an additional AUD 123.5 million over 4 years. The program has a comprehensive approach to supporting the development of solar projects and their maintenance, and in assisting in overall community energy planning.

Bushlight uses incentives, direct technical assistance, and education to increase small remote indigenous communities' access to affordable, consistent, and reliable renewable energy services. The program is implemented as a quasi-commercial venture with the Centre for Appropriate Technology and has three objectives, notably to improve reliability, ensure indigenous communities have access to an integrated energy service network, and to build confidence in renewable energy systems among participants.[46]

Bushlight has been subject to boom/bust cycles based on federal government focus. The 2005 evaluation found that "Bushlight remains relevant against current federal government policies." However, the program has undergone numerous renewals as the initial funding covered a 4-year commitment, followed by a subsequent 2-year commitment and two 6-month extensions. Despite this funding uncertainty, the program has continued for over a decade.

In addition to providing grants for renewable energy projects, Bushlight directly addresses barriers that are specific to remote and rural communities by focusing appropriate technologies and maintenance agreements. It directly addresses the "softer" barriers such as lack of skilled labor or effort needed to understand technologies and process applications as well as providing training programs on installation and maintenance of the solar systems. The 2005 review of the Bushlight program recommended that Bushlight "extend its role in supporting the Regional Industry and technical capacity development, and in particular to consider opportunities for indigenous people" as well as noting that the approval process can be a "severe bottleneck" to project implementation. As of 2011, the Bushlight program provided ongoing support to 220 communities and 265 renewable energy systems. While aggregated data are not collected, summaries of over 120 projects illustrated as case studies ranged from community energy planning, to small solar installations for individual buildings, to full community energy projects.[47]

Mandating Generation Portfolios

Rather than finding support mechanisms to foster renewable energy systems, governments can simply mandate that they be implemented. A renewable portfolio standard is a common approach to mandating clean energy development and is simply a specified target of renewable electricity that needs to be delivered in a given jurisdiction. Targets can be voluntary, as was the case of Alberta,[48] or legally binding with associated penalties for failure to comply, as was the case in Nova Scotia.[49] While Alberta achieved its modest voluntary target in 2008, the proportion of renewable electricity was lower in both 2009 and 2010 than it was in 2008.[50] In Nova Scotia, the proportion of renewable electricity has continued to grow from 10 percent in 2009,[51] to 13 and 17 percent in 2010 and 2011, respectively.[52] The standard can be the minimum amount of electricity that must be provided as a portion of the total electricity sales or generation, or simply an installed capacity target (regardless of whether that capacity actually generates electricity). This approach is popular in the United States as well as in Australia. Jurisdictions often allow the trade of renewable energy credits so that companies that exceed their minimum requirements can choose to sell credits to companies that are below the standard that year.

For such a standard to work in remote Canadian communities, it would require that the quota be made specific to diesel-powered communities, as all provinces and territories with the exception of Nunavut have significant renewable energy systems (typically hydro), the production from which dwarfs the power consumed in remote communities. As such, it would be difficult to set a target that would spur development in remote communities because very small changes in the larger systems could more easily and more economically meet the target.

As a compliance mechanism for portfolio standards, or other climate change mitigation policies, emissions credits created for renewable energy projects can be sold in either mandated or voluntary markets. The ability to sell the offsets essentially monetizes the value of reducing emissions, effectively becoming an additional revenue stream for clean energy projects and an additional cost to polluting sources.

One difficulty that is particularly acute for the small populations and relatively small levels of overall pollution resulting from remote communities compared to large industries would be the relatively small amounts of credits that they could generate, and equally challenging would be the accounting and auditing of the credits themselves, which may outweigh the potential value of the credits themselves. One option that remote communities could pursue in such a system would be to bundle their respective credits in a similar way to what was allowed for small projects in the Kyoto Protocol's Clean Development Mechanism.[53]

POLICY RECOMMENDATIONS FOR CANADA'S REMOTE COMMUNITIES

Renewable energy systems in remote communities face unique barriers. These barriers include financial obstacles such as difficulty attracting investment capital, difficulty in fostering local project ownership, high capital costs, and small-scale production. Other development barriers include limited local human capacity as well as difficult planning logistics in remote communities. Even when there are policies to support or enable clean energy alternatives, such policies may have short life spans, limited resources, or be easily subject to cancellation due to political or fiscal pressures. Stability and certainty are important steps for any long-term industrial decision-making process. Many renewable energy policies have been in the form of budgetary incentives and are subject to continual review and potential renewal, thereby creating business development and growth uncertainty. Finally, the local government, developers, or provincial/federal governments may misunderstand aspects of a relatively new suite of renewable technologies.

Additionally, remote and rural communities with limited technical or financial capacity may particularly benefit from support for feasibility studies or community energy planning as a component of support.

Policies that provide incentives to develop locally owned projects help to keep the financial support in the community, ideally leading to respending of these benefits to other local businesses. It is also important to note that some rural or remote communities may not have the capacity to develop renewable energy projects, so if policies do not help to build that capacity, local ownership requirements might prove to be an impediment to project development rather than an incentive.

It is prudent to balance community economic benefits with environmental performance of technologies, since community-owned projects may be smaller in scale than facilities owned by large developers. However, recognizing and valuing the impacts of increased economic activity from community-owned renewable energy projects can serve as an important driver to develop policies that further incentivize renewable energy in rural communities that may be economically depressed or lack economic diversity.

Long-term and stable policies are needed for renewable energy programs in rural communities. This is a result of additional challenges that these communities face in attracting financing from outside or generating the financing from within. Long-term support helps reduce the apparent risk for potential project investors, while allowing projects to unfold at their own rate rather than struggling to meet looming deadlines, which can be difficult in remote communities, where projects may evolve at a slower pace.

Administrative assistance programs or policies may help communities on a range of aspects from system design to applying for federal funding to developing service agreements for maintenance of systems.

For remote communities to be successful in developing renewable energy projects, the policies that are put in place need to be specific to remote communities, and not simply part of overall provincial or federal programs; otherwise they will be overrun by larger, more lucrative projects.

Wind energy projects in Canada's northern, remote, and Aboriginal communities to date have not been able to benefit from federal power production incentive programs for wind energy because these incentive levels do not reflect the higher costs as well as other technical and nontechnical barriers in off-grid communities. While wind-diesel systems are increasingly being deployed globally, they remain rare in Canada despite its role as an early leader in research and deployment of the technology, while being home to close to 90 suitable communities.

Given the federal government's jurisdiction with respect to Aboriginal peoples as well as northern communities in Canada, it is appropriate that a federal policy framework be developed to assist in their development and deployment. Of the policy options available to the government, a combination of capital grants and production incentives can address two of the key barriers to deploying wind-diesel systems in Canada, notably capital as well as operations and maintenance costs.

In the past, many remote wind energy projects have focused on communities with the strongest local wind resource. Alaska has been successful in developing multiple remote community projects in large part because Kotzebue, a relatively large community, was among the first to develop a project and has been able to service many of the smaller surrounding communities. This is often described as a "hub-and-spoke" model. The NWT have tried to replicate this success by starting with the community of Tuktoyaktuk for their pilot project, even though it has the weakest wind resources of the four Beaufort communities. Tuktoyaktuk is the largest of the four communities, has significant technical capacity with offshore gas exploration in the region, and is the only community with winter road access. Local capacity to support such projects can significantly lower the operations and maintenance costs and increase local community pride in the project, compared with building, operating, and servicing the project solely from outside the community. Dowland Contracting Ltd was working with the community and the territorial government to complete this project and as of 2010 reported wind studies and environmental screening had been completed, and that foundation and electrical design, as well as power purchase agreements, were still outstanding.[54] At the time of writing this chapter, the project had not been built.

While there is an obvious temptation to optimize every individual project, specific equipment, such as wind turbine sizes can significantly alter overall project design. When looking at a project in isolation, one particular type of equipment might outperform one other. However, thinking regionally and using standard equipment can facilitate long-term parts availability and regional technician training.

Past federal incentive programs have focused on capital cost grants. Such mechanisms do not reward the long-term operations of renewable systems. In contrast, Ontario's FIT payments are for actual production and the now fully allocated federal ecoEnergy for Renewable Power Program was a successful production-based top-up. The ecoEnergy program resulted in over 4,500 MW of renewable energy installations across Canada in its 4 years of existence, while Ontario's FIT has contracted 4,600 MW of renewable energy in its first 2 years, representing over $20 billion in investment.[55] These programs ensure that incentives are tied to long-term efficient operation of systems. This is also an appropriate model for remote communities, as the diesel costs can vary significantly between communities based on accessibility and diesel plant sizes. Production-based top-ups would also recognize the inherent variability in electricity supply costs between different communities.

Remote community policy development needs to be cognizant of the fact that grant money alone will not likely succeed in deploying wind-diesel systems in Canada. Successful jurisdictions that have supported renewable power in remote and off-grid communities, notably Australia and Alaska, have had comprehensive community engagement and support structures that have been put in place in conjunction with monetary incentives. Prefeasibility and feasibility costs can be difficult for small communities who have limited understanding of these types of projects or limited resources for such a project.

Early adoption and strategic deployment of alternatives such as wind-diesel systems in remote Canadian communities will be increasingly important in enabling these communities to remain viable before price shocks or steady annual price increases force a more costly rapid technological deployment of systems that may not be as well field tested as they could have been through a more deliberate approach.

Many Canadian remote communities are disadvantaged economically and are also exposed to environmental and health risks as a result of reliance on imported diesel fuel to supply their energy needs. Strategically investing in sustainable energy sources will help mitigate environmental and social risks associated with continued reliance on rising fossil fuels. To quote Barring-Gould and Dabo, "the option of waiting for another 10 years to 'see how the technology matures' just guarantees that in 10 years, hundreds of diesel plants will have been installed or upgraded without consideration of alternatives, and little new information will have been gained."[56]

NOTES

1. K. Ah-You and G. Leng, *Renewable Energy in Canada's Remote Communities*, CETC Number 1999-26-27/1999-06-10, Natural Resources Canada, Accessed May 23, 2013 http://fnbc.info/sites/default/files/documents/Renewable%20Energy%20in%20Remote%20Communities.pdf

2. Power Equipment Department of Ontario Hydro (PEDOH), *Fort Severn Wind/Diesel Project* (Ottawa, Canada: The CANMET Energy Technology Centre, Energy Technology Branch, Energy Sector, Department of Natural Resources Canada, 1995).

3. J. Royer, Status of Remote/Off-Grid Communities in Canada, Natural Resources Canada, 2011, accessed July 2, 2013 http://canmetenergy.nrcan.gc.ca/renewables/smart-grid/publications/3213.

4. T. Weis and K. Zarowny, *Wapekeka First Nation Community Energy Map, 2005 Energy Baseline Study* (Toronto, Canada: The Pembina Institute, 2006).

5. P. Cobb and R. Wong, *Ontario Community Energy Baselines, Summary Report* (Toronto, Canada: The Pembina Institute, 2009).

6. R. Reid and J. P. Laflamme, *Case Study: High Penetration No Storage Wind-Diesel System For Inukjuak, Northern Quebec* (presentation, 1995 AWEA-CanWEA Wind-Diesel Workshop, Hanover, New Hampshire, June 5–7).

7. J. P. Pinard and T. M. Weis, *Pre-Feasibility Analysis of Wind Energy for Inuvialuit Region in Northwest Territories* (report, Aurora Research Institute, Inuvik, Northwest Territories, 2003).

8. T. M. Weis and T. Lambert, *Kyuquot Community Energy Planning: Long-Term Electrical Supply Options* (technical report, Ka:'yu:'k't'h'/Che:k:tles7et'h' NationKa:'yu:'k't'h'/Che:k:tles7et'h', The Pembina Institute and Mistaya Engineering, Toronto, Canada, 2004).

9. T. M. Weis and P. Cobb, *Aboriginal Energy Alternatives*, Pembina Institute, accessed May 1, 2013, http://www.pembina.org/pub/1850.

10. *Case Study: Biomass Heating Project*, RETScreen International, accessed May 1, 2013, http://www.retscreen.net/download.php/fi/79/3/BIOH03-C.pdf

11. *Sharing the Story: Sustainable Initiatives in First Nations*, Centre for Indigenous Environmental Relations, Accessed on May 23, 2013 http://www.broadwayarchitects.com/downloads/Sharing_the_Story_Sustainable_Initiatives_in_First_Nations_INAC.pdf

12. M. S. Chappell, *Program Report: Wind Energy Research and Development at the National Research Council of Canada 1975-1985*, (NRCC no. 27459, National Research Council of Canada, Division of Energy,Ottawa, Canada, 1986).
13. T. M. Weis and A. Ilinca, "The Utility of Energy Storage to Improve the Economics of Wind-Diesel Power Plants in Canada," *Renewable Energy* 33, no. 7 (2008): 1544–57.
14. *Canada reaches milestone as wind energy now produced in every province* press release, Canadian Wind Energy Association (CanWEA), accessed May 1, 2013, http://www.canwea.ca/media/release/release_e.php?newsId=70.
15. Cobb and Wong, *Ontario Community Energy...*
16. Assembly of First Nations, *Challenges to Implementing...*
17. C. P. Underwood et al., "Renewable-Energy Clusters for Remote Communities," *Applied Energy* 84 (2007): 579–98.
18. G. St. Denis and P. Parker, "Community Energy Planning in Canada: The Role of Renewable Energy," *Renewable and Sustainable Energy Reviews* 13 (2008): 2088–95.
19. Assembly of First Nations, *Challenges to Implementing...*
20. E. Martinot and O. McDoom, *Promoting Energy Efficiency and Renewable Energy: GEF Climate Change Projects and Impacts*, (Washington, DC: Global Environment Facility, 2000).
21. RETScreen Report on Canadian Remote Communities, Natural Resources Canada, CANMET-Varennes, Quebec, 1999.
22. Weis and Ilinca, "The Utility of Energy Storage..."
23. Martinot and McDoom, *Promoting Energy Efficiency...*
24. J. F. Maissan, *Wind Energy for Small Communities, Leading Edge Projects Inc.*, (report, Inuit Tapiriit Kanatami, Ottawa, Canada, 2006).
25. W. Carpenter (Alternative Energy Specialist, Department of Environment and Natural Resources, Government of the Northwest Territories), interview September 29, 2009.
26. J. F. Maisson, *Wind Power Development in Sub-Arctic Conditions with Severe Rime Icing* (presentation, Circumpolar Climate Change Summit and Exposition, Whitehorse, Yukon, March 19–21, 2001).
27. K. Keith, *Alaska High Penetration Wind Diesel Systems* (presentation, 2009 Wind-Diesel Workshop, The Pembina Institute, Ottawa, Canada), accessed May 1, 2013, http://www.pembina.org/docs/arctic/Wind-Diesel-1-Katherine%20Keith.pdf.
28. T. Laakso et al., *State-of-the-Art of Wind Energy in Cold Climates, International Energy Agency R&D Wind Programme Annex XIX*, Accessed May 23, 2013 http://arcticwind.vtt.fi/reports/StateOfTheArtOfColdClimatesWindEnergy2009-VTT-W152.pdf
29. M. Mendonça et al., "Stability, Participation and Transparency in Renewable Energy Policy: Lessons from Denmark and the United States," *Policy and Society* 27 (2009): 379–98.
30. B. Sovacool, "The Importance of Comprehensiveness in Renewable Electricity and Energy-Efficiency Policy," *Energy Policy* 37 (2009): 1529–41.
31. *Safe Drinking Water on First Nation Reserves: Roles and Responsibilities*, Indian and Northern Affairs Canada (INAC) in collaboration with Health Canada, accessed May 1, 2013, http://collection.nlc-bnc.ca/100/200/301/inac-ainc/safe_drinking_water-e/wqr_e.pdf, 5Sept05.
32. J. Lipp, "Lessons for Effective Renewable Electricity Policy from Denmark, Germany and the United Kingdom," *Energy Policy* 35 (2007): 5481–95.

33. *Sharing the Story – Aboriginal and Northern Energy Experiences: Energy Efficiency and Renewable Energy*, Indian and Northern Affairs Canada (INAC), accessed October 20, 2008, http://www.ainc-inac.gc.ca/clc/tp/shar_e.html

34. Centre for Indigenous Environmental Research, *Sharing Knowledge for a Better Future: Adaptation and Clean Energy Experiences in a Changing Climate* (summary report, Indian and Northern Affairs Canada, Ottawa, Canada, 2010).

35. Weis and Ilinca, "The Utility of Energy Storage…"

36. *Renewable Energy Fund Grant*, Alaska Energy Authority (AEA). accessed October 23, 2009, http://www.akenergyauthority.org/RE_Fund.html

37. M. Dabo, J. Jensen, and J. Smith, *Regional Economic Wind Development in Rural Alaska—Part I Technical Potential* (presentation, Arctic Energy Summit, Anchorage, Alaska, October 15-18, 2007).

38. I. Barring-Gould and M. Dabo, *Technology, Performance, and Market Report of Wind-Diesel Applications for Remote and Island Communities* (National Renewable Energy Paper NREL/CP-500-45810, Ottawa, Canada, 2009).

39. M. Mendonça, *Feed-in Tariffs. Accelerating the Deployment of Renewable Energy* (London, England: Earthscan, 2007).

40. P. Gipe, *Renewables Without Limits: Moving Ontario to Advanced Renewable Tariffs by Updating Ontario's Groundbreaking Standard Offer Program*, Ontario Sustainable Energy Association, accessed January 23, 2008, http://www.ontario-sea.org/Storage/22/1375_RenewablesWithoutLimits.pdf

41. *ecoENERGY for Renewable Power Program*, Natural Resources Canada, accessed March 20, 2012, http://www.ecoaction.gc.ca/ecoenergy-ecoenergie/power-electricite/index-eng.cfm

42. Northwest Territories Power Corporation, *Wind Generation in the Northwest Territories: Request for Proposals* (RFP no. 20804, Hay River, Northwest Territories, 2008).

43. St. Denis and Parker, "Community Energy Planning…"

44. Centre for Indigenous Environmental Research, *Sharing Knowledge…*

45. B. Lloyd, D. Lowe, and L. Wilson, *Renewable Energy in Remote Australian Communities* (Perth, Australia: Australian CRC for Renewable Energy, Murdoch University, 2000).

46. *Bushlight Evaluation Final Report* (ITP/Ref: A0004, IT Power), Bushlight, Accessed May 23, 2013 http://www.icat.org.au/wp-content/uploads/2012/05/BL-evaluationreport-2005.pdf

47. *Case Studies*, Bushlight Center for Appropriate Technology, accessed April 2, 2012, http://www.bushlight.org.au/default.asp?action=article&ID=38

48. Clean Air Strategic Alliance, *Renewable and Alternative Energy as a Source of Electricity in Alberta* (report to the CASA Board, Calgary, Alberta 2005).

49. Bill 146: Environmental Goals and Sustainable Prosperity Act, 60th Nova Scotia General Assembly, 1st Session, Royal Assent April 13, 2007.

50. *2010 Annual Market Statistics*, Alberta Electricity System Operator, accessed May 1, 2013, http://www.aeso.ca/downloads/2010_Annual_Market_Stats_Data_File.xls

51. *National Inventory Report 1990–2009, Greenhouse Gas Sources and Sinks in Canada Part 3* (Tables A13-1:A13-12), Environment Canada, accessed May 1, 2013, http://www.ec.gc.ca/Publications/A07097EF-8EE1-4FF0-9AFB-6C392078D1A9%5CNationalInventoryReportGreenhouseGasSourcesAndSinksInCanada199020 09ExecutiveSummary.pdf

52. *Q & A Fuel Mix Update*, Nova Scotia Power, accessed May 1, 2013, http://cleaner.nspower.ca/post/QA-Fuel-Mix-Update.aspx.

53. R. Peters, L-A. Roberson, and C. Brunt, *A User's Guide to the CDM- Clean Development Mechanism* (Drayton Valley, Canada: Pembina Institute, 2003).
54. J. Macgillivray, *Tuktoyaktuk Wind Farm* (proceedings, Canadian Wind Energy Association 2010 Annual Conference, Montreal, Canada, November 1-3, 2010).
55. F. Amin, *Ontario's Feed-in Tariff Program Building Ontario's Clean Energy Future Two-Year Review Report*, Accessed on May 23, 2013 http://www.energy.gov.on.ca/docs/en/FIT-Review-Report.pdf
56. Barring-Gould and Dabo, *Technology, Performance,...*

CHAPTER 13

Remote Indigenous Populations and Climate Change

Reducing the Impacts on Health and Well-Being

JAMES FORD AND PETER ADAMS

The global climate is changing and will continue to change even with policy intervention.[1,2,3,4] Research is only beginning to examine the potential health implications and indicates significant vulnerabilities. The World Health Organization (WHO) estimates that climate change could already be causing over 150,000 deaths and the loss of approximately 5 million disability-adjusted life years per year.[5] Costello et al. argue that climate change is the biggest health threat of the 21st century,[6] while the American Public Health Association and American Medical Association have publically drawn attention to the significant challenges posed by climate change.[7] Key risks include increasing exposure to infectious diseases, exacerbated water and food insecurity, natural disasters, and population displacement.[8,9,10]

Populations will be differentially vulnerable to climate change impacts. Those at highest risk include populations with an existing high burden of ill health, who are sensitive to climate-related health risks, and live in nations with limited technological capacity, weak institutions, high levels of poverty, and political inequality.[11,12] It is developing nations, particularly the least developed countries (LDCs) and small island developing states (SIDS), who are commonly believed to have the highest vulnerability, where climate change is expected to compromise progress toward meeting the Millennium Development Goals.[13] Recent studies have also indicated significant health vulnerabilities in developed nations.[14,15,16,17,18] Largely neglected in the literature on health and climate change, however, are indigenous populations.[19,20,21,22,23]

This research deficit leaves indigenous peoples often labeled as vulnerable to the health effects of climate change but with little information on the nature of this vulnerability. While there has been limited research on climate change and indigenous health, there is a substantial body of scholarship on indigenous health outcomes and determining factors, which will affect, to a large extent, vulnerability and resilience to climate change. This chapter uses this broader scholarship to identify the underlying factors that are likely to determine how climate change is experienced and responded to among remote indigenous populations. It is noteworthy that the extent to which these factors are relevant to specific populations will differ widely depending on geographic location, livelihood characteristics, history, socioeconomic-political conditions, and interaction with nonindigenous peoples and governance structures, reflected in differential vulnerability and resilience to climate change at regional to local levels. Our aim here then is not to generalize determinants of vulnerability across groups, but rather to document and categorize key factors identified as relevant in different contexts. Herein, and to complement the review and provide examples of how underlying determinants of vulnerability and adaptation might play out locally, recently completed fieldwork conducted with remote indigenous populations in the Arctic (Inuit), Peruvian Amazon (Shawi and Shipibo people), and Uganda (Batwa pygmies) is drawn upon.[24,25,26,27,28,29] These study locations capture the diversity of socio-cultural-economic and geographical contexts in which remote indigenous populations inhabit, providing examples from high-, middle-, and low-income nations. The identification of drivers of vulnerability is then used to explore opportunities for adaptation intervention. Specifically, we use examples of successful policy intervention in a general health/environment context to examine lessons for climate adaptation in remote indigenous communities.

DETERMINANTS OF VULNERABILITY

In this section, six factors that are likely to result in remote indigenous population being disproportionately vulnerable to the health effects of climate change are identified, noting these factors will differ widely at various scales.

Indigenous Livelihood Characteristics

Many indigenous populations face unique sensitivities to climate-related risks and climate change, a function of the close relationships with and dependence on land, sea, and natural resources, livelihoods, and culture. The scope for climate change to affect health, therefore, is much broader than altering the incidence and prevalence of disease, with risks profiles that often differ significantly from nonindigenous populations, and within and between indigenous groups.

First, food systems in remote regions are typically dual in nature, combining elements of traditional subsistence hunting, farming, and fishing, and the consumption of market foods. In dual food systems, food security is often highly climate dependent. Thus, for Arctic indigenous populations, the access and availability of traditional foods is linked to sea/lake ice conditions for access to hunting locations and the health and availability of wild animals. Compromised food security has already been documented due to a changing climate in Alaska, northern Canada, and Greenland.[30,31,32,33,34,35,36] As noted by a community member in Igloolik, Nunavut, one consequence is that "some people go without food for days...it really takes its toll when you cannot [get the traditional] food which to us is cheaper than [the] store [food]."[37]

Food quality is also sensitive to climate change, with consumption of raw meats increasing the risk of foodborne diseases associated with the storing and preparation of traditional foods (e.g., gastroenteritis, foodborne botulism), and zoonotic diseases (e.g., Giardia).[38,39] For Shawi and Shipibo populations in the Amazon, climatic conditions are important for subsistence agriculture, with regional warming documented. Warming trends have been linked to reduced yields, increased pests and weeds, with implications for local food availability and the ability to earn cash income. As reported by a community member in Panaillo, "My rice is yellowing (...) when the river flooded it brought sand rather than mud (...) I'm afraid I'll have [less food] this year."[40]

Secondly, in many instances, indigenous conceptualizations of health capture not just physical well-being but accord significant weight to interpersonal and environmental relationships, stewardship, life experience and balance, spiritual considerations, family, and oral history.[41,42,43,44,45,46,47] While a significant factor in underpinning indigenous adaptive capacity to changing environmental conditions, this broad conceptualization of health also increases the scope for climate change impacts. Thus, the loss of traditional plants and medicines, reduced access to hunting grounds, compromised food availability, weakening social networks, ability to engage in traditional activities—all of which have been linked to climate change in various indigenous contexts—could have significant ramifications for mental health. Indeed, in the Arctic and for Aboriginal Australians, mental health effects (depression, feelings of loss, anxiety) have already been documented and associated with cultural loss.[48,49,50,51,52] Concern is particularly acute where indigenous settlements and heritage sites are threatened by climate change impacts (e.g., low-lying coastal areas). In such instances, relocation could lead to an exacerbation of loss of culture and disconnection from the land, with implications for depression, anxiety, and substance abuse.[53,54]

Geography

Remote indigenous populations inhabit regions that are experiencing some of the most dramatic climate change. At a global scale, this is particularly pertinent in the Arctic and sub-Arctic, where temperatures are increasing at twice the global average and all models project accelerated change in the future.[55] The implications here of geography are magnified by the close relationship to the environment maintained by many Arctic indigenous populations.[56,57] At a regional scale, indigenous populations often inhabit high-risk areas, a function of historical patterns of settlement or relocation, sometimes forced, by the state to marginal environments. Australia's Aboriginal population in the Northern Territory faces a number of climatic exposures, including cyclones, flooding, and high temperature,[58,59,60,61,62] along with susceptibility to sea level rise and infectious diseases (e.g., dengue, Murray Valley encephalitis, malaria).[63,64] For Uganda's Batwa pygmies, location in marginal environments reflects eviction from their traditional forest homelands due to the creation of a national park, and into areas at high risk of malaria.[65,66] As Batwa community members reported: "Malaria is rampant here and all the time we are going to Kihembe clinic [for treatment]."[67]

Geography also affects adaptive capacity to manage changes in climate-related health outcomes. Remote populations by their very definition are difficult to reach (e.g., Amazonian communities that can only be accessed by boat or by walking, fly-in fly-out communities in the Arctic), and this creates significant challenges (and costs) for the provision of health care services, with implications for diagnosis, treatment, and provision of information—key activities for climate adaptation.[68]

Socioeconomic Disadvantage

Social and economic disadvantage are evident in significant health inequalities among many indigenous populations, which experience some of the highest rates of infant mortality, nutritional deficiency, and rates of infectious and parasitic disease globally, while access to education, housing, and employment are typically well below nonindigenous populations.[69,70] These conditions can increase sensitivity to climate-related health outcomes through a number of pathways, including forcing people to live in suboptimal conditions, engage in dangerous activities, live in areas of high risk, and engage in unhealthy behaviors. Inadequate water infrastructure common in many remote communities, for example, increases the likelihood of outbreaks of temperature-related waterborne diseases, including diarrheal disease and parasitic infections. The challenges are particularly pronounced in developing countries where water for household use is sourced directly and often untreated from local water sources, exposing individuals to waterborne pathogens, including leptospirosis, schisto-somiasis, and typhoid fever. While populations are typically aware of the risks posed, there are often few alternatives, and while boiling is important, research has indicated various barriers from lack of firewood to perceptions of taste. As noted by a Shipibo participant in a study in the Peruvian Amazon, "I know this water makes my baby sick, it's yellow and smells like iron, but we have no alter-native,"[71] and among Uganda's Batwa, "We have no clean water. We use the stag-nant water that kids play and bathe in. Every dry season it dries up and we must go somewhere else to fetch water. When that dries up, we go even further."[72]

Particularly in frontier zones being affected by rapid resource development, indigenous livelihoods and habitation characteristics are being transformed rapidly, with implications for sensitivity to climate-related health outcomes. Among Uganda's Pygmy communities, eviction from traditional forest lands to high-density fixed settlements with poor sanitation and limited access to water has increased exposure and sensitivity to climate-related risks that could be exacerbated by climate change, including malaria and parasitic infec-tions.[73,74,75] In the Amazon, a resurgence of hydrocarbon-related resource development and deforestation is challenging access to and ownership of traditional lands, introducing new diseases and creating conditions for the spread of existing diseases, which have a strong link to climate (e.g., dengue, malaria, leishmaniasis, cholera).[76,77,78,79,80]

Socioeconomic disadvantage also translates to affecting adaptive capacity of indigenous communities and their health systems to prevent, prepare for, and manage climate-related health risks. Indigenous populations in poorer nations face substantial challenges herein, particularly in remote regions experiencing significant resource development pressure. In the Peruvian Amazon, deforestation is resulting in loss of medicinal plants, while indus-trial development in general is an additional stress on fish resources impor-tant in local subsistence and water quality. For the Batwa, health systems and social relationships were fundamentally transformed when they were evicted from their traditional forest homes in the 1990s. Transitioning to an agricul-tural way of life has been challenging, with associated acculturation linked to problems of addiction, suicide, and a weakening of social networks and tradi-tional health knowledge, which underpin adaptive capacity.[81,82] The erosion and in some case loss of traditional knowledge is a concern that transcends many remote indigenous populations and will have significant implications for future generations as they experience and respond to changing conditions.

Political Inequality

Remote indigenous populations face unique political challenges to achieving a range of social, economic, environmental, and health goals, with implications for sensitivity and adaptive capacity to climate change effects on health. Inequality is evident in the neglect of indigenous rights globally, which in developed nations and also some developing nations (e.g., Peru) are protected in theory by the state and international human rights (e.g., UN Charter of Human Rights, UN Declaration on the Rights of Indigenous Populations).[83] The reality is often somewhat different, as evidenced by the marginalization often faced by indigenous populations to outright land eviction. The Batwa in Uganda, for instance, were evicted from their traditional lands to make way for a wildlife reserve, while in North America lands were expropriated during colonization and legal title to large areas of traditional territory was extinguished.

Political inequality links to climate change vulnerability in a number of ways. First, political inequality—ranging from exclusion in decision making, to historical injustices surrounding land expropriation, to failure of nations to recognize the special rights of indigenous peoples, to discrimination—has been linked to a range of negative social, economic, and health outcomes, which increase sensitivity to climate change.[84,85] Illegal logging is a major issue faced by Shipibo peoples in the Amazon. As noted by a community member in Hofmeijer's study, "Illegal loggers steal our big trees from our territory (...) we are going to run out of medicinal trees (...) our children won't be able to recognize the different species, all they see is [a medicinal tree with no commercial value]."[86] Among Uganda's Batwa, concentration on small plots of land and lack of legal title are major challenges: "We continuously dig on the same land, so it gets exhausted. We have small portions of land and the crops don't grow very well."[87]

Second, inequality reduces the political power of indigenous populations to draw attention to pressing issues and develop interventions to manage emerging threats, including climate change. This is evident in the neglect of indigenous issues in research and lack of international research programs focusing on indigenous health in a changing climate.[88] It is also evident in climate policy debates internationally where indigenous issues, up until recently, have been overlooked in negotiations, and at a national level where specific programs for indigenous adaptation are lacking.[89,90]

Institutional Capacity

Indigenous health systems are frequently composed of multiple institutions, including formally provided health care through the state and/or nongovernmental organizations, and informal traditional health networks. These institutions are important for health prevention, preparedness, and response, particularly during times of change, and are essential for moderating the effects of climate change. Concerns have already been noted regarding the weakening of traditional knowledge systems, which could result in the loss of a highly localized and specialized knowledge base essential for adaptation.

As voiced by a Shipibo community member in Peru: "The children don't know about our trees and their spirits, all they see in the community is [a medicinal tree with no commercial value] and that is the only tree they recognize (...) kids don't know big trees like lupuna. When I was a child, our grandfathers told us that only the juice of the lupuna could be taken, cutting the tree would kill someone. (...) but the teachers don't know our stories and the kids don't learn."[91]

This is compounded by the challenges allopathic health provision experiences across remote indigenous populations. In developed nations, for example, the cost of servicing remote regions, lack of personnel, difficulties of providing culturally appropriate care and advice, and conflicting health jurisdictions all present serious challenges for providing the kind of health servicing provided to nonindigenous populations. In the Canadian Arctic, for instance, most communities only have a nursing station and require individuals to travel to regional centers or down south for more advanced diagnosis and treatment, necessitating time away from family and community. In low- and middle-income nations the challenges are more acute, ranging from outright absence of health services, vagaries in support dependent upon aid or other resource challenges, constraints of accessing health services from remote and/or inaccessible locations, to discrimination and sometimes oppression through the allopathic health system. In Amazonian communities, for instance, while some communities will have nursing stations, they are only in operation periodically, with enhanced services demanded locally.[92]

These challenges have direct implications for sensitivity and adaptive capacity to climate change because local capacity is important for identifying and managing risks: evidence from multiple contexts has shown that well-developed local health capacity increases the likelihood that policies and actions will be appropriate, effective, and acceptable.[93,94] Difficulty in recruiting and retaining human health resources has been widely noted among indigenous populations in developed nations.[95,96,97,98] High staff turnover has been noted to present barriers to developing relationships with community members and stakeholders and creates problems for basic service delivery with employees often overworked and fatigued, key positions vacant, and inexperienced personnel undertaking responsibilities for which they do not have the necessary training or expertise. In this context, action on climate change is often undermined by other priorities, dependent on personnel, subject to sudden change, with long-term planning often absent.

If the health of indigenous peoples is to be improved, with sensitivity to climate change reduced and adaptive capacity enhanced, there is a need to build health systems that work well and provide adequate health education.[99] In developed nations, policy discussion has focused on numerous ways to address institutional problems, including resolving land claims, consolidating fragmented funding, adapting health programs to local priorities, giving indigenous people a direct voice in health planning, making indigenous health the responsibility of provincial and territorial governments, and increasing self-reliance.[100,101,102,103] The increase in self-government, self-determination, and community-level health initiatives reported in many developed nations is indicative of progress being made. In developing nations the needs are more basic, and in many instances they reflect the need for primary local health care facilities in remote regions where indigenous populations live, providing medical care and advice targeted to the needs of local populations, and giving populations secure title to their traditional lands.

Information Deficit

As Fankhuaser and Tol note, "Successful adaptation requires a recognition of the necessity to adapt, knowledge about available options, the capacity to assess them, and the ability to implement most suitable ones."[104] Without such information, anticipatory interventions are less likely. Vulnerability and adaptation assessments are an important first step herein, yet for many indigenous populations they have not been conducted. Few international research programs or specific funds are directed toward indigenous populations through the international climate regime or international bodies. This likely reflects the fact that indigenous peoples as subnational groups are not explicitly referred to in the text of the United Nations Framework Convention on Climate Change (UNFCCC) or recent Copenhagen Accord. Addressing this research deficit is a priority for identifying key health risks in a changing climate for indigenous populations and necessary policy interventions.

HOW CAN THESE DETERMINANTS OF VULNERABILITY BE ADDRESSED?

Given the inevitability of some degree of future climate change and experience of changing conditions today, adaptation has become an important component of climate policy alongside mitigation,[105,106] where adaptation refers to efforts to reduce or moderate vulnerability to climate change and take advantage of new opportunities.[107] Identifying determinants of vulnerability is an important step for adaptation, and the previous section outlines at a general level key socioeconomic-political conditions and processes that offer entry points for intervention. In this section we draw upon examples of successful policy interventions designed to address general health and environment concerns affecting remote indigenous communities, with the aim of identifying key considerations and opportunities for future adaptation action.

Intervention Case Studies

"Caring for Country" Projects to Enhance the Health of Aboriginal Australians

The social, physical, and emotional well-being of Aboriginal Australians is intricately tied to "country," a multidimensional concept that includes "people, animals, plants, Dreamings...earth, soils, minerals, waters, air."[108] Yet similar to many remote indigenous populations, historic disenfranchisement has limited their access to the land with negative ramifications for community health, and it has been linked to a significantly higher morbidity and mortality among Aboriginal peoples compared to European Australians. Land dispossession has also had environmental implications, as Aboriginal populations have less opportunity to care for the country. This ancient relationship encompasses many practical ecological services, including control of invasive weeds and feral animals, wildfire management, water management, and conservation. The loss of these services has had a growing impact on Australian ecosystems and species, which is being exacerbated by climate change.

To address the health concerns associated with a loss of traditional linkages to the land, communities and researchers have called for initiatives to address this. Such calls mirror similar developments in the Canadian Arctic, where the teaching of traditional hunting skills has been identified as essential for enhancing well-being and climate adaptation.[109] In this context, Burgess investigated whether increasing caring for country opportunities for Aboriginal Australians was associated with improved health outcomes.[110] Their cross-sectional study involved ~300 subjects, and tracked a wide range of health indicators and social behaviors in the cohort for over 2 years. During this period, individuals were given opportunities to participate in six core "caring for country" activities: time on country; burning of annual grasses; gathering of food and medicinal resources; ceremony; protecting sacred areas; and producing artwork. Results indicated significant and substantial associations between caring for country and health outcomes, including lower body mass index, less diabetes, lower systolic blood pressure, and better diet,[111] with the intervention enhancing livelihoods, tackling socioeconomic disadvantage by strengthening cultural, traditional and social networks, and increasing local decision-making power. In this way, it is hoped that the intervention will strengthen communities to manage the health effects of climate change.

Traditional Knowledge to Protect Soils and Watersheds in Coastal Honduras

Coastal Honduras is a region highly vulnerable to hurricanes, an increasing number of which have been recorded in recent decades, and which could increase in magnitude and frequency with future climate change.[112] Crops in coastal regions are affected by these storms, which can destroy harvests and erode topsoil, exacerbated by unsustainable land use activities, including slash-and-burn agriculture and deforestation. In this context, indigenous Honduran farmers are organizing communities and mobilizing local resources to favor more sustainable land use practices, reducing reliance on slash-and-burn techniques and large-scale industrial agriculture, to focus on traditional Quezungal farming systems that involve planting crops under trees whose roots anchor the soil, pruning vegetation to provide nutrients to the soil and conserve soil water, and terracing to reduce soil erosion.[113] Farmers are also organizing community-based agricultural research teams that are finding ways to diversify the genetic resources of their crops and develop hardier plant varieties that grow well on their soils.[114] While these interventions are not intended to address future climate change impacts, by reducing vulnerability to present-day climatic risks they can serve to moderate sensitivity and enhance adaptive capacity to manage future changes.

Adopting indigenous Quezungal techniques has saved crops and preserved topsoil in recent hurricanes, seen, for example, during Hurricane Mitch in 1998 when those villages adopting such land management approaches were considerably less affected.[115] These successes—based on the mobilization of local decision making, leveraging of traditional knowledge, and confrontation of historic inequalities—have been recognized and are now being actively shared with other communities in Honduras and beyond by the national government and the FAO.[116] Over a decade after this initiative began, Honduras has seen the regeneration of 60,000 ha of secondary forest, improved topsoil quality, and better crop yields.[117] Similarly, efforts to increase genetic variation have resulted in improved varieties of maize that are capable of withstanding the physical trauma brought by the hurricanes.

Artificial Glacier Cultivation to Manage Water Scarcity in Himalayan India

The glacier-dependent Ladakh region in Himalayan India—inhabited largely by ethnic Tibetans—is facing rapid depletion of water supply as glaciers recede and demand for water increases with warming temperatures. This is having implications for subsistence farming activities, which rely on water diverted by a network of irrigation channels, and is projected to accelerate in the future with climate change. In this context, the ancient practice of harvesting melt-water and collecting it in artificial glaciers is being revived as a modern adaptation. These frozen reservoirs are built above villages by diverting natural stream flow from glacial melt across depressed, shadowed valleys. In the fall, water accumulates behind dams, gates, and other scattered obstacles (often rock or wood debris), freezing in patches, which naturally accumulate and grow into a larger ice body. Cultivated "glaciers" then melt in the spring, with runoff channeled downstream into the town and toward fields using existing narrow rock canals.[118] These artificial glaciers can be cultivated year by year, continuing to naturally extend and provide an ongoing source of water. In Leh, the largest city in Ladakh, 10 artificial glaciers have been created so far, with more under construction. On average each provides enough water to irrigate 250 acres, or enough for about 200 families,[119] and represents a low-cost response to changing water availability built upon traditional practices, increasing adaptive capacity to manage changing hydrological regimes.

Managing Health Risks in the Swinomish Indian Reservation

The Swinomish Indian Reservation is located on an island near Puget Sound in the northwestern United States. This small, coastal community faces a wide array of climate-related health problems, both directly through exposure to natural hazards (such as flooding and heat waves) and indirectly through the weakened connection between spiritual well-being and the environment. For the Swinomish, health is measured at the community rather than at the individual level, where it "consist[s] of inseparable strands of human health, ecological health, and cultural health woven together, all equally important."[120] This increases the scope for climate change and other stresses to affect health, and the reservation is believed to be particularly vulnerable to climate change due to higher than average levels of accidental injuries, substance abuse, hypertension, obesity, and diabetes,[121] with heat-related illnesses and food insecurity identified as key potential future impacts.

Working with the University of Washington and local stakeholders, the Swinomish Indian Tribal Community led an extensive, multiyear Climate Change Initiative that examined current and future impacts of climate change, applying risk management techniques to establish funding priorities and address points of vulnerability.[122] Though co-run by community members, further Swinomish participation was solicited through regular community consultations and extensive outreach campaigns. After climate vulnerabilities were identified, an adaptation action plan was developed that ranked each problem's impact and likelihood and offered direct responses to each, many of which are already under way. Increased temperatures and heat wave events are being countered with public education campaigns, a heat alert warning system, construction of community cooling centers, and retrofitting old houses and designing new houses to use passive cooling systems. Concerns over toxins in shellfish (an important local food) with rising temperatures are being addressed through the promotion of traditional knowledge on food safety, and development of upland aquaculture where conditions can be controlled and shellfish can be cultivated as traditional sources become unsafe. As such, the project used principles of community-based participatory research to engage and empower local people to understand and prepare for climate impacts, addressing a lack of knowledge on climate vulnerability and altering livelihood conditions to moderate sensitivity.

The Xeni Gwet'in Community-Based Adaptation Plan

Located in British Columbia, Canada, the Xeni Gwet'in live in one of the few intact ecosystems on the east side of the Chilcotin Mountains. This small indigenous community is affected by a number of climate-related risks, including forest fires, and it is dependent on climate-sensitive resources for its livelihood and cultural well-being, including fisheries and forestry.[123] Recognizing these current and future challenges, the community commissioned a study to identify impacts and potential adaptations to climate change. Numerous scientific experts and a sustainable development consulting firm were brought in to the community to discuss climatology, forestry, hydrology, public health, and economics, comparing their insights and forecasts with the local observations and concerns of the community.[124] Adaptation recommendations were jointly made by planners, scientists, and community members to address several immediate and long-term concerns in conservation, livelihoods, infrastructure, health, and safety. Several of these recommendations have been implemented since the plan was created, with fire protection built around homes and water conservation initiatives developed. Education programs have also worked toward heightening household water conservation, and there has been increased research into stream and groundwater restoration. Strategies directed at improving food security and strengthening food self-sufficiency include the building of a community greenhouse, training in gardening and food preservation, along with agricultural diversification. All of these strategies have been implemented with the full support of the community and integrate traditional knowledge and community forums in planning and implementation processes.

Case Study Lessons for Adaptation

A number of lessons can be drawn from these examples with regard to adaptation to climate change in remote indigenous communities, including both the process of policy development and the nature of interventions.

First, outside facilitation and/or expertise may be necessary, and in some cases desirable, to initiate adaptation planning where there is limited institutional and financial capacity at a local level. In such cases, the earlier examples indicate that success is most likely when policy development occurs through a process of continuous engagement of community members and local stakeholders, with the aim of building local ownership. Without local owner-ship and buy-in, and in absence of formal planning mechanisms, adaptations are unlikely to be adopted. Even in cases where interventions are locally led, multiple forms of outreach, education, and capacity building were identified as important for success.

Second, incorporating traditional indigenous cultural values, practices, and knowledge were consistently identified as essential for intervention suc-cess. As the Australian "care for country" project highlighted, interventions based on traditional values are essential not only for improving health and environmental management, but they can also help empower communities in the context of a history of disenfranchisement and colonialism, key drivers of climate change vulnerability. Interventions based on traditional knowledge not only build upon and leverage detailed place-based knowledge developed and tested over generations but are also cost effective. In the Honduran exam-ple, for instance, adoption of traditional farming practices to conserve soil resources and fertility has been more effective and cheaper than moderating the impacts of land management practices through the application of chemi-cal fertilizers. In the Himalayan example, the cultivation of glaciers offers an alternative to centralized water management systems involving dam con-struction. The value of traditional knowledge for adaptation is increasingly recognized in the climate change scholarship, although less so among interna-tional and national bodies providing adaptation financing.[125,126,127]

Third, science can play a central role in helping communities address prob-lems and plan for climate change. Indeed, many of the examples documented earlier integrated scientific insights to identify future challenges, enhance planning, and evaluate the success of policy interventions. In some cases sci-entists were invited by communities to participate; in other cases scientists initiated the projects. For both cases, the process through which research-ers work with communities is essential, with principles of community-based participatory research essential to building trust, interest, and understand-ing in science.[128] Herein, understanding local attitudes and experience with planning is a fundamental consideration for policy intervention when out-side led. In some instances, for example, there is distrust of researchers and government given past (and even current) links to colonialism and parachute research practices, while local notions of planning and intervention may dif-fer considerably from Western notions.[129] Failure to reconcile these challenges is likely to limit the effectiveness of adaptation interventions, and it further highlights the importance of allowing ample time for facilitators to be present in the community, build relationships, and learn about local conditions.

Fourth, these examples highlight the importance of linking policy to present-day challenges facing communities, particularly given the high bur-den of ill health already experienced and other pressing issues. This is per-tinent in a climate change context where adaptation policy has tended to be framed in terms of avoided future impacts,[130] typically using timescales used in climate modeling (e.g., 2020, 2050, 2080). Framed in this way, adaptation would likely have limited local interest and buy-in, and emphasizes the importance of "normalization" or "mainstreaming" of adaptation where interventions are linked to present-day processes and planning.[131]

DISCUSSION

This chapter utilizes the indigenous health scholarship and recently completed pilot research to identify the upstream or distal processes and conditions that are likely to affect the vulnerability and adaptability of remote indigenous populations to the health effects of climate change. Clearly there are a lot of gaps in understanding, and developing a greater knowledge of the nature of health vulnerabilities and opportunities for intervention should be a priority for future research. This is beginning to be recognized. At a global level, the WHO and UN Permanent Forum on Indigenous Peoples have noted the special needs of indigenous populations in a changing climate. A UN-organized meeting was also held in summer 2011 and aimed to inform the IPCC on indigenous issues, which have been neglected in previous assessments.[132] These developments are to be welcomed, but they need to be complemented by the development of a global workplan by a relevant international organization designed to tackle the indigenous health vulnerability deficit. The engagement of indigenous populations and their organizations in driving the research agenda at global to local levels is essential to this end.

There is evidence from some developed nations that indigenous health is beginning to be prioritized in climate change research initiatives.[133] In Canada, for instance, the Indigenous Health Adaptation to Climate Change project (http://www.ihacc.ca) represents a 5-year investment by the federal government to examine indigenous health and climate change in remote regions as part of the IRIACC initiative. The federal government, through the department of Aboriginal Affairs and Northern Development and Health Canada, has also supported research projects on climate change adaptation. These include funds targeted directly at communities to assess their vulnerabilities, build local capacity, and begin to integrate climate change into their long-term planning.[134,135] Some of these projects have developed formal adaptation plans, usually targeted at enhancing community sustainability in general in light of climate change. Other projects have sought to strengthen community adaptive capacity in general to manage risks, including but not limited to climate change.

While more research is needed to understand the vulnerability of indigenous health systems to climate change to inform adaptation policy development, this should not be used as a cover for inaction. This chapter highlights how the underlying determinants of indigenous vulnerability to climate change are linked to ongoing social, economic, cultural, and political factors, many of which are not climate related but nevertheless determine sensitivity and adaptive capacity to changing conditions. Many of these stresses have to be understood within the marginalized context in which many indigenous populations find themselves, including lack of secure land title, forced acculturation, lack of political voice, land expropriation, limited self-determination, and discrimination in access to state-supplied services. As such, these inequalities can be tackled by policy interventions in ways we know how; failure to do so reflects political factors at international to local levels. Progress toward addressing these broader factors is slow, but the adoption of the United Nations Declaration on the Right of Indigenous Peoples by the UN General Assembly, the rising political voice of indigenous peoples globally, and progress in land claims negotiations in developed nations indicate that change is happening. Climate change may provide additional impetus toward the recognition of indigenous rights, with indigenous issues prominent in UNFCCC meetings.

While addressing these broader challenges is important for improving indigenous well-being in general, there are opportunities for communities to plan for adaptation. Indeed, many are already doing so. Herein, the experience of policy intervention in a general health/environment context holds a number of important lessons about the process of policy development. The examples reviewed here indicate that central to success has been community leadership and engagement in identifying opportunities for intervention, the identification of responses based on traditional knowledge and local cultural values, linking policy to present-day problems, and integrating science through local collaboration.

NOTES

1. J. Rogelj et al., "Analysis of the Copenhagen Accord Pledges and Its Global Climatic Impacts-A Snapshot of Dissonant Ambitions," *Environmental Research Letters* 5, no. 3 (2010): 034013.
2. M. Parry, J. Lowe, and C. Hanson, "Overshoot, Adapt and Recover," *Nature* 458, no. 7242 (2009): 1102–3.
3. M. New et al., "Four Degrees and Beyond: The Potential for a Global Temperature Increase of Four Degrees and Its Implications," introduction, *Philosophical Transactions of the Royal Society a-Mathematical Physical and Engineering Sciences* 369, no. 1934 (2011): 6–19.
4. H. M. Fussel, "An Updated Assessment of the Risks from Climate Change Based on Research Published Since the IPCC Fourth Assessment Report," *Climatic Change* 97, nos. 3–4 2009): 469–82.
5. A. McMichael et al, "Climate Change," in *Comparative Quantification of Health Risks: Global and Regional Burden of Disease Due to Selected Major Risk Factors*,

eds. M. Ezzati et al. (Geneva, Switzerland: World Health Organization, 2004), 1543–1649.

6. A. Costello et al., "Managing the Health Effects of Climate Change," *Lancet* 373 (2009): 1693–733.

7. G. Watts, "Leaders of US Medicine Speak Out on Health Effects of Climate Change," *British Medical Journal* 342 (2011): d1339.

8. S. S. Myers and J. A. Patz, "Emerging Threats to Human Health from Global Environmental Change," *Annual Review of Environment and Resources* 34 (2009): 223–52.

9. Costello et al., "Managing the Health Effects..."

10. U. Confalonieri et al., "Human Health," in *Climate Change 2007: Impacts, Adaptation and Vulnerability. Working Group II contribution to the Fourth Assessment Report of the Intergovernmental Panel on Climate Change*, eds. M. Parry et al. (Cambridge, England: Cambridge University Press, 2007), 391–431.

11. Costello et al., "Managing the Health Effects..."

12. S. C. Walpole, K. Rasanathan, and D. Campbell-Lendrum, "Natural and Unnatural Synergies: Climate Change Policy and Health Equity," *Bulletin of the World Health Organization* 87, no. 10 (2009): 799–801.

13. S. Friel et al., "Global Health Equity and Climate Stabilisation: A Common Agenda," *Lancet* 372, no. 9650 (2008): 1677–83.

14. K. Ebi et al., *Regional Impacts of Climate Change: Four Case Studies in the United States,* ed. E. Claussen (report, The Pew Center on Global Climate Change, Arlington, VA (2007).

15. K. L. Ebi, "Public Health Responses to the Risks of Climate Variability and Change in the United States," *Journal of Occupational and Environmental Medicine* 51, no. 1 (2009): 4–12.

16. R. S. Kovats and K. L. Ebi, "Heatwaves and Public Health in Europe," *European Journal of Public Health* 16, no. 6 (2006): 592–9.

17. S. Hajat, M. O'Connor, and T. Kosatsky, "Health Effects of Hot Weather: From Awareness of Risk Factors to Effective Health Protection," *Lancet* 375, no. 9717 (2010): 856–63.

18. J. D. Ford and L. Berrang-Ford, *Climate Change Adaptation in Developed Nations: From Theory to Practice* (Dordrecht, The Netherlands: Springer, 2011).

19. J. Salick and N. Ross, "Traditional Peoples and Climate Change Introduction," *Global Environmental Change-Human and Policy Dimensions* 19, no. 2 (2009): 137–9.

20. J. Trostle, "Anthropology Is Missing: On the World Development Report 2010: Development and Climate Change," *Medical Anthropology* 29, no. 3 (2010): 217–25.

21. M. Macchi, *Indigenous and Traditional Peoples and Climate Change* (Gland, Switzerland, issues paper, International Union for Conservation of Nature: 2008).

22. J. Salick and A. Byg, *Indigenous Peoples and Climate Change* (Oxford, England: Tyndall Centre for Climate Change Research, 2007).

23. J. D. Ford et al., "Climate Change Policy Responses for Canada's Inuit Population: The Importance of and Opportunities for Adaptation," *Global Environmental Change* 20 (2010): 177–91.

24. S. Harper, *"Green Christmas, Full Graveyard": Government and Community Identified Climate Change and Health Priorities in Nunatsiavut, Canada* (report supporting the development of the IHACC Research Program, University of Guelph, Canada, 2010).

25. K. Dingle, *"Our health needs a health environment": Community Identified Climate Change and Health Priorities among the Batwa of Uganda* (report supporting the development of the IHACC Research Program, McGill University, Montreal, Canada, 2010).

26. I. Hofmeijer, *"The Lakes are Drying and the Fish are Scarce": Community Identified Climate Change and Health Priorities in Panaillo* (report supporting the development of the IHACC Research Program, McGill University, Montreal, Canada, 2010).

27. L. Berrang-Ford et al., "Vulnerability of Indigenous Health to Climate Change: A Case Study of Uganda's Batwa Pygmies," *Social Science and Medicine (1982)* 75, no. 6 (2012): 1067–77.

28. I. Hofmeijer et al., "Community Vulnerability to the Health Effects of Climate Change Among Indigenous Populations in the Peruvian Amazon: A Case Study from Panaillo and Nuevo Progreso," *Mitigation and Adaptation Strategies for Global Change* (2012): doi 10.1007/s11027-012-9402-6.

29. M. Sherman et al., "Balancing Indigenous Principles and Institutional Research Guidelines for Informed Consent: A Case Study from the Peruvian Amazon," *American Journal of Bioethics: Primary Research* 3, no. 4 (2012): 53–68.

30. M. Beaumier and J. Ford, "Food Insecurity among Inuit Females Exacerbated by Socio-Economic Stresses and Climate Change," *Canadian Journal of Public Health* 101, no. 3 (2010): 196–201.

31. J. D. Ford, "Dangerous Climate Change and the Importance of Adaptation for the Arctic's Inuit Population," *Environmental Research Letters* 4, no. 2 (2009):024006.

32. J. D. Ford and M. Beaumier, "Feeding the Family during Times of Stress: Experience and Determinants of Food Insecurity in an Inuit Community," *Geographic Journal* 177, no. 1 (2011): 44–61.

33. C. Furgal, D. Martin, and P. Gosselin, "Climate Change and Health in Nunavik and Labrador," in *The Earth is Faster Now: Indigenous Observations of Climate Change*, eds. I. Krupnik and D. Jolly (Fairbanks, AK: Arctic Research Consortium of the United States, 2002), 266–300.

34. C. M. Furgal and J. Seguin, "Climate Change, Health and Community Adaptive Capacity: Lessons from the Canadian North," *Environmental Health Perspectives* 114, no. 12 (2006): 1964–70.

35. T. L. Nancarrow and H. C. Chan, "Observations of Environmental Changes and Potential Dietary Impacts in Two Communities in Nunavut, Canada," *Rural Remote Health* 10, no. 2 (2010): 1370.

36. C. Goldhar, J. Ford, and L. Berrang-Ford, "Prevalence of Food Insecurity in a Greenlandic Community and the Importance of Socio-Economic-Environmental Stressors," *International Journal of Circumpolar Health* 69, no. 3 (2010): 285–303.

37. J. D. Ford, "Vulnerability of Inuit Food Systems to Food Insecurity as a Consequence of Climate Change: A Case Study from Igloolik, Nunavut," *Regional Environmental Change* 9, no. 2 (2009): 83–100.

38. A. J. Parkinson and J. C. Butler, "Potential Impacts of Climate Change on Infectious Diseases in the Arctic," *International Journal of Circumpolar Health* 64, no. (2005): 478–86.

39. A. J. Parkinson and B. Evengard, "Climate Change, Its Impact on Human Health in the Arctic and the Public Health Response to Threats of Emerging Infectious Diseases," *Glob Health Action* 2 (2009).

40. Hofmeijer et al., "Community Vulnerability to the Health Effects..."

41. D. Pedersen and V. Baruffati, "Health and Traditional Medicine Cultures in Latin-America and the Caribbean," *Social Science and Medicine* 21, no. 1 (1985): 5–12.
42. Ibid.
43. M. King, A. Smith, and M. Gracey, "Indigenous Health Part 2: The Underlying Causes of the Health Gap," *Lancet* 374, no. 9683 (2009): 76–85.
44. M. Gracey and M. King, "Indigenous Health Part 1: Determinants and Disease Patterns," *Lancet* 374, no. 9683 (2009): 65–75.
45. R. A. Montenegro and C. Stephens, "Indigenous Health 2—Indigenous Health in Latin America and the Caribbean," *Lancet* 367, no. 9525 (2006): 1859–69.
46. C. Stephens et al., "Indigenous Health 4—Disappearing, Displaced, and Undervalued: A Call to Action for Indigenous Health Worldwide," *Lancet* 367, no. 9527 (2006): 2019–28.
47. C. A. M. Richmond and N. A. Ross, "The Determinants of First Nation and Inuit Health: A Critical Population Health Approach," *Health and Place* 15, no. 2 (2009): 403–11.
48. H. Berry, "Pearl in the Oyster: Climate Change as a Mental Health Opportunity," *Australasian Psychiatry* 17, no. 6 (2009): 453–6.
49. H. L. Berry, K. Bowen, and T. Kjellstrom, "Climate Change and Mental Health: A Causal Pathways Framework," *International Journal of Public Health* 55, no. 2 (2010): 123–32.
50. H. L. Berry et al., "Mind, Body, Spirit: Co-Benefits for Mental Health from Climate Change Adaptation and Caring for Country in Remote Aboriginal Australian Communities," *New South Wales Public Health Bulletin* 21, no. 6 (2010): 139–45.
51. J. Kellogg et al., "Alaskan Wild Berry Resources and Human Health under the Cloud of Climate Change," *Journal of Agricultural and Food Chemistry* 58 (2010): 3884–900.
52. A. Consolo-Willox et al., "'The Land Enriches Our Soul:' On Environmental Change, Affect, and Emotional Health and Well-Being in Nunatsiavut, Canada," *Emotion, Space and Society* 6 (2013): 14–24.
53. J. J. Hess, J. N. Malilay, and A. J. Parkinson, "Climate Change: The Importance of Place," *American Journal of Preventive Medicine* 35, no. 5 (2008): 468–78.
54. S. Kvernmo and S. Heyerdahl, "Acculturation Strategies and Ethnic Identity as Predictors of Behavior Problems in Arctic Minority Adolescents," *Journal of the American Academy of Child and Adolescent Psychiatry* 42, no. 1 (2003): 57–65.
55. IPCC, *Climate Change 2007: The Physical Science Basis* (contribution of Working Group I to the Fourth Assessment Report of the Intergovernmental Panel on Climate Change, Geneva, Switzerland, 2007).
56. ACIA, *Arctic Climate Impacts Assessment*. Cambridge, England: Cambridge University Press, 2005.
57. J. D. Ford et al., "Climate Change in the Arctic: Current and Future Vulnerability in Two Inuit Communities in Canada," *Geographical Journal* 174 (2008): 45–62.
58. D. L. Green et al., "An Assessment of Climate Change Impacts and Adaptation for the Torres Strait Islands, Australia," *Climatic Change* 102, nos. 3–4 (2010): 405–33.
59. D. Green, J. Billy, and A. Tapim, "Indigenous Australians' Knowledge of Weather and Climate," *Climatic Change* 100, no. 2 (2010): 337–54.

60. E. Hunter, "'Radical Hope' and Rain: Climate Change and the Mental Health of Indigenous Residents of Northern Australia," *Australasian Psychiatry* 17, no. 6 (2009): 445–52.
61. G. D. Cook and E. Woodward, "Climate Change and Indigenous Communities of the Kakadu Region," in *Kakadu National Park Landscape Symposia Series 2007–2009, Symposium 4: Climate Change*, ed. S. Winderlich (Darwin, Australia: Department of the Environment, Waterm Heritage and the Arts, 2008), 42–46.
62. A. Leigh, *A Review of the Vulnerabilities and Potential Health Risks to the Australian Indigenous Population Associated with Global Warming* (Melbourne, Australia: University of Melbourne, School of Philosophy, Anthropology, and Social Inquiry, 2008).
63. F. H. Johnston et al., "Ambient Biomass Smoke and Cardio-Respiratory Hospital Admissions in Darwin, Australia," *BMC Public Health* 7 (2007): 240.
64. Leigh, *A Review of the Vulnerabilities...*
65. Dingle, *"Our health needs a health environment...*
66. Berrang-Ford et al., "Vulnerability of Indigenous Health..."
67. Ibid., 1072.
68. J. D. Ford, et al., "Vulnerability of Aboriginal Health Systems in Canada to Climate Change," *Global Environmental Change-Human and Policy Dimensions* 20, no. 4 (2010): 668–80.
69. Stephens et al., "Indigenous Health 4—Disappearing..."
70. N. Ohenjo et al., "Indigenous Health 3—Health of Indigenous People in Africa," *Lancet* 367, no. 9526 (2006): 1937–46.
71. Hofmeijer et al., "Community Vulnerability to the Health Effects..."
72. Berrang-Ford et al., "Vulnerability of Indigenous Health...," 1072
73. Ohenjo et al., "Indigenous Health 3..."
74. Minority Rights Group International, *World Directory of Minorities and Indigenous Peoples—Uganda: Batwa* (London: Minority Rights Group International, 2008).
75. A. Namara, "GEF Case Study of Creation and Implementation of National Parks and of Support to Batwa on Their Livelihoods, Wellbeing and Use of Forest Products," in *GEF Impact Evaluation*, (New York: Global Environment Facility, United Nations Development Programme, 2007).
76. D. Napolitano, "Towards Understanding the Health Vulnerability of Indigenous Peoples Living in Voluntary Isolation in the Amazon Rainforest: Experiences from the Kugapakori Nahua Reserve, Peru," *Ecohealth* 4, no. 4 (2007): 515–31.
77. Montenegro and Stephens, "Indigenous Health 2..."
78. M-L. Foller, "Interactions between Global Processes and Local Health Problems. A Human Ecology Approach to Health among Indigenous Groups in the Amazon," *Cadernos de Saude Publica* 17, supp. (2001): 115–26.
79. M. Finer and M. Orta-Martinez, "A Second Hydrocarbon Boom Threatens the Peruvian Amazon: Trends, Projections, and Policy Implications," *Environmental Research Letters* 5, no. 1 (2010): 014012.
80. M. Maheu-Giroux et al., "Risk of Malaria Transmission from Fish Ponds in the Peruvian Amazon," *Acta Tropica* 115, nos. 1–2, SI (2010): 112–18.
81. Berrang-Ford et al., "Vulnerability of Indigenous Health..."
82. Dingle, *"Our health needs a health environment...*
83. Ford, "Dangerous Climate Change and the Importance..."

84. N. Adelson, "The Embodiment of Inequity—Health Disparities in Aboriginal Canada," *Canadian Journal of Public Health-Revue Canadienne De Sante Publique* 96 (2005): S45–S61.

85. Richmond and Ross, "The Determinants of First Nation..."

86. Hofmeijer et al., "Community Vulnerability to the Health Effects..."

87. Berrang-Ford et al., "Vulnerability of Indigenous Health...," 1072

88. Macchi, *Indigenous and Traditional Peoples...*

89. J. D. Ford, L. Berrang-Ford, and J. Patterson, "A Systematic Review of Observed Climate Change Adaptation in Developed Nations," *Climatic Change Letters* 106 (2011): 327–36.

90. J. D. Ford, "Indigenous Health and Climate Change," *American Journal of Public Health* 102, no. 7 (2012): 1260–6.

91. Hofmeijer et al., "Community Vulnerability to the Health Effects..."

92. Hofmeijer, *"The Lakes are Drying...*

93. E. Blas et al., "Addressing Social Determinants of Health Inequities: What Can the State and Civil Society Do?" *Lancet* 372, no. 9650 (2008): 1684–9.

94. J. D. Ford et al., "Reducing Vulnerability to Climate Change in the Arctic: The Case of Nunavut, Canada," *Arctic* 60, no. 2 (2007): 150–66.

95. M. Boyle and H. Dowlatabadi, "Anticipatory Adaptation in Marginalised Communities within Developed Countries," in *Climate Change Adaptation in Developed Nations: From Theory to Practice*, ed. J. D. Ford and L. Berrang-Ford (Dordrecht, The Netherlands: Springer, 2011), 461–73.

96. J. Bird, "Feds Tried to Bypass Inuit on Polar Bears," *Nunatsiaq News* November 28th, 2008.

97. S. Marrone, "Understanding Barriers to Healthcare: A Review of Disparities in Health Care Services among Indigenous Populations," *International Journal for Circumpolar Health* 66, no. 3 (2007): 188–98.

98. B. Minore et al., "Addressing the Realities of Health Care in Northern Aboriginal Communities Through Participatory Action Research," *Journal of Interprofessional Care* 18, no. 4 (2004): 360–8.

99. Adelson, "The Embodiment of Inequity..."

100. R. Romanow, *Building on Values: The Future of Health Care in Canada* (Ottawa, Canada: Commision on the Future of Public Health Care in Canada, 2002).

101. M. MacKinnon, "A First Nations Voice in the Present Creates Healing in the Future," *Canadian Journal of Public Health-Revue Canadienne De Sante Publique* 96 (2005): S13–6.

102. J. Richards, "Indian/Non-Indian Life Expectancy: Why the Gap?" *Inroads* January (2003): 48–59.

103. Public Health Agency of Canada, *The Chief Public Health Officer's Report on the State of Public Health in Canada 2008* (Ottawa, Canada: PHAC, 2008).

104. S. Fankhuaser and R. S. J. Tol, "The Social Costs of Climate Change: The IPCC Second Assessment Report and Beyond," *Mitigation and Adaptation Strategies for Global Change* 1 (1997): 385–403.

105. L. Berrang-Ford, J. D. Ford, and J. Patterson, "Are We Adapting to Climate Change?" *Global Environmental Change* 21, no. 1 (2011): 25–33.

106. Ford and Berrang-Ford, *Climate Change Adaptation in Developed...*

107. B. Smit and J. Wandel, "Adaptation, Adaptive Capacity, and Vulnerability," *Global Environmental Change* 16 (2006): 282–92.

108. C. P. Burgess et al., "Healthy Country, Healthy People: The Relationship between Indigenous Health Status and 'Caring for Country'," *Medical Journal of Australia* 190, no. 10 (2009): 567–72.

109. Ford et al., "Climate Change Policy Responses for Canada's..."
110. Burgess et al., "Healthy Country, Healthy People..."
111. Ibid.
112. D. Mijatovic, "The Use of Agrobiodiversity by Indigenous and Traditional Agricultural Communities in Adapting to Climate Change," *Satoyama Initiative*, accessed December 1, 2011, http://satoyama-initiative.org/en/case_studies-2/group_agriculture-2/the-use-of-agrobiodiversity-by-indigenous-and-traditional-agricultural-communities-in-adapting-to-climate-change/
113. Macchi, *Indigenous and Traditional Peoples...*
114. Mijatovic, "The Use of Agrobiodiversity..."
115. Macchi, *Indigenous and Traditional Peoples...*
116. Ibid.
117. Mijatovic, "The Use of Agrobiodiversity..."
118. A. A. Sudhalkar, *Adaptation to Water Scarcity in Glacier-Dependent Towns of the Indian Himalayas: Impacts, Adaptive Responses, Barriers, and Solutions* (Cambridge, MA: DSpace@MIT, 2010).
119. Ibid.
120. Swinomish Tribal Community Office of Planning and Community Development, *Climate Adaptation Action Plan, October 2010,* accessed May 4, 2013, http://www.swinomish-nsn.gov/climate_change/project/reports.html
121. Ibid.
122. Ibid.
123. J. Lerner, *Xeni Gwet'in Community-Based Climate Change Adaptation Strategy,* accessed May 4, 2013, http://www.cakex.org/case-studies/3753
124. Ibid.
125. J. D. Ford, T. Smith, and L. Berrang-Ford, "Canadian Federal Support for Climate Change and Health Research Compared with the Risks Posed," *American Journal of Public Health* 101, no. 5 (2011): 814–21.
126. J. D. Ford, W. Vanderbilt, and L. Berrang-Ford, "Authorship in IPCC AR5 and Its Implications for Content: Climate Change and Indigenous Populations in WGII," *Climatic Change* 113, no. 2 (2012): 201–13.
127. M. Hulme, "Problems with Making and Governing Global Kinds of Knowledge," *Global Environmental Change-Human and Policy Dimensions* 20, no. 4 (2010): 558–64.
128. T. D. Pearce et al., "Community Collaboration and Climate Change Research in the Canadian Arctic," *Polar Research* 28, no. 1 (2009): 10–27.
129. Sherman et al., "Balancing Indigenous Principles..."
130. R. A. Pielke et al., "Climate Change 2007: Lifting the Taboo on Adaptation," *Nature* 445 (2007): 597–8.
131. S. Dovers, "Normalizing Adaptation," *Global Environmental Change* 19, no. 1 (2009): 4–6.
132. Ford et al., "Authorship in IPCC AR5..."
133. Ford et al., "Canadian Federal Support..."
134. Indian and Northern Affairs Canada, *Sharing Knowledge for a Better Future: Adaptation and Clean Energy Experiences in a Changing Climate* (Ottawa, Canada: INAC, 2010).
135. *Understanding the Health Effects of Climate Change,* Health Canada, accessed May 1, 2010, http://www.hc-sc.gc.ca/ewh-semt/climat/impact/index-eng.php

INDEX

AANDC. *see* Aboriginal Affairs and
    Northern Development
    Canada (AANDC)
ABAPP, 210
Aboriginal Affairs and Northern
    Development Canada
    (AANDC), 285
Aboriginal and Northern Climate Change
    Program (ANCCP), 285
ACCA. *see* Coalition for Community
    Action Programme (ACCA)
Adams, P., xiii, 299
Africa
    AIDS in, 252
    HIV in, 252
    malaria in, 252
    road death rate in, 143
    solid fuel use mortality rates in, xxiii
    sub-Saharan. *see* sub-Saharan Africa
    urbanization in
        slum development, xx
African Americans
    achieving environmental equity for,
        48–68
African Population and Health Research
    Centre, xx
agriculture
    healthy and sustainable, 189–220
    in LMICs, 259
    in sub-Saharan Africa
        water demand related to, 249
    water usage in, 259
        strategies for increasing, 267–8
Agroecological Producer Association
    TAMIA, 207
AIDS
    in Africa and Asia, 252

air pollution
    in Hong Kong, xxiii
    local
        sustainable urban transport impacts
            on, 141–3
    in Mexico City, xxiii
    road traffic and, xxiii–xxiv
air quality
    impact on low-income populations,
        xxiii
    inequalities in
        energy poverty related to, xxiii–xxiv
airport(s)
    in low-income communities, 58
Alameda County, California
    community health guidelines from, 53
Alaska
    Renewable Energy Grant Program in,
        287
Alaska Energy Authority, 287
Albany, New York
    racial health disparities in, 52
Alperovitz, G., 6
alternative energy
    in remote communities in Canada
        constraints to, 278–84. *see also*
            remote communities in
            Canada, constraints to alterna-
            tive energy in
American Medical Association
    on climate change, 299
American Public Health Association
    on climate change, 299
American Recovery and Reinvestment
    Act, 139–40
American YouthWorks (AYW), 102, 107
    mission of, 95

ANCAP. *see* Northern Community Action Program (ANCAP)

ANCCP. *see* Aboriginal and Northern Climate Change Program (ANCCP)

anchor institutions
  in Austin, Texas, 9–10
  colleges as, 10
  as community-stabilizing entities, 9–12
  in generating local jobs, 10
  in local community and economic development, 10
  types of, 9–10

Andes
  central
    peri-urban vegetable farm households in MRs of, 192–4, 193*t*
  of Latin America
    healthy and sustainable agriculture in, 189–220. *see also specific countries and* Latin America

Arctic
  indigenous populations in
    climate change effects on, 299–319

Arthur Kroeger College Award
  from Carleton University, 74

Artificial Glacier Cultivation to Manage Water Scarcity in Himalayan India, 308–9

Asia
  AIDS in, 252
  HIV in, 252
  motor vehicle use in, 167–8
  urbanization in
    slum development, xx

Asian Coalition for Community Action, 40

Asian Coalition for Housing Rights, 40, 41

Austin, Texas
  anchor institutions in, 9–10
  CBV in, 92–111. *see also* Casa Verde Builders (CVB)
  poverty rate in, 93–4

Austin Energy, 14, 97

Australia
  Bushlight program in, 290–1

Avery, R., 20

AYW. *see* American YouthWorks (AYW)

Baan Mankong (secure housing) program, 37

Badami, M., xiii, xxvii, 167

Baldwin Hills, California
  creating park in, 49

Bangalore, India
  road traffic accidents in, xxiv
  water services control in
    PAC on, 265

Bangalore Water Supply & Sewerage Board services, 265

Bangladesh
  water decision-making approaches in, 249

Banister, D., xiii, xxvii, 135

BAPE. *see* Bureau d'audiences publiques sur l'environnement (BAPE)

Barrera, M., xi, xix

Barring-Gould, 295

Barrios Unidos
  in Santa Cruz, California, 57–8

Batwa pygmies
  climate change effects on, 299–319. *see also* remote indigenous populations, climate change effects on

Berliner Wasserbetriebe (BWB) utility company, 265

Bertrand, L., xiv, xxvii, 221

BEST 4 Buildings (B4B), 97, 98, 104

BEST Academy, 92–111
  in fostering social and economic development, 100–2
  history and mission of, 96–7
  keys to success, 105–9
    caring and dedicated staff, 109
    strong case management before and after graduation, 106–7
    thorough participant selection process, 107–8
  limitations of, 104–5
  in merging social and environmental goals, 102–4
  methodology of, 94–5
  of SSBx, 92–111
    context of, 93–4
    described, 92–3
    raison d'être for, 93–4

teaching environmentally friendly
skills and raising awareness at,
98–9
BetterFuture, 127
B4B. see BEST 4 Buildings (B4B)
Bhopal disaster, xxi
binner(s)
in DTES, 73–4
binning
in DTES, 73–4
United We Can in support of, 83
binning community
social marginalization of, 73
"Biols," 200
Blackwell, A.G., xiv, xxvii, 48
Bloomington, Indiana
poverty rate in, 6
Brandeis, J., Justice, 5
BRIC-countries
water-stressed areas in, 248, 249f
Bronx Environmental Stewardship
Training (BEST) program,
92–111. see also BEST Academy
BRT systems. see bus rapid transit (BRT)
systems
Buenos Aires
environmental health in, 30
Buffalo, New York
poverty rate in, 6
Bureau d'audiences publiques sur
l'environnement (BAPE), 266
bus depots
in low-income communities, 58
bus rapid transit (BRT) systems
in India, 181–2
Bushlight program
in Australia, 290–1
BWB utility company, 265

California Air Resources Board, 58
California Rural Legal Assistance, Inc.,
61–2
California Rural Legal Assistance
Foundation, 61–2
Cameroon
Waza Logone Floodplain in, 262–3
Canada
Minister of Natural Resources of, xxvi
motor vehicle ownership in, 175
remote communities in

potential of clean energy for equity
in, 275–98. see also remote
communities in Canada
"Canada's poorest postal code,"
69, 71–3
cancer(s)
lung
solid fuel use and, xxiv
capital
types of, 191, 191f
car dependence
sustainable urban transport effects
of, 140
"Caring for Country" Projects to Enhance
the Health of Aboriginal
Australians, 307
Carleton University
Arthur Kroeger College Award from,
74
Carson, R., 50
Casa Verde Builders (CVB)
academic component of, 95
context of, 93–4
described, 92–3
fostering social and economic development, 99–102, 99t
history and mission of, 95–6
keys to success, 105–9
caring and dedicated staff, 109
strong case management before and
after graduation, 106–7
thorough participant selection
process, 107–8
limitations of, 104–5
merging social and environmental
goals of, 102–4
methodology of, 94–5
on-site component of, 95–6
raison d'être for, 93–4
teaching environmentally friendly
skills and raising awareness,
97–8
Catskill Mountains
water supply from, 264
CD-IPO. see community-development
initial public offering (CD-IPO)
CDCs. see community development
corporations (CDCs)
CDFIs. see community development
financial institutions (CDFIs)

CEI. *see* Community Equity Initiative
    (CEI)
Center for Public Health Policy, 55
Centre for Appropriate Technology, 290
children
    diarrheal diseases in, 252
China
    water conservation in, 267
    water consumption in, 261
    water imported by, 261
    water in
        available *vs.* demanded, 249
    water pollution in
    cost of, 251
chronic obstructive pulmonary disease
        (COPD)
    solid fuel use and, xxiv
city(ies)
    health outcomes in, 27–8, 28f
    inequalities within
        categories deserving attention,
            33–5
    in LMICs
        environmental health inequalities
            within, 29–31, 32f
    struggling
        in high-income countries, 3–25. *see*
            also specific cities
    sustainable transport in, 135–66.
        see also sustainable urban
        transport
    "throw-away," 4
    U.S.
        declining populations in, 6
    water stress in
        price disparity within, xxiii
city governments
    as anchor institutions, 9–10
Cleveland, Ohio
    declining population of, 6
    Evergreen Corporation of, 5, 15–18
    poverty rate in, 6
"Cleveland model," 15–18
climate change
    American Medical Association on, 299
    American Public Health Association
        on, 299
    dwindling water resources and increas-
        ing demand related to, 250–1
    effects on LDCs, 299

effects on remote indigenous
    populations, 299–319. *see also*
    remote indigenous popula-
    tions, climate change effects on
effects on SIDS, 299
effects on water resources, 247–8,
    248f
environmental impacts of, xxi-xxii
health impact of, xxii
impact on cities, 138
impact on ensuring environmental
    sustainability, xxi-xxii
impact on rainfall variability and
    intensity, 258
low-income populations
    effects of, xxii
mortality related to, 299
natural disasters resulting from, xxvi
populations most impacted by,
    299–300
in South Asia
    effects of, 251
sustainable urban transport impact
    on, 139–40
water stress related to, xxiii
WHO on, 299
climate-change action
    financial issues impact on, xxvi
Climate Change Community
    of United Nations, 117
CLSC (centre local de services commu-
        nautaires), 224
CNG. *see* compressed natural gas (CNG)
CO$_2$ emissions
    global levels of, 139
Coalition for Community Action
        Programme (ACCA), 41–2
Code of Conduct on the Distribution and
        Use of Pesticides
    of FAO, 211
CODI. *see* Community Organization
        Development Institute (CODI)
Cole, D., xiv, xxvii, 189
college(s)
    as anchor institutions, 10
Commoner, B., 3
community(ies)
    binning
        social marginalization of, 73
    remote

in Canada, 275–98. *see also* remote communities in Canada
defined, 276
community action
in informal settlements, 26–42. *see also* informal settlements
community-anchoring jobs, 9
community development
United We Can in support of, 83–4
community development corporations (CDCs), 7–8
community development finance industry, 7
community development financial institutions (CDFIs), 8
community-development initial public offering (CD-IPO), 21
community energy needs
in remote communities in Canada, 277–8
Community Equity Initiative (CEI), 61–2
Community Organization Development Institute (CODI), 37
community stability
bolstering economic core of cities in enhancing
elements in, 4
community-supportive economic enterprises
new forms of, 7
community transformation
framework for, 53–62
economic environment in, 53–6
physical environment in, 58–9
service environment in, 60–2
social environment in, 56–8
community wealth building, 7–9
anchor institutions in, 9–12
described, 7
national policy promoting activities and processes in, 8
new direction in
principles for, 18–21
strategies for, 7
challenges facing, 8–9
compressed natural gas (CNG)
in India, 169
Conference of Mayors, 13
congestion
transport-related

imperative and strategies related to, 169
Cooperative Home Care Associates, 20–1
cooperative networks
developing, 15
COPD. *see* chronic obstructive pulmonary disease (COPD)
Copenhagen Accord, 306
Cosgrove, W., xiv–xv, xxvii, 246
Costa Rica
water use tax in, 264
Costello, A., 299
crop management
in Latin America, 197–201, 199*f*
CSSS Lucille-Teasdale area
in Montreal
fruits and vegetables availability in, 233–4, 234*f*
CVB. *see* Casa Verde Builders (CVB)
Cycle 2.2 Nutrition, 228
cyclist accessibility
imperative and strategies related to, 170–1

Dabo, 295
deficient housing
injuries and high health care costs associated with, 59
Delhi, India
average annual income in, 175
BRT systems in, 182
flyovers in, 172
motor vehicle ownership in, 175
demographics
in equity imperative, 53
Département de santé publique (DSP)
of Montreal, 223–6
mandate of, 223
2010–2015 Action Plan for, 223–6
Urban Environment and Health sector of, 231
Department of Aboriginal Affairs, 312
Department of Science and Technology
in New Delhi, India, 116–17
depression
among people living in deficient housing, 59
Detroit, Michigan
declining population of, 6
poverty rate in, 6

development
  water for, 246–74. *see also* water, for
    development
diabetes mellitus
  type 2
    health disparities related to, 52
diarrheal diseases
  in children, 252
  interventions for
    impacts of, 252, 253*t*
  mortality data, 252
dietary habits
  changes in
    impact on environmental health, xxi
Doha Round of the World Trade
    Organization, 262
Dominican Republic
  road death rate in, 143
Dowland Contracting Ltd., 294
Downtown Eastside (DTES)
  binning in, 73–4
    United We Can in support of, 83
  described, 69
  hard drug addiction in, 72
  lessons from, 69–91
  mental illness in, 72
  population of, 71
  poverty levels in, 72
  unemployment in, 72–3
Drinking Water and Sanitation Decade
  of 1980s, 261
Drinking Water Plan, 62
drought(s)
  floods and
    cycle of, 258
  in Malawi, 251
drug(s)
  in DTES, 72
DSP. *see* Département de santé publique
  (DSP)
DTES. *see* Downtown Eastside (DTES)
Dublin Principles and Chapter 18 of
    Agenda 21
  from Earth Summit, 261

Earth Summit
  Dublin Principles and Chapter 18 of
    Agenda 21 of, 261
EBO Group, 15
ECL. *see* Evergreen Cooperative Laundry
  (ECL)

ecoENERGY for Renewable Power
    Program (eERP), 288, 294
ecology
  first law of, 3
  in LMICs
    inequalities in, 32–3
economic environment
  in community transformation, 53–6
economic growth
  dwindling water resources and
    increasing water demands
    related to, 250
  environmental protection *vs.*,
    xxv–xxvi
  water and, 257–60
economic impacts
  of poor sanitation, 255, 255*b*
Economic Mobility Project, 51
economy
  environment and, xix–xxxii
    barriers to action, xxv–xxvi
  green. *see* green economy
eERP. *see* ecoENERGY for Renewable
    Power Program (eERP)
EIQ. *see* Environmental
    Impact Quotient (EIQ)
El Salvador
  road death rate in, 143
electricity
  in remote communities in Canada
    high prices of, 276–7
emission(s)
  CO_2
    global levels of, 139
  global, 137–8, 138*t*
employee-owned companies
  in U.S., 7–8
employee-owned company assets
  leveraging existing, 15
employee stock ownership
    plan (ESOP) companies, 15
Encorp Pacific, 78
energy
  availability of
    quality of life effects of, xxiii
  community needs for
    in remote communities in Canada,
    277–8
  renewable
    in remote communities in Canada,
    285–92, 286*t*. *see also* remote

communities in Canada,
renewable energy in
energy consumption
  imperative and strategies related to,
    170
energy demands
  urbanization and, xx
energy poverty
  inequalities in air quality and,
    xxiii–xxiv
entrepreneurship
  social
    as poverty-reduction strategy, 112–
      32. *see also* TIDE (Technology
      Informatics Design Endeavour)
environment. *see also* social environ-
    ment; *specific types, e.g.,*
    economic environment
  climate change effects on, xxi–xxii
  economy and, xix–xxxii
    barriers to action, xxv–xxvi
    financial issues impact on, xxv–xxvi
    impact on healthy foods, xxi
    (in)equity and, xx–xxiv
    as luxury, xxvi
environmental degradation
  economic costs of, 262–3
  economic threats posed by, xxvi
  prevalence of, xxvi
environmental equity
  achieving, 48–68
    guideposts for action, 63–4
    framework for community trans-
      formation, 53–62. *see also*
      community transformation,
      framework for
    learning from effective examples,
      xxvi–xxviii
    seeking solutions to, xix–xx
environmental health
  within cities
    inequalities in, 29–31, 32f
  in LMICs, 26–47
    inequalities in, 28–9, 28f, 35–9,
      36t, 38b
    TIDE in improving, 115–17. *see also*
      TIDE (Technology Informatics
      Design Endeavour), environ-
      mental health benefits of
  urbanization's impact on, xxi
environmental health differentials

described, 26–7, 27f
  in LMICs, 26–7, 27f
Environmental Impact Quotient (EIQ),
    199
environmental protection
  economic growth and
    perceived tradeoff between, xxv
  economic growth *vs.*, xxv–xxvi
environmental sustainability
  climate change effects on, xxi–xxii
  community stabilization and equitable
    development and
    in struggling cities in high-income
      countries, 3–25
  United We Can in, 76–8
equity
  challenges,
    environmental health and, 26–34
  clean energy and, 275–98
  environment and, xx–xxiv
  environment, place, and, 35
  environmental
    achieving, 48–68
    guideposts for action, 63–4
    framework for community trans-
      formation, 53–62. *see also*
      community transformation,
      framework for
    learning from effective examples,
      xxvi–xxviii
    seeking solutions to, xix–xx
  four principles of, 63–64
  gender
    TIDE's impact on, 123–5
  health outcomes and, 26–27
  improved environmental health and,
    26–47
  social
    through urban sustainability,
      69–91
  sustainable urban transport impacts
    on, 141–51, 144f, 148f. *see also*
    sustainable urban transport,
    health and equity impacts of
  water
    policy approaches for, 260–9, 263f
    governance, 264–6
    need for global action, 260–4,
      263f
    public and private sector invest-
      ments, 266–9

equity (*Cont.*)
  water governance and, 264–6
  see also environmental equity, health
      equity, social equity, the equity
      imperative
equity imperative, 50–3
  demographics in, 53
  health crisis in, 51–2
  inequity in, 50–1
ESOP companies, 15
essential connection
  among environmental sustainability,
      community stability, and equi-
      table development, 3–25
Europe
  air pollution in, 141–2
Evergreen Cooperative Corporation, 18
Evergreen Cooperative Initiative, 15–16
Evergreen Cooperative Laundry (ECL),
      17
Evergreen Corporation
  of Cleveland, Ohio, 5, 15–18
Evergreen Initiatives, 21
extreme weather
  low-income populations effects of, xxii

Fankhuaser, S., 306
FAO
  Code of Conduct on the Distribution
      and Use of Pesticides of, 211
  Global IPM facility of, 198
farm household health
  in Latin America, 201–4
farmer field schools (FFSs)
  in Latin America, 192, 195, 199–200,
      202–3
Federal Deposit Insurance Corporation,
      54
feed-in tariff (FIT), 14, 288
fertilizer(s)
  environmental and health impacts of
      in Latin America, 191–2
FFFI. *see* Fresh Food Financing Initiative
      (FFFI)
FFSs. *see* farmer field schools (FFSs)
financial capital
  defined, 191, 191*f*
FIT. *see* feed-in tariff (FIT)
flood(s)
  droughts and

cycle of, 258
  impact on cities, 138
  in Malawi, 251
  in Nepal
      mortality associated with, xxii
food production
  water use in, 259
food system
  in Montreal
      public health and, 223–8, 226*f*,
          227*f*. *see also* Montreal, food
          system in
Ford, J., xv, xxvii, 299
Fresh Food Financing Initiative (FFFI),
      56
fruit and vegetable consumption
  in Montreal, 221–45. *see also* Montreal
Fullerton, J., 5

GBD study. *see* Global Burden of Disease
      (GBD) study
gender equity and empowerment
  TIDE's impact on, 123–5
GIS. *see* Global Information Systems
      (GIS)
Gita
  TIDE entrepreneur, 120
Global Burden of Disease (GBD) study
  of WHO, 141, 147–51, 148*f*
global climate change
  mortality associated with, xxii
global emissions, 137–8, 138*t*
Global Information Systems (GIS), 268
Global Integrated Pest Management
      (IPM) facility
  of FAO, 198
Global Water Partnership (GWP), 261
Godtland, E., 199
Good Agricultural Practice Guide, 210
governance
  in tackling inequalities in wealth and
      power between countries and
      blocks of countries, 208–11
  in water equity, 264–6
grassroots organizations
  channelling aid to
      importance of, 39–42
Great Depression, 50, 60
Great Recession, 50
Greater University Circle, 15–16

Greater University Circle Initiative, 16–17
Green City Growers, 17–18
green economy
  emerging, 13
  growth of, 12–15
  in improving economic, environmental, and health inequalities, 92–111
  new skills for, 92–111. *see also* BEST Academy; Casa Verde Builders (CVB)
  taxpayer-financed public investment in, 13
Green Economy Report
  of UNEP, 258
green jobs
  examples of, 14–15
  to green ownership, 12–15
green ownership
  from green jobs to, 12–15
green social enterprises
  focus of, 112–13
green social entrepreneurship
  as poverty-reduction strategy, 112–32
    TIDE, 112–32. *see also* TIDE (Technology Informatics Design Endeavour)
green water credit
  in Tana River Basin, Kenya, 264
greenhouse gas mitigation
  in transport sector
    health benefits from, 151–4
Guangzhou City, 138
Guybourg
  in Montreal, 233*f*, 234–6
GWP. *see* Global Water Partnership (GWP)

Harlem Children's Zone, 50
health
  climate change effects on, xxii
  environmental. *see* environmental health
  farm household
    in Latin America, 201–4
  lack of access to safe water, basic sanitation, and good hygiene practices and, 252

sustainable urban transport impacts on, 141–51, 144*f*, 148*f*. *see also* sustainable urban transport, health and equity impacts of
health crisis
  in equity imperative, 51–2
health outcomes
  in LMICs
    differentials in, 26–7, 27*f*
    influences on, 26–7, 27*f*
healthy communities
  in U.S.
    movement to build, 48–68
Healthy Development Measurement Tool
  in San Francisco, 59
Healthy Food Financing Initiative (HFFI), 56
healthy foods
  living environment effects on, xxi
  in Montreal. *see* Montreal, healthy foods in
  in urban settings, 221–45
heart disease
  health disparities related to, 52
heat waves
  mortality associated with, xxii
Heredia, Costa Rica
  water use tax in, 264
Heymann, J., xi, xix
HFFI. *see* Healthy Food Financing Initiative (HFFI)
high-income countries
  struggling cities in
    environmental sustainability, community stability, and equitable development in, 3–25
highways
  in low-income communities, 58–9
HIV
  in Africa and Asia, 252
Hoffman, 209
Hofmeijer, 304
Homeless People's Federation of the Phillipines
  partnerships with municipal governments, 38, 38*b*
Hong Kong
  air pollution in, xxiii
HortiSana project, 192–220

hospital(s)
    as anchor institutions, 10
housing
    inadequate
        in U.S., xxi
housing deficiency
    injuries and high health care costs
        associated with, 59
Houston, Texas
    expansion in, 6
Howard, T., xv, xxvii, 3
"hub-and-spoke" model, 293–4
human capital
    defined, 191, 191f
Hurricane Katrina
    in New Orleans
        impact on low-income populations,
            xxii–xxiii
hygienic sanitation facilities
    global lack of access to, 247

"ice-breaker" activities, 124
ICEF. see India-Canada Environment
    Facility (ICEF)
IIN. see Institute for Nutritional
    Research (IIN)
IISc. see Indian Institute of Science (IISc)
IIT. see Indian Institute of Technology
    (IIT)
Iloilo City
    city government of
        partnership with community orga-
            nizations, 38b
INAC. see Indian and Northern Affairs
    Canada (INAC)
income
    through urban sustainability, 69–91
India. see also specific cities and regions
    agricultural production in
        through groundwater depletion,
            251
    CNG in, 169
    cycling in, 148–9
    literacy rates in, 113
    NMT in, 178–80
    poverty rates in, 113
    road traffic accidents in, xxiv
        imperative and strategies related to,
            168–9
    road traffic deaths in, 168–9

savings groups formed by slum and
    shack dwellers in, 37–8
SHGs in, 123–4
stove-building entrepreneur in,
    119–22
urban transport in, 167–88
    BRT systems, 181–2
    characteristics of, 174–7
    congestion-related, 169
    considerations related to, 174–7
    cost-effective, quality public transit
        provision, 180–2
    cyclist accessibility, 170–1
    energy consumption–related, 170
    imperatives and strategies for,
        167–88
    nonmotorized, 178–80
    pedestrian accessibility, 170–1
    policy imperatives and strategies,
        178–83, 179f
    poverty and, 175–6
    rational pricing of road use, 182–3
    resource allocation and, 176–7
    road traffic deaths–related, 168–9
    urban geography and, 176
    vehicle emissions–related, 169
    vehicle ownership, 174–5
    why "business as usual" is futile,
        171–4
water in
    available vs. demanded, 249
water services control in
    PAC on, 265
water stress in, xxiii
India-Canada Environment Facility
    (ICEF), 114
Indian and Northern Affairs Canada
    (INAC), 283, 285
Indian Institute of Science (IISc), 121
Indian Institute of Technology (IIT), 121
Indigenous Health Adaptation to
    Climate Change project, 312
indigenous populations
    remote
        climate change effects on, 299–319.
            see also remote indigenous
            populations, climate change
            effects on
industrial sites
    in remote communities in Canada, 276

inequalities
  access to healthy foods reflection of, 253
  communities facing rise in, 36–38, 80–82
  green economy and improving economic, environmental, and health, 92–111
  in air quality and energy poverty, xxiii–xxiv
  income, 50–51
  in ecology
    in LMICs, 32–3
  in environmental health
    within cities, 29–31, 32f
  in LMICs, 28–9, 28f, 35–9, 36t, 38b
  in wealth and power between countries and blocks of countries, 208–11
  remote indigenous populations
    climate change effects on
    political, 303–4
  strategy to improve food environment and reduce, 230–6, 231f–6f
  within cities
    categories deserving attention, 33–5
inequity
  environment and, xx–xxiv
  in equity imperative, 50–1
infant(s)
  mortality rates in
    in informal settlements in Nairobi, xx
informal settlements
  community action in, 26–42
  extreme weather events effects on, xxii
  in Nairobi
    child health outcomes related to, xx
Inhofe, J., Sen., xxvi
Institute for Nutritional Research (IIN), 202
Integrated Pest Management (IPM) facility
  global
    of FAO, 198
Intergovernmental Panel on Climate Change (IPCC), 258
  4th assessment report, xxii

International Potato Center, 197
intestinal worm diseases
  high-intensity, 252
Inuit
  climate change effects on, 299–319. see also remote indigenous populations, climate change effects on
IPCC. see Intergovernmental Panel on Climate Change (IPCC)
IPM facility. see Global Integrated Pest Management (IPM) facility
IRIACC initiative, 312

Jackson, F., Mayor, 21
Jacobs, J., 5
Japan
  water consumption in, 261
J.P. Morgan, 5

"Katalysis" projects, 196–7
Kenya
  cycles of floods and droughts in, 258
  green water credit in, 264
Kuglutuk, 279
Kyoto Protocol's Clean Development Mechanism, 292

Lake Victoria, 268–9
Lake Victoria Region Water and Sanitation Initiative, 268
Lalita Bai
  TIDE entrepreneur, 119, 126
Lanare, California
  dysfunctional water system in, 49
Lanes Cleaning Project
  of United We Can, 76, 84, 85
Latin America
  central Andrean region in
    access to clean (enough) water in, 195–7
    access to fertile land in, 194–5
    agriculture in, 190–4, 191f, 193t
    capital assets in, 191, 191f
    crop management in, 197–201, 199f
    farm household health in, 201–4
    FFSs in, 192, 195, 199–200, 202–3
    food production in
      appropriate governance in, 208–11

Latin America (*Cont.*)
    market influences and opportuni-
        ties, 204–8, 205f, 208f
    working with farmers to transform,
        189–220
Latino(s)
    achieving environmental equity for,
        48–68
LDCs. *see* least developed countries
        (LDCs)
"Le café citoyen," 239
lead
    in peeling paint, 59
Leadership Council on Civil and Human
        Rights, 55
least developed countries (LDCs)
    climate change effects on, 299
l'Éco-quartier Maisonneuve-Longue-
        Pointe, 236, 236f
les ilôts St-Jacques, 239
life expectancy
    demographic variations in, 31
    in sub-Saharan Africa, 252
"lifestyle" conditions
    health disparities related to, 52
literacy rates
    in India, 113
living standards
    dwindling water resources and increas-
        ing water demands related to,
        250
LMICs. *see* low- and middle-income
        countries (LMICs)
Local Health Services Center, 234
Lockhart, S., xv, xxvii, 112
logging field camps
    in remote communities in Canada, 276
Logue, J., 20
low- and middle-income countries
        (LMICs)
    agriculture in, 189–220, 259
    ecological impacts in
        inequalities in, 32–3
    energy efficiency characteristics for
        transport modes in, 140t
    environmental health in
        addressing inequities in, 35–9, 36t,
            38b
        inequalities in, 28–9, 28f, 35–9,
            36t, 38b

improved environmental health and
        equity in, 26–47
    inequalities within cities in
        categories deserving attention,
            33–5
    moving toward sustainable urban
        transport in, 136–40, 138t,
            140t
    secure access to productive land in, 194
    water problems in, 246–74
low-income communities
    in Montreal
        comprehensive strategy for, 221–45
low-income countries. *see also* low- and
        middle-income countries
        (LMICs)
    poor-quality housing in, xxi
low-income populations
    air quality effects on, xxiii
    burden disproportionately felt by,
        xx–xxiv
    channelling aid to grassroots organiza-
        tions and federations formed
        by
        importance of, 39–42
    climate change effects on, xxii
    extreme weather events impact on,
        xxii–xxiii
    Hurricane Katrina impact on,
        xxii–xxiii
lung cancer
    solid fuel use and, xxiv
Lyotier, K., 85

Madhav
    TIDE entrepreneur, 126
Mahila Milan, 37–8
malaria
    prevalence of, 252
Malawi
    droughts and floods in, 251
Managing Health Risks in the Swinomish
        Indian Reservation, 309–10
manufacturing jobs
    loss of
        poverty due to, 6
Mar del Plata Declaration, 261
market(s)
    influences of food production in
        in Latin America, 204–8, 205f, 208f

Market Creek Plaza
  in San Diego, 21
Matheny Tract
  CEI in, 62
MDD. *see* Montreal Diet Dispensary
      (MDD)
MDGs. *see* Millennium Development
      Goals (MDGs)
mental illness
  in DTES, 72
Mercier-Quest
  in Montreal
    mobilization for better access to
        healthy foods in, 233–4, 233*f*,
        234*f*
"Mercier-Quest Quartier en Santé," 234,
      235*f*, 236*f*
Meritorious Service Medal
  from Canada's Governor General, 74
metropolitan regions (MRs)
  defined, 192
Mexico City
  air pollution in, xxiii
middle-income countries. *see also* low-
      and middle-income countries
      (LMICs)
  poor-quality housing in, xxi
military outposts
  in remote communities in Canada,
      276
Millennium Development Goals (MDGs),
      42–3, 265, 268–9, 299
  on drinking water supply and sanita-
      tion, 246, 253–6
  Target 7 of, xx
mine(s)
  resource extraction
    in remote communities in Canada,
        276
Minister of Natural Resources
  of Canada, xxvi
Ministry of Economic and Social
      Inclusion, 210
Montreal
  DSP of, 223–6. *see also* Département
      de santé publique (DSP), of
      Montreal
  food initiative in
    integration with other development
        approaches, 239–40

food system in
  access to health foods, 226–7, 227*f*
  consumption of healthy foods, 225,
      226*f*
  food insecurity, 224–5
  minimum cost of nutritious food
      basket, 225
  public health and, 223–8, 226*f*, 227*f*
  success of program objectives,
      236–9, 238*t*
healthy foods in
  access to, 226–7, 227*f*
  consumption of, 225, 226*f*
  increasing access to, 237–9, 238*t*
  measuring disparities in access to,
      228–36, 229*f*–36*f*
  in Mercier-Quest, 233–4, 233*f*, 234*f*
  mobilization for better access to,
      233–4, 233*f*, 234*f*, 239
  strategies to improve, 230–6,
      231*f*–6*f*
  viability of solutions identified for,
      240
low-income communities in
  comprehensive strategy for, 221–45
  mandate of public health departments
      of, 223
region of
  described, 222
strategy to improve food environment
      and reduce inequalities in,
      230–6, 231*f*–6*f*
Montreal Diet Dispensary (MDD), 225
Montreal Protocol on Substances That
      Dilute the Ozone Layer, 262
motor vehicles
  global use of, 167
  per thousand population
    road traffic deaths related to, 144,
        144*f*
  use among countries in OECD, 167
  use in Asia, 167–8
MRs. *see* metropolitan regions (MRs)
Mumbai, India
  flyovers in, 172
  rail-based transit in, 182
  savings groups formed by slum and
      shack dwellers in, 37–8
Muthurajawela Marsh
  in North Sri Lanka, 263–4, 263*f*

Nairobi
  informal settlements in
    child health outcomes related to, xx
Namasté Solar, 14
National Center for Employee
    Ownership, 7–8
National Public Affairs Centre (PAC), 265
National Slum Dwellers Federation
  in Mumbai, India, 37–8
National Urban Poor Funds, 43
National Urban Transport Policy, 172
National Water Strategy
  of Québec, 266
natural capital
  defined, 191, 191f
natural disasters
  economic effects of, xxvi
  impact on cities, 138
  impact on low-income populations,
    xxii
natural gas
  compressed
    in India, 169
Navigation Canada, 283
Nepal
  flood-related mortality in, xxii
Netherlands
  water decision-making approaches in,
    248–9
network building, 15
New Deal, 50
New Delhi, India
  Department of Science and
    Technology in, 116–17
New Orleans
  Hurricane Katrina in
    impact on low-income populations,
      xxii–xxiii
New York City
  drinking water supply for, 264
1999 Brookings Institution report, 10
NMT. see nonmotorized transport
    (NMT)
Noah, T., 6
nonmotorized transport (NMT)
  in India, 178–80
    accessibility and infrastructure for,
      179–80
nonrenewable fuels
  in sustainable urban transport, 139

North Sri Lanka
  Muthurajawela Marsh in, 263–4, 263f
Northern Community Action Program
    (ANCAP), 285
Northern Development and Health
    Canada, 312
Northern Ontario
  Wapekeka First Nation in
    social, technical, and economic
      frameworks in, 276
Northern Québec
  Oujé-Bougoumou biomass project in,
    278
Northwest Territories Power
    Corporation, 289
Nova Scotia
  renewable energy in, 291

Obama administration
  initiatives to improve lives of low-
    income people, 49–50
Oberlin College, 12
obesity
  health disparities related to, 52
  sustainable urban transport impacts
    on, 146–51, 148f
Occupy Wall Street, 6
OCS. see Ohio Cooperative Solar (OCS)
OECD. see Organization for Economic
    Cooperation and Development
    (OECD)
Office municipal d'habitation, 239
Ohio Cooperative Solar (OCS), 17
Ohio Employee Ownership Center, 20
Ontario
  Wapekeka First Nation in
    social, technical, and economic
      frameworks in, 276
Organization for Economic Cooperation
    and Development (OECD), 256
  motor vehicle use among countries
    in, 167
  water-stressed areas outside of, 248, 250
Ottawa Health Promotion Charter, 226
Oujé-Bougoumou biomass project
  in Northern Québec, 278
overweight people
  sustainable urban transport impacts
    on, 146–51, 148f
OXFAM, 209

PAC. *see* National Public Affairs Centre
    (PAC)
Paduraru, C., xv–xvi, xxvii, 92
paint
  peeling
    lead in, 59
Pakistan
  cycles of floods and droughts in, 258
Pan-India CII-Bharti Woman Exemplar
    Award, 119
Paredes, M., 197
Parks Opportunity Program, 101
particulate matter levels
  WHO guidelines on, 169
Partnership for Sustainable
    Communities
  of U.S. Department of Housing
    and Urban Development,
    Department of Transportation,
    and Environmental Protection
    Agency, 50
pedestrian accessibility
  imperative and strategies related to,
    170–1
peeling paint
  lead in, 59
Pennsylvania Fresh Food Financing
    Initiative (FFFI), 56
Peruvian Amazon
  climate change effects in, 299–319
pesticide(s)
  environmental and health impacts of,
    191–2
Pesticide Action Network, 211
Pew Charitable Trust
  2009 study by, 13
Phillipines
  Homeless People's Federation partner-
    ships with municipal govern-
    ments in, 38, 38*b*
Phoenix, Arizona
  expansion in, 6
physical activity
  sustainable urban transport impacts
    on, 146–51, 148*f*
physical capital
  defined, 191, 191*f*
physical environment
  in community transformation,
    58–9

place-based enterprises
  anchor institutions as, 9–12
PolicyLink, 55, 61–2
pollutant(s)
  air. *see* air pollution
  in low-income communities, 58–9
poor. *see* low-income populations
poor-quality housing
  in middle- and low-income
    countries, xxi
poor sanitation
  economic impacts of, 255, 255*b*
Poplar Hill First Nation
  social, technical, and economic frame-
    works in, 276
port(s)
  in low-income communities, 58–9
poverty
  decline of America's cities due to,
    5–6
  energy
    inequalities in air quality and,
      xxiii–xxiv
    as factor in access to transportation,
      xxiv
    as factor in urban transport in India,
      175–6
  reduction of
    water and, 257–60
  in U.S.
    US Census Bureau on, 5
poverty rate
  in Austin, Texas, 93–4
  in South Bronx, New York, 94
poverty reduction
  green social entrepreneurship in,
    112–32. *see also* TIDE
    (Technology Informatics
    Design Endeavour)
Pradel, W., xvi, xxvii, 189
Prain, G., xvi, xxvii, 189
prison rehabilitation
  in community transformation, 61
Program to Support the Development of
    Food Security
  framework for, 231, 231*f*
Promise Neighborhoods program, 50
psychiatric patients
  in Vancouver
    deinsitutionalization of, 72

public health department (DSP)
  of Montreal. *see* Département de santé
    publique (DSP), of Montreal
Pune, India
  four-lane elevated highway in, 172

quality of life
  air quality effects on, xxiii
Québec
  National Water Strategy of, 266
  Oujé-Bougoumou biomass project in,
    278
Québec Water Policy, 266
Quennell, K., xvi, xxvii, 92
Quezungal farming systems, 308

race
  health disparities related to, 51–2
Rain Water Harvesting, 118
rainfall
  climate change effects on, 258
Ranveer
  TIDE entrepreneur, 120, 129
rapid urban growth
  new challenges of, 167–88
"recent progress in the [Human
    Development Index] has come at
    the cost of global warming," xxv
Recology, 14–15
recycling
  employee ownership in, 14–15
reentry programs
  in community transformation, 61
rehabilitation
  prison
    in community transformation, 61
remote communities
  defined, 276
remote communities in Canada
  clean energy for equity in
    potential of, 275–98
  constraints to alternative energy in,
    278–84
    cold weather, 284
    competition for access to resources,
      282
    difficulty of quantifying environ-
      mental costs, 283
    high costs of developing new infra-
      structure and market institu-
      tions, 284

high front-end capital costs/lack of
    credit, 281
institutional mismatch of capital
    costs and fuel price risks, 283
institutional mismatch of energy
    costs and capital costs, 281
lack of detailed geographic resource
    data, 283
lack of government support, 284
lack of information, 280
lack of legal framework for indepen-
    dent power production, 281
lack of technical or commercial
    skills, 281
lack of utility acceptance of tech-
    nologies/prejudice against a
    technology due to poor perfor-
    mance, 282
lack of utility grid access to remote
    sites, 282
opposition of existing interest
    groups, 284
perceived technology performance
    uncertainty and risk, 281
restrictions on siting and construc-
    tion, 282
risks of permit process, 283
subsidized or average cost energy
    prices, 280
transaction costs, 280
cost and limited access to affordable
    energy in, 275
electricity in
  high prices of, 276–7
energy needs in, 277–8
policy recommendations for,
    292–5
population of, 276
renewable energy in, 285–92, 286t
  capacity development, 289–91
  capital cost reductions, 286–8
  described, 285–6, 286t
  mandating generation portfolios,
    291–2
  production incentives, 288–9
social, technical, and economic frame-
    works in, 276
wind power in
  problems related to, 279
remote indigenous populations
  climate change effects on, 299–319

addressing vulnerability, 306–12
discussion, 312–13
geography and, 302
information deficit and, 306
institutional capacity, 304–6
intervention case studies related to,
    307–12
livelihood characteristics and,
    300–1
political inequality and, 303–4
socioeconomic disadvantage and,
    302–3
vulnerability determinants,
    300–306
renewable energy
public and co-op power company
    procurement of, 14
in remote communities in Canada,
    285–92, 286t. see also remote
    communities in Canada,
    renewable energy in
Renewable Energy Grant Program
in Alaska, 287
Renewable Remote Power Generation
    Program (RRPGP), 290
Resettlement Monitoring Task Force
after Typhoon Frank, 38b
resource allocation
as factor in urban transport in India,
    176–7
resource extraction mines
in remote communities in Canada,
    276
respiratory infections
solid fuel use and, xxiv
Rest of the World (ROW) countries
described, 248
water decision-making approaches in,
    248–9
retail
in community transformation,
    54–6
Right to Food, 211–12
Rio Summit, 135
road traffic
air pollution due to, xxiv
injuries related to
sustainable urban transport impacts
    on, 143
road traffic accidents
in Bangalore, India, xxiv

growth in
imperative and strategies related to,
    168–9
road traffic deaths
in India, 168–9
RRPGP. see Renewable Remote Power
    Generation Program (RRPGP)
rural communities
economic opportunities in
TIDE in, 117–22. see also TIDE
    (Technology Informatics
    Design Endeavour)
in U.S.
underinvestment and government
    neglect in, 61
Russia
cycles of floods and droughts
    in, 258

Samson
TIDE entrepreneur, 118
San Diego, California
Market Creek Plaza in, 21
San Francisco, California
Healthy Development Measurement
    Tool in, 59
San Joaquin Valley, California
CEI in-2, 61
sanitation
deficiencies in provision for
    in low-income nations, 31, 32f
poor
economic impacts of, 255, 255b
Santa Catalina women farmers' associa-
    tion, 200–1
Santa Cruz, California
Barrios Unidos in, 57–8
Sarala stove-building program, 116, 126,
    129
Satterthwaite, D., xvi, xxvii, 26
Savir
TIDE entrepreneur, 120–2
school facilities
in underfunded, overcrowded dis-
    tricts, 59
SDI. see Slum/Shack Dwellers
    International (SDI)
sea level
average rate of rise of, xxii
self-confidence
TIDE's impact on, 125–7

self-help groups (SHGs)
  in rural India, 123–4
service environment
  in community transformation, 60–2
Setting an Economic Value on
       Environmental Services Water,
       262
Shawi
  climate change effects on, 299–319.
       see also remote indigenous
       populations, climate change
       effects on
SHGs. see self-help groups (SHGs)
Shilpa
  TIDE entrepreneur, 120, 126
Shipibo
  climate change effects on, 299–319.
       see also remote indigenous
       populations, climate change
       effects on
SIDS. see small island developing states
       (SIDS)
Silent Spring, 50
single-room occupancy (SRO) hotels
  in DTES, 71–2, 82, 89
SJF Ventures, 21
slum development
  in low and middle-income
      countries, xx
Slum/Shack Dwellers International
      (SDI), 35–6, 36t, 40
small island developing states (SIDS)
  climate change effects on, 299
smallholders
  water dependence of, 259
Smith, A., 246
social capital
  concept of, 57
  defined, 191, 191f
social development
  TIDE's impact on, 122–7. see also
      TIDE (Technology Informatics
      Design Endeavour)
  water and sanitation impact on,
      256–7
social enterprise(s)
  green
      focus of, 112–13
social enterprise projects
  of United We Can, 74–7
social entrepreneurship

green technology with, 112–32.
      see also TIDE (Technology
      Informatics Design Endeavour)
  as poverty-reduction strategy, 112–32
social environment
  in community transformation, 56–8
social equity
  through urban sustainability, 69–91
Social Exclusion Unit
  of United Kingdom, xxiv
solar energy
  employee ownership in, 14–15
SOLEfood Urban Farm
  of United We Can, 76, 85, 87
solid fuels
  prevalence of, xxiii
  WHO on, xxiv
South Asia
  climate change effects in, 251
  MDG target on sanitation in, 247–8,
      248f
South Bronx, New York
  BEST Academy in, 92–111. see also
      BEST Academy
  poverty rate in, 94
South-East Asia
  solid fuel use mortality rates in, xxiv
SRO hotels. see single-room occupancy
      (SRO) hotels
SSBx. see Sustainable South Bronx
      (SSBx)
Stern Report, 258
stove-building entrepreneur
  in India, 119–22
stress
  among people living in deficient hous-
      ing, 59
  water-related
      climate change and, xxiii
sub-Saharan Africa
  agriculture in
      water demand related to, 249
  environmental degradation in
      economic effects of, xxvi
  investments in water in, 267
  life expectancy in, 252
  MDG target on sanitation in, 247–8,
      248f
  water and sanitation deficiencies in,
      31, 32f
      annual costs to country, 251

water collection in
    girls and women in, 257
sustainable development
    in Montreal
        food security and, 231, 232f
Sustainable Development Commission
    in United Kingdom, xxiv
Sustainable Mobility Paradigm, 156–60,
        157f, 158t
Sustainable South Bronx (SSbx)
    BEST Academy of, 92–111. *see also*
        BEST Academy
    described, 92–3
sustainable urban transport
    car dependence effects on, 140
    climate change effects on, 138–40
    current investment in transport infra-
        structure and services, 137
    efficient technologies in, 140, 140t
    environmental and public health
        needs, 137
    global emissions, 137–8, 138t
    health and equity impacts of, 141–51,
        144f, 148f
        health, 151
        local air pollution, 141–3
        physical activity, overweight, and
            obesity, 146–51, 148f
        road traffic injuries, 143–6, 144f
    as investment, 138–9
    issues impacting, 139–40, 140t
    leadership requirements, 138–9
    moving toward, 135–66
        described, 136–40, 138t, 140t
        in LMICs, 136–7
        Sustainable Mobility Paradigm in,
            156–60, 157f, 158t
    natural hazards effects on, 138
    nonrenewable fuels in, 139
    research in planning for, 151–6
        cost–benefit analysis, 153–4
        health impact modeling of increas-
            ing active transport and reduc-
            ing greenhouse gas emissions
            from transport, 151–4
        turning research into policy, 154–6
    strong city-level governance and, 138–9
    supply not meeting demand, 137
    world population of urban dwellers
        and, 136
Swinomish Indian Tribal Community

multiyear Climate Change Initiative
    of, 309–10

TAMIA, 207
Tana River Basin, Kenya
    green water credit in, 264
tariff
    feed-in, 14, 288
Thailand
    savings groups formed by slum and
        shack dwellers in, 37
"The Great Divergence," 6
The Pew Charitable Trusts, 51
The Province, 85
The Xeni Gwet'in Community-Based
        Adaptation Plan, 310
Thompson, M., xvi–xvii, xxvii, 69
"throw-away cities," 4
TIDE (Technology Informatics Design
        Endeavour), 112–32
    in creating economic opportunities in
        rural communities, 117–22
    described, 112–14
    entrepreneurs of, 118–22
    environmental health benefits of,
        115–17
        household benefits, 116–17
        outdoor benefits, 115–16
    goal of, 115
    impact on social development, 122–7
        promoting gender equity and
            empowerment, 123–5
        promoting self-confidence and goals
            for better future, 125–7
    lessons for successful dissemination,
        127–30
    as poverty-reduction strategy
        enterprising in new markets, 120–1
        in income generation, 118–20
        multiplier effect of economic oppor-
            tunity, 121–2
    technologies associated with
        guidelines for selecting, 114
        testing of, 114–15
Tol, R.S.J., 306
Traditional Knowledge to Protect Soils
        and Watershed in Coastal
        Honduras, 307–8
transport
    sustainable urban, 135–66. *see also*
        sustainable urban transport

Transport Canada, 283
Tropp, H., xvii, xxvii, 246
2010–2015 Action Plan for Montreal's
    DSP, 223–6
2004 Canadian Community Health
    Survey, Cycle 2.2 Nutrition,
    228
2008 economic crisis
    environmental issues taking backseat
        to, xxv–xxvi
2011 Human Development report
    of United Nations Development
        Program, xxv
Typhoon Frank, 38b

Uganda
    climate change effects in, 299–319
    use of inland water resources in, 264
UIS. see Urban Inequities Survey (UIS)
UN Conference on Sustainable
        Development (2012), 262
UN Convention on the Law of the
        Non-navigational Uses of
        International Watercourses,
        261
UN Economic Commission for
        Europe Convention on the
        Protection and Use of Trans-
        boundary Watercourses and
        International Lakes, 262
UN Environment Programme (UNEP),
        262
    Green Economy Report of, 258
UN-HABITAT, 268
UNDP, 262
UNEP. see UN Environment Programme
        (UNEP)
UNFCCC. see United Nations Framework
        Convention on Climate Change
        (UNFCCC)
United Kingdom
    cycling in, 147–8, 148f
    move from active to motorized trans-
        port in, 147–8, 148f
    road traffic accidents in, xxiv
    Social Exclusion Unit of, xxiv
    Sustainable Development Commission
        in, xxiv
United Nations
    Climate Change Community of, 117

United Nations Development Program
    2011 Human Development report of,
        xxv
United Nations Environmental Program,
        xxv
United Nations Framework Convention
        on Climate Change (UNFCCC),
        306, 313
United States (U.S.)
    cities in
        declining populations in, 6
    decline of cities in
        poverty related to, 5–6
    employee-owned companies in, 7–8
    inadequate housing in
        prevalence of, xxi
    median weekly wage in, 93
    movement to build healthy communi-
        ties in, 48–68
    poverty in
        US Census Bureau on, 5
    road infrastructure development in
        example, 172–3
    rural
        underinvestment and government
            neglect in, 61
United We Can, 69–91. see also
        Downtown Eastside (DTES)
    case study
        methodology, 70–1
    in creating environmental, economic,
        and social change, 74–6
    described, 69–70
    in economic development, 78–81
    founding of, 69, 73
    grassroots approach to community
        empowerment and engage-
        ment, 75–6
    impact of, 76–84
        community development, 83–4
        employee development, 78–83
        environmental sustainability, 76–8
        personal and social development,
            81–3
        supporting binning community, 83
    lessons from, 84–9
        build and maintain relationships,
            85–6
        challenge not-in-my-backyard atti-
            tudes, 86–7

financial survival takes planning,
84–5
integrate workforce issues into business model, 87–8
redefine poverty, 88–9
main objective of, 74
social enterprise projects of, 74–7
university(ies)
as anchor institutions, 10
University Hospitals, 10–12
University of California, Los Angeles,
55
University of Pennsylvania
as anchor institution, 10
Urban Binning Unit program, 87
urban dwellers
world population of, 136
Urban Environment and Health sector
of Montreal DSP, 231
urban growth
rapid
new challenges of, 167–88
Urban Inequities Survey (UIS), 268
Urban Poor Fund International, 40–2
funding for members of, 40
urban sustainability
building income and social equity
through, 69–91
urban transport
sustainable, 135–66. see also sustainable urban transport
urbanization
in Asia and Africa, xx
challenges related to, xx
impact on environmental health, xxi
natural resources effects of, xx
US Census Bureau
on poverty in U.S., 5, 6

Vancouver
deinsitutionalization of psychiatric
patients in, 72
described, 71
DTES of, 69–91. see also Downtown
Eastside (DTES)
housing costs in, 71
SROs in, 71–2, 82, 89
vegetable consumption
in Montreal, 221–45. see also Montreal
vegetable farm households

peri-urban
in MRs in central Andes, 192–4,
193t
vehicle emissions
imperative and strategies related to,
169
vehicle ownership
as factor in urban transport in India,
174–5
Vision 2010, 10–12
Vision and Plan for Integrated Economic
Development of the Region of
Junin for 2011–2014, 210

W. Hayward Burns Institute for Juvenile
Justice Fairness and Equity, 61
WAGES. see Women's Action for Gains in
Economic Security (WAGES)
Wapekeka First Nation
in Northern Ontario
social, technical, and economic
frameworks in, 276
water. see also water resources
in agriculture
strategies for increasing, 267–8
in central Andrean region in Latin
America
access to, 195–7
deficiencies in provision for
in low-income nations, 31, 32f
dependence on
of poor smallholders, 259
for development, 246–74
cost–benefit approach to improved
water services in, 253–6, 255b,
256t
economic growth and poverty
reduction, 257–60
human health and, 252, 253t
importance of, 251–7, 253t, 255b,
256t
social development, 256–7
distribution of, 246
as essential, 246
as global resource
policy approaches for equity, 260–4,
263f
indispensableness of, 259–60
largest users of, 259
in LMICs

water. *see also* water resources (*Cont.*)
  problems, 246–74
  low investments in
    dwindling water resources and
      increasing demand related to,
      249–51
  management of
    water governance framework in,
    261
  for New York City
    supply for, 264
  safe drinking
    global lack of access to, 247–8, 248f
  in sub-Saharan Africa
    collection by girls and women, 257
    investments in, 267
*Water: A Resource to Be Protected, Shared
  and Enhanced,* 266
Water: Our Life, Our Future, 266
water conservation
  in China, 267
water consumption
  in Japan, 261
water demands
  increasing
    factors in, 249–51
water equity
  policy approaches for, 260–9, 263f
    governance, 264–6
    need for global action, 260–4, 263f
    public and private sector invest-
    ments, 266–9
water pollution
  in China
    cost of, 251
water resources. *see also* water
  current state of, 247–51, 248f, 249f
  dividing of
    international boundaries and,
    260–1
  dwindling
    factors in, 249–51
  inland
    use in Uganda, 264
  overexploitation and pollution of
    dwindling water resources and
      increasing demand related to,
      251
water services
  in Bangalore, India

PAC on, 265
  improved
    cost–benefit approach to, 253–6,
    255b, 256t
water stress
  in BRIC-countries, 248, 249f
  in cities
    price disparity within, xxiii
    climate change and, xxiii
  severe
    described, 248
water systems
  dysfunctional
    in Lanare, California, 49
water usage
  in agriculture, 259
  in food production, 259
  lack of efficiency in
    dwindling water resources and
      increasing demand related to,
      250
  on national level
    policy approaches for equity, 260–4,
    263f
  tax for
    in Heredia, Costa Rica, 264
Waza Logone Floodplain
  in Cameroon, 262–3
wealth
  in American society
    escalating concentration of, 5–6
  concentration of
    "medievalness" of, 6
  inequity of
    decline in America's cities due to,
    5–6
wealth building
  community, 7–9. *see also* community
    wealth building
Wealth of Nations, 246
Weis, T., xvii, xxvii, 275
WHO. *see* World Health Organization
  (WHO)
WHO HEAT tool, 152, 154
wind power
  for remote communities in
    Canada
      problems related to, 279
Wind Power Producer Incentive (WPPI),
  288

wind production
  community ownership of, 14
Women's Action for Gains in Economic
        Security (WAGES), 15
Woodcock, J., xvii, xxvii, 135, 152
World Bank, 112
World Health Organization (WHO)
  on climate change, xxii, 299
  GBD study of, 141, 147–51, 148*f*
  HEAT tool of, 152, 154
  on lack of sanitation and access to
        safe and clean water, 252,
        254
  particulate matter guidelines of, 169
  on road traffic–related deaths, xxiv
  on solid fuels, xxiv
  World Report on Road Traffic Injury
        Prevention, 143

World Report on Road Traffic Injury
        Prevention
  of WHO, 143
World Trade Organization, 209, 211
  Doha Round of, 262
World Water Council, 261
worm diseases
  intestinal
    high-intensity, 252
WPPI. *see* Wind Power Producer
        Incentive (WPPI)

Y'a quelqu' un l'aut'bord du mur (YQQ),
        236, 236*f*
YouthBuild federal program, 99
  success of, 109
YQQ. *see* Y'a quelqu' un l'aut'bord du mur
        (YQQ)